The Community as an Epidemiologic Laboratory

A Casebook of Community Studies

EDITED BY
IRVING I. KESSLER
AND
MORTON L. LEVIN

THE JOHNS HOPKINS PRESS
BALTIMORE AND LONDON

Copyright © 1970 by The Johns Hopkins Press
All rights reserved
Manufactured in the United States of America

The Johns Hopkins Press, Baltimore, Maryland 21218
The Johns Hopkins Press Ltd., London

Library of Congress Catalog Card Number 79-109096

Standard Book Number 8018-1119-8

LIST OF CONTRIBUTORS

Helen Abbey, Sc.D.
Department of Biostatistics
The School of Hygiene and Public
    Health
The Johns Hopkins University
Baltimore, Maryland

Guillermo Arbona, M.D.
Department of Preventive Medicine
    and Public Health
University of Puerto Rico School of
    Tropical Medicine
San Juan, Puerto Rico

Robin F. Badgley, Ph.D.
Department of Behavioural Science
Faculty of Medicine
University of Toronto
Toronto, Canada

Robert C. Benfari, Ph.D., S.M. Hyg.
Department of Behavioral Sciences
Harvard School of Public Health
Boston, Massachusetts

George W. Comstock, M.D., Dr.P.H.
Department of Epidemiology
The School of Hygiene and Public
    Health
The Johns Hopkins University
Baltimore, Maryland

Lila R. Elveback, Ph.D.
Department of Medical
    Statistics, Epidemiology and
    Genetics
Mayo Clinic
Rochester, Minnesota

Frederick H. Epstein, M.D.
Cardiovascular Research Center
Department of Epidemiology
The University of Michigan
Ann Arbor, Michigan

Sidney Goldstein, Ph.D.
Department of Sociology and
    Anthropology
Brown University
Providence, Rhode Island

Tavia Gordon
Biometrics Research Branch
National Heart and Lung Institute
Bethesda, Maryland

Paul W. Haberman, M.B.A.
Division of Sociomedical Sciences
Columbia University School of Public
    Health and Administrative Medi-
    cine
New York City, New York

Joseph R. Hochstim, Ph.D.
Human Population Laboratory
California State Department of Pub-
    lic Health
Berkeley, California

August deB. Hollingshead, Ph.D.
Department of Sociology
Yale University
New Haven, Connecticut

Benjamin C. Johnson, M.D., Dr.P.H.
Cardiovascular Research Center
Department of Epidemiology
The University of Michigan
Ann Arbor, Michigan

William B. Kannel, M.D.
Framingham Heart Study
National Heart and Lung Institute
Framingham, Massachusetts

Richard V. Kasius, M.P.H.
Milbank Memorial Fund
New York City, New York

Irving I. Kessler, M.D., Dr.P.H.
Department of Chronic Diseases
The School of Hygiene and Public
Health
The Johns Hopkins University
Baltimore, Maryland

Leonard T. Kurland, M.D.
Department of Medical Statistics,
Epidemiology and Genetics
Mayo Clinic
Rochester, Minnesota

Alexander H. Leighton, M.D.
Department of Behavioral Sciences
Harvard School of Public Health
Boston, Massachusetts

Morton L. Levin, M.D., Dr.P.H.
Department of Chronic Diseases
The School of Hygiene and Public
Health
The Johns Hopkins University
Baltimore, Maryland

Frank E. Lundin, Jr., M.D., Dr.P.H.
Occupational Studies Unit
National Institute of
Environmental Health Sciences
Bethesda, Maryland

Raúl A. Muñoz
Department of Social Services
Commonwealth of Puerto Rico
Santurce, Puerto Rico

John A. Napier, B.A.
Cardiovascular Research Center
Department of Epidemiology
The University of Michigan
Ann Arbor, Michigan

Fred T. Nobrega, M.D.
Department of Medical Statistics,
Epidemiology and Genetics
Mayo Clinic
Rochester, Minnesota

Harold N. Organic, Ph.D.
Department of Sociology and
Anthropology
Brown University
Providence, Rhode Island

O.K. Sagen, Ph.D.
National Center For Health Statistics
Department of Health, Education,
and Welfare
Rockville, Maryland

Herman A. Tyroler, M.D.
Department of Epidemiology
School of Public Health
University of North Carolina
Chapel Hill, North Carolina

Alfonso Mejía Vanegas, M.D.
Department of Social and Preventive
Medicine
National University
Bogotá, Colombia

CONTENTS

PREFACE

Human communities have long concerned the historian, the anthropologist, and the sociologist. In more recent years, they have also engaged the interest of the epidemiologist, the basic scientist of preventive medicine. Knowledge of the distribution of disease and disability in communities is important not only for making proper medical decisions in a local situation but also for the light which may be shed on causal factors of possible general significance. To serve the latter function, it is essential that community studies be designed and executed in accordance with valid epidemiological principles. The studies presented in this casebook illustrate the wide range of methods and objectives which can be encompassed.

In spite of the importance of this subject, no systematic presentation of community studies from an epidemiological viewpoint has yet appeared. We hope that this need will be served by the present volume. While not comprehensive, many of the different types of community studies—medical, social, and psychiatric—are represented. Although these studies were not infrequently planned and conducted by social scientists, they are of considerable value to medical epidemiologists as well. We should like to emphasize that the accompanying editorial discussion and evaluation is always from the epidemiological point of view.

We are indebted to all the contributors to this volume for their cooperation in the seminar presentations as well as in the preparation of this volume. Dr. Abraham M. Lilienfeld was very generous with his timely advice and encouragement and Dr. James Silvan of the Johns Hopkins Press offered many helpful suggestions. Thanks are also due Janice Hume for her editorial assistance and John C. Clarke for his meticulous typing of the manuscript.

I.I.K.
M.L.L.

FOREWORD

Epidemiologic methods have contributed significantly to our under-standing of the communicable diseases and are now increasingly em-ployed in the elucidation of etiological factors in the chronic diseases such as cancer, cardiovascular diseases, and mental diseases. During the past several decades, an interest has developed in utilizing geographically defined communities as units for epidemiologic study. This holistic ap-proach contrasts sharply with the more traditional methods of hypothesis testing, and differences of opinion persist among epidemiologists as to the relative merits of these contrasting research strategies.

In order to provide an overview of community-based studies, the Department of Chronic Diseases of The Johns Hopkins University School of Hygiene and Public Health, in 1968, sponsored a series of seminars at which individual investigators discussed the background, methodology, and pertinent findings of their community studies. A majority of recent and planned population studies in the United States, Puerto Rico, and Colombia were presented and subjected to critical evaluation.

The seminar series afforded an opportunity to assemble, in a sys-tematic fashion, detailed descriptions of these studies, including material which has heretofore not been available in published form. This case-book, based upon the seminars, provides the necessary background for the interpretation and evaluation of research findings which have been reported from these and other community laboratories. Drs. Kessler and Levin have performed a valuable service for epidemiologists, research administrators, and other investigators who are concerned with studies on the etiology of human disease and related problems. Their casebook will facilitate the review and critical assessment of community-based studies of health and health-related variables. It will thus enable the reader to make an independent judgment as to the future research potential of this important investigational strategy.

ABRAHAM M. LILIENFELD

INTRODUCTION

The development of community studies, beginning with the social surveys and sanitary surveys of the last century, is reviewed in this chapter and the interests of social scientists and epidemiologists in geographically defined populations are contrasted. Some important methodological considerations in the epidemiological investigation of communities are discussed, and criteria for the evaluation of community studies are suggested. Finally, the principle features of the studies in this Casebook are tabulated and commented upon.

THE COMMUNITY AS AN EPIDEMIOLOGIC LABORATORY

Irving I. Kessler and Morton L. Levin

Medical practitioners are interested directly in the health of their patients, but only indirectly in the health of their communities, which is the legally defined responsibility of public officials. In addition to the latter, two other scientific groups are concerned with community patterns of health and disease, viz., social scientists and epidemiologists. To these researchers the community is akin to a laboratory where data on health-related phenomena may be collected under controlled conditions.

The systematic and objective collection of health information relating to defined populations may be considered to have its roots in the social survey and sanitary survey movements of the eighteenth and nineteenth centuries, beginning, perhaps, with the studies of conditions within English and Welsh prisons by John Howard (1777). The increasingly sophisticated social surveys of life among the laboring classes by Le Play (1855), Booth (1892), and Rowntree (1908) encouraged the establishment of settlements for community studies in Chicago's Hull House (Addams 1895) and in Boston's South End House (Woods 1898). With the incorporation of the Russell Sage Foundation, in 1906, and its sponsorship of the Pittsburgh Survey (Kellogg 1909) the modern era of the scientific, sociologic study of communities may be said to have begun.

The pioneering social surveys of the last century have their epidemiological counterpart in the sanitary surveys of that era, the most significant being those of Chadwick (1842) in London and Shattuck (1850) in Boston. These studies were primarily descriptive in nature, comprising tabular presentations of data rather than more sophisticated statistical tests of pertinent hypotheses. The statistical methods which underlie modern epidemiologic research owe their development to such workers as Graunt (1662) and Farr (1885), as well as to the founders of mathematical biostatistics, including Galton (1889), Pearson (1938), and Fisher (1958).

The patterns and problems of life in the urban environment have increasingly engaged the attention of social scientists since Robert E. Park first described "the city as a social laboratory" (Smith and White 1929). Today there are not only individual researchers but entire institutes and academic centers devoted to urban studies. All facets of urban living have come under scrutiny: health, poverty, environmental pollution, education, housing, transportation, and the interactions of these factors with each other, as well as with other variables of interest.

For epidemiologists, by way of contrast, communities are not usually of primary interest in and of themselves. Their concerns are mainly with elucidating pathogenetic mechanisms: identifying risk factors in disease and, to the extent possible, etiologic agents. Nevertheless, it is clear that epidemiologic investigations are best conducted on subjects who are selected from clearly defined populations in order to insure the validity of inferences drawn from the experimental findings.

Populations may be selected for study in various ways. They may consist of all diagnosed cases of a given disease who were seen in a particular hospital or hospitals over a stated period of time. Alternatively, they may comprise a random or systematic sample of such cases. In order to evaluate the suspected pathogenetic role of a given attribute of these cases, parallel observations must be made on both the cases and a comparison, or control, group of persons free of the disease in question. Besides hospitals and clinics, cases and controls may be obtained from rosters of industrial workers, labor union members, school classes, insurance holders, military veterans, death certificates, and the like.

In unbiased and well-designed "case-control" studies, differences between cases and controls in the distribution of suspected risk factors may legitimately be attributed solely to the disease itself, or to chance. By their nature, case-control studies are retrospective in orientation with respect to time. Subjects are selected after the onset of their diseases and the prevalence of a suspected risk factor is then ascertained by inquiry, observation, or direct measurement. A possible weakness in this approach is that the investigator's or the subject's awareness of the disease might influence the responses given or the observations made. For example, the responses of a lung cancer patient to questions on smoking habits might be influenced by his beliefs concerning the relationship between smoking and lung cancer. Similarly, the intensity with which an interviewer probes a subject's smoking pattern (and, perhaps, his interpretation of the response) might be affected by his prior knowledge of whether the respondent were a case or a control. Another problem inherent in the retrospective approach is that it may be difficult, or impossible, to establish whether the dependent variable of interest (the suspected risk factor) antedates or follows the onset of the disease. In clinical studies of patients with endometrial cancer, for example, an unexpectedly high prevalence of diabetes mellitus has sometimes been reported (Garnet 1958; Way 1954), but it was not possible to identify the disease as antecedent to the onset of cancer.

Another type of study design, and one which is common to many of the studies in this volume, encompasses the community-based, cross-sectional approach. Panum's (1846) study of measles in the Faroe Islands and Snow's (1855) observations on cholera in London are illustrative of this method. Instead of selecting a group of cases and suitable controls, a population (in this instance, a geographically defined community) is chosen for study, without reference to presence or absence of the disease or of the suspected etiologic factors. The status of all subjects with respect to these variables is then determined—cross-sectionally—at the same point in time, and comparisons are made between those found to have the disease and those who are free of it. Although the independent and dependent variables of interest are ascertained cross-sectionally, this type of study is essentially retrospective in nature. As with the case-control study, there is an inherent difficulty in ascertaining the temporal relationships between suspected disease factors and onset of disease. The possibility that knowledge of who is and who is not a case may affect one's assessment of the presence or absence of risk factors can also not be entirely eliminated.

In contradistinction to *retrospective* and *cross-sectional* studies, biases in identification of associations and of temporal relationships between disease and suspected factors are not usually serious problems in *prospective* studies. In this approach, one classifies the members of a population according to the presence or absence of a particular characteristic and then ascertains the incidence of disease among both groups at some later point in time. In general, such studies are limited by practical, rather than theoretical, considerations. Because significant periods of time must intervene between exposure to risk factor and development of disease, prospective studies tend to be protracted and expensive. A not uncommon by-product of the lengthy observation period is attenuation of the study sample through death, migration, and withdrawal. Unfortunately, one cannot always be certain that the study outcome has not been affected by such losses. The Framingham and Tecumseh studies are representative of this genre.

It is probably not unfair to assert that epidemiologic studies which are or which claim to be "community studies" tend to be enveloped in what may be described as an aura of authenticity. There may be two reasons for this: first, that a community-based population is being studied and, second, that the prospective approach is being utilized. While this type of study design may, indeed, be advantageous in some circumstances, other approaches may sometimes be preferable. Consider, for example, the presumed advantage of studying a total community or representative sample thereof as compared with a population of hospitalized patients. A frequently cited example of the alleged bias in hospital-based populations is the study of Pearl (1929). Among hospitalized patients who were autopsied, the frequency of tuberculous lesions in patients dying of cancer was compared with that in patients of comparable age, sex, race, and autopsy date who died of all other diseases. The author's conclusions regarding the negative association between tuberculosis and cancer were generally conceded to be invalid. In fact, they led some investigators to acquire a distrust of hospital-based studies in general. Actually, the fault lay not in the study population utilized, but in the invalid group comparisons which were made. Lilienfeld (1967) has pointed out that the proportion of tuberculosis cases found among Pearl's autopsy series who were free of cancer was "a grossly biased estimate of the prevalence of tuberculous lesions in a living population." An alternate explanation would be that Pearl's comparison suffers from an error in logic or in the selection of a suitable comparison group. When one observes a given degree of association between two diseases (say, cancer and tuberculosis), the logical question to ask in evaluating this association is whether the observed association differs (a) from that between the disease of interest (here, tuberculosis) and any other, presumably unrelated, disease or (b) from its prevalence in the general population. The prevalence of the disease in one segment of a particular hospital population is not relevant here. We would, accordingly, suggest that the studies in this casebook be evaluated on the basis of the appropriateness of the methods to the investigational goals, rather than in terms of the extent to which they are adjudged to be "community studies."

Fifteen community studies and one hospital-based study are described in the present volume. All were discussed during 1968 at a series of seminars sponsored by the Department of Chronic Diseases of the Johns Hopkins University School of Hygiene and Public Health. Though by no means exhaustive, it is believed that most of the recent health-related community studies are represented. They encompass a wide spectrum of communities, ranging from a rural area of 7,000 persons to a nation of 200,000,000. Just as diverse are the objectives of the various studies: three being concerned with a variety of medical conditions, four with cardiovascular disease, four with social factors in health, two with psychiatric symptoms, and three with the collection of comprehensive health-related data on a national basis. The study instruments include private censuses, personal interviews, interviewer observations, mailed questionnaires, physical examinations, screening examinations, and reviews of existing medical and vital records. In some studies the entire community was surveyed; in others, samples were chosen; while in a few both methods were utilized in various circumstances.

STUDY OBJECTIVES

Some of the community studies presented in this volume, including all three national surveys, were designed to collect descriptive data for a variety of purposes. None of the studies was expressly intended to test one specific etiologic hypothesis, but it is clear that many were undertaken in the hope of uncovering new leads to the pathogenesis of particular diseases. Although few genuinely new hypotheses were, in fact, generated, a number were strengthened by being tested on a community-wide basis.

It is possible to speculate on explanations for the paucity of etiological hypotheses which have been generated by community-based studies. One rather obvious explanation is that community studies constitute a very small proportion of the total number of epidemiologic investigations undertaken. Therefore, relatively few of the promising epidemiologic leads might be expected to have been derived from them in any case. Another possible explanation is that hypotheses are more readily developed by synthesizing the results of many different studies than from individual studies, even large community-based investigations. Thus, the great number and variety of case-control studies and of analyses based upon national or international mortality statistics may lend themselves more easily to hypothesization.

The prospective approach taken by some community laboratories, while advantageous in many ways, may be more suitable for testing than for generating hypotheses. This stems from the possibility that too few etiologically suggestive contrasts between the diseased and the healthy may be derived from prospective studies of relatively small and presumably healthy population groups. By contrast, the likelihood of finding a new clue to a disease may be enhanced when one observes large numbers of patients with that disease, as, for example, in hospital-based case-control studies. In any event, it remains true that there are no hard and fast rules for generating etiological hypotheses.

In addition to their general utility in studies of disease etiology, population laboratories often collect descriptive data that are of value to the local communities themselves. Measurements of the utilization of existing medical services, unmet medical needs, and responses to health education programs exemplify the potential service functions of community laboratories. An occasional by-product of community studies is a residual mass of data, unused and unanalyzed long after its collection. Hospital-based studies are by no means immune to this problem, but the larger size and greater time-span of most community studies may render them particularly susceptible. Some use can almost always be made of such data, as material for classroom lectures or laboratory exercises, for example. However, one is obliged to ask whether a sizable amount of residual data reflects a satisfactory degree of precision in the specification of study objectives.

This raises the question of whether the administrative advantages of some community studies (long-term funding, ease of staff recruitment, etc.) may not be realized at the expense of their potential disadvantages. Among the latter may be included a built-in deterrent to the periodic review and modification of investigational procedures. The fact that the aims of community studies are sometimes only vaguely defined makes it difficult or impossible to subject them to objective periodic evaluation. Thus, the decision as to when a population laboratory has out-lived its usefulness cannot always be made readily.

Relatively few of the community studies reviewed here were designed to investigate a specific disease, risk factor, or population attribute. The four laboratories studying cardiovascular disease are exceptions. Evans County, Charleston County, and North Carolina were selected for study because of their unusual risk of cardiovascular disease, as indicated primarily from mortality statistics. On the other hand, Framingham was chosen for reasons unrelated to the presumed incidence of heart disease there. Most of the other population studies were undertaken to investigate multiple diseases, outcomes, or characteristics. A number of relatively rare conditions were also surveyed; some by the smaller community laboratories.

SELECTION OF THE COMMUNITY

The selection of a community for study must, at least in part, be a function of the study objectives. If one is interested in a particular disease, for example, then one might select a community in which the reported prevalence of the disease is high. This would assure an adequate number of cases for statistical analysis. Equally important, the chances of identifying multiple-risk factors or etiological agents may be enhanced in areas of high prevalence. Of course, the association between an etiological factor and a disease need not be altered in areas of high prevalence.

The elucidation of the pathogenesis of a disease may also require studies in communities of unusually low disease prevalence, where exposure to risk factors may be diminished or immunity is increased. In fact, if a suitable degree of co-ordination between laboratories could be accomplished, it might be feasible to establish two companion population studies: one in a community of high prevalence and the other in an otherwise comparable community of low prevalence. Another possibility might be the selection of a "control" community to serve for a comparison of outcomes with a study community. This would control for the effects of the study procedures themselves upon ascertainment of disease, or other characteristic of interest.

If many diseases, or risk factors, are to be investigated simultaneously, a sizable and heterogeneous community is needed, especially if relatively infrequent conditions are of interest. A number of advantages and disadvantages are inherent in large community studies. Medical and scientific resources are usually close by, and the recruitment and maintenance of trained personnel is facilitated. On the other hand, the costs of operating population laboratories are often higher in metropolitan areas and greater efforts are required to maintain favorable public relations. By the same token, it is sometimes difficult to attract suitably trained research personnel to small communities, and it may be impossible to justify the expense of establishing clinical and laboratory facilities which are to be employed only for the duration of the study. A peculiarity of some studies, to which the small community may be especially prone, is the "Hawthorne effect" (Homans 1941). By this is meant the effect upon subjects of the knowledge that they are taking part in an experiment of some sort. The 10,000 residents of Tecumseh, for example, have undergone periodic interview and examination for a number of years. One can conceive of ways in which the responses and health behavior of this intensively studied community might be affected by the research facility in its midst. The use of a "control" community, mentioned above, would help to deal with this potential problem.

In general, one should attempt to select communities in which optimal response rates and response validity can be anticipated. Ideally, these would be relatively stable communities with little migration and with self-contained medical care systems (see below). A useful, though not essential, factor in choosing a community for study is the availability of existing demographic data relating to it. Prior knowledge of the distribution of the population according to such variables as age, sex, occupation, and education will facilitate the choice of appropriate sampling methods, stratification schemes, and so forth. This information can be obtained ad hoc as well, though at additional cost.

Finally, there are circumstances in which a community may be chosen for study although it fails to satisfy any of the above criteria. Primarily these arise when substantive data on a particular community are needed for a public health service program as contrasted with epidemiological research purposes. In this case, the interest lies primarily in the identification of unmet health needs and other problem areas rather than in disease etiology.

To summarize, six criteria have been suggested for selecting a community:

1. Unusual prevalence of disease
2. Unusual prevalence of suspected risk factor
3. Administrative convenience
4. Favorable community relations
5. Availability of demographic data on the community
6. Needs of public health service programs

The argument sometimes used that community studies are somehow superior to other methodologies because they permit the "study of disease in its natural setting" is difficult to accept as a criterion in the selection of a community for study. One might ask, what is the "natural setting" of a disease. If by this is implied a place where both the disease and its associated predisposing factors coexist, then one should require a sufficiently high prevalence of the disease and its risk factors in any community which is selected for study. Thus, in studying a neoplasm suspected of being related to an environmental factor one would select a community where the incidence of the neoplasm or of the suspected factor was relatively high. Conversely, a low-risk community would be chosen in a study of cancer immunity. In point of fact, few of the community laboratories appear to have been established on this basis.

The most compelling considerations in the selection of the communities appear to have been pragmatic or administrative, rather than theoretical or methodologic. Proximity to a university health center, ease of staff recruitment, favorable community relations, and similar features seem to have been the important criteria for some laboratories. To researchers who are concerned with quality of interviews, nonresponse rates, accessibility of clinical and data-processing facilities, and so forth, these are no mean advantages. However, one may ask whether shorter-term special studies might not better justify the allocation of limited research funds in a community which has no uniquely compelling rationale for intensive and long-term epidemiologic investigation.

In the three national studies and in several of the others reviewed here, collection of substantive data for public health and social welfare purposes was an essential objective. Such community laboratories which are engaged in applied epidemiology have an inherent self-justification which lies beyond the purview of the other considerations discussed here.

In appraising the selected communities, one wonders whether the researches of population laboratories might not be better co-ordinated than they are at present. Should the location of each be determined without reference to the location of the others? Should study methodologies be devised without concern for comparability of results? To a degree, these questions might be directed at all health researchers, regardless of their investigational strategies. On the other hand, community laboratories are so durable, expensive, and few in number that they might be held to a higher standard of methodological quality than the smaller and more numerous ad hoc investigations.

Some precedents can be found for collaboration between research centers. A recent example is the Pooling Project for Cardiovascular Disease Studies which is sponsored by the National Heart Institute and the American Heart Association (Karunas 1969). Investigators from a number of epidemiological studies of cardiovascular disease in Albany, Framingham, Chicago, Minneapolis, and Los Angeles are meeting in an effort to pool the data from their studies and thereby increase the sample size substantially. Despite the many advantages of such co-operative ventures, there would be even greater merit in joint decision-making on case definition and operational criteria *before* studies are actually undertaken.

If a greater degree of co-ordination between community laboratories could be accomplished, it might become feasible to establish companion studies: one in a community of high risk of disease or risk-factor prevalence; the other in an otherwise comparable community of low risk. Another possibility might be the selection of a "control" community, already alluded to.

SIZE OF THE COMMUNITY

To some extent there is a relationship between the size of a community laboratory and the study methodology employed. Once a community of a given size is decided upon, the methodological options are immediately limited. Conversely, if a given method is to be employed, the optimal community or sample size is thereby determined. Studies to be conducted in large metropolitan areas, for example, must employ population samples and, usually, teams of interviewers. On the other hand, surveys requiring repeated follow-up of total populations would necessitate the selection of small, relatively stable, communities.

The size of a community in which a specific hypothesis is to be tested should be such that statistically adequate numbers of cases would be available. As already noted, however, the community laboratories presented here were not established primarily to test specific hypotheses, and this criterion for community size has not been applied. As a matter of fact, sample sizes were sometimes fixed according to estimates of a study staff's capacity for collecting data. Moreover, these estimates were in some instances lowered for budgetary or administrative reasons, even before the magnitude of the nonresponse had been ascertained. One would surmise that major modifications in study procedures are more likely to occur in the descriptive type of investigation, where specific etiological hypotheses have not been stated in advance.

In general, four factors can be suggested for consideration in determining the optimal size of a community for study:

1. The nature of the problems to be investigated
2. Whether total ascertainment or sampling is proposed
3. The confidence level and power of the statistical test to be employed
4. The capacity of the study staff to collect and analyze the data

TYPES OF STUDY DESIGN

A number of population laboratories, especially the relatively permanent ones, utilize the prospective approach. All residents of a community, or a statistically selected sample thereof, are identified at a point in time, interviewed, and, perhaps, examined. Thereafter, efforts are made to ascertain all important events of medical significance occurring to members of the "cohort." If ascertainment of such events is complete and accurate then the true risks of disease morbidity or mortality can be measured in groups of people who share relevant characteristics in common.

As already intimated, some investigators believe that the prospective approach increases the likelihood of generating new etiological hypotheses. This view stems, in part, from a unique feature of longitudinal studies: that among the subjects being examined there are some who are or will soon be in the developmental stages of their disease. Unfortunately, with the exception of the most prevalent conditions, relatively few cases of a given disease can be expected to develop in populations of the usual size during the usual periods of observation. Thus, a population of 10,000 Americans, followed for one year, would yield no more than about two cases of stomach cancer. Another difficulty in prospective studies involves case follow-up. In no epidemiologic studies is it easy to persuade all subjects to co-operate; in prospective studies the investigator must continually expose himself to the risk of nonresponse. Consequently, all prospective studies suffer from attrition of the cohort through nonresponse as well as through migration and death. The costs of minimizing such losses are high and sometimes not easily justified to funding agencies. As a result, nonresponding or migrating subjects are ignored in some community studies; in others, unduly modest efforts are made to trace them. The extent of the effort to reduce nonresponse is, perhaps, the hallmark of the well-executed prospective community study. The advantages of this approach, as well as its disadvantages, have been well-documented (MacMahon et al. 1960; Lilienfeld et al. 1967).

The Framingham and Tecumseh studies are prospective in design, with a closed panel being utilized in the former and an essentially open-ended cohort in the latter. Some features of the longitudinal approach are also incorporated in the Washington County, Alameda County, and Rhode Island laboratories. The Evans County Cardiovascular Survey will acquire some characteristics of prospective studies when the screening is repeated in the near future. Prospective elements were also initially incorporated into both the Washington Heights and the Puerto Rico surveys but were later eliminated for various reasons. The Rochester studies, by virtue of their reliance on existing medical records, are at present retrospective (or retrospective-prospective) in approach. With the development of a self-administered patient inventory questionnaire and with the possible initiation of multiphasic screening in community-based samples, prospective investigations may become feasible there as well.

The remaining studies are essentially cross-sectional in design. As such, they are characterized by measurements of health parameters at a given point or over a relatively short period of time. The resulting data thus pertain to the prevalent rather than the incident cases of disease. The distinction between these two statistics is important to the epidemiologist who is basically interested in disease etiology. Prevalence is a function of both incidence and duration of disease (or survivorship) over time. Thus, prevalent cases of cervical cancer, for example, would tend to be older than newly incident cases. Long-surviving cases would be over-represented among prevalent cases and early decedents would be under-represented. In general, a variable interval of time would have elapsed between their disease onset and their selection for study. The longer this time interval the more likely their exposure to other (extraneous) environmental factors and the greater the difficulty in differentiating between these factors and those of possible etiological significance.

The above notwithstanding, it should be noted that, historically, most of the epidemiological contributions to the etiology of acute and chronic disease have come from cross-sectional or retrospective studies of essentially prevalent cases. Of course, it is possible to distinguish incident cases by collecting information on dates of disease onset or clinical diagnosis.

Cross-sectional community studies are sometimes made necessary by the difficulties in obtaining long-term funds for prospective investigations. It is easier to propose a one- or two-year study to test a specific hypothesis than to justify an expensive ten-year search for risk factors which may or may not be discovered. This also has the advantages of encouraging the investigator to clarify his objectives and to complete his work in a reasonable period of time. Prospective studies often leave one with the difficult problem of deciding when they have outlived their scientific usefulness.

It is sometimes possible to combine advantageous features of both the prospective and the cross-sectional approaches. For example, the study design of the Rhode Island Population Research Laboratory incorporates a clustered community sample with five successive annual surveys. Each survey will yield prevalence data for the particular year, but comparisons between the results for successive years will provide longitudinal data.

Even if the advantages of the longitudinal study are assumed to outweigh the disadvantages (which is by no means certain), the rationale for developing community laboratories on this basis is still not clearly evident. One might suggest, for example, the alternative of a well-designed prospective follow-up of a population defined on some basis other than geographic residence. Selected ethnic groups, familial groups, or exposure groups of various types might be followed with respect to a particular variable of interest. Of course, the choice of a cohort is not easily made if specific hypotheses have not been formulated.

MEDICAL CARE PATTERNS

Many community laboratories utilize existing medical data from hospitals and other institutions; the Rochester studies at present depend entirely upon this source of information. Since the pattern of medical care in Rochester is centripetal, an essentially complete record of the population's morbidity is to be found in the central record file of the local affiliated hospitals. This has made it feasible to conduct a number of community health surveys with the existing data, rather than by cross-sectional or prospective survey.

In many communities, however, the patterns of seeking medical care are not centripetal but centrifugal or diffuse, thus making it unwise to depend upon local hospital records for investigational purposes. In Washington Heights or Alameda County, for example, residents commonly seek medical services outside the community, and surveys of local hospital records would be impractical. This may explain the failure of these laboratories to secure independent validation of interview responses on questions relating to health and illness. If the prevalence of disease rather than the perception of illness is of interest, an objective measure of morbidity is essential. Thus, in a community with a centrifugal pattern of medical care, one must either survey the hospital records of the entire catchment area or else ascertain disease directly, perhaps by sample screening. Otherwise, one is left with unvalidated, and therefore inconclusive, information.

The retrospective approach would also not be suitable for the study of conditions which do not invariably lead to hospitalization or clinic visit. Unless interviews with patients are contemplated, this method must be limited to variables of interest which are routinely entered in the medical record: appendectomy history, circumcision status, detailed smoking habits, and similar items, for example, are generally not recorded in hospital charts in the United States.

CRITERIA FOR EVALUATION

Evaluation of community studies should be in terms of their stated objectives. For studies undertaken in the hope of generating new hypotheses, the number and quality of such hypotheses may provide a benchmark. However, the failure of a study to generate a new hypothesis need not lead to disappointment. Negative findings are often valuable, provided that they are based upon well-designed and well-executed procedures.

Studies conducted for the purpose of testing an existing etiological hypothesis can also be valuable. A single prospective study may obviate the need for several retrospective (case-control) studies which, together, may equal or exceed its cost. The prospective study also provides a measure of the *actual* risk of disease in contrast with the *relative* risk estimates deriving from retrospective studies.*

* Absolute estimates of risk can also be derived from retrospective studies if the entire community is studied, or if the total community incidence as well as the distribution of the risk factor are known.

A negative criterion for the evaluation of community studies may be the volume of data collected but still unutilized after a reasonable period of time. One can visualize such a problem with large prospective community surveys in which study objectives have been imprecisely defined. It is true, of course, that some use can almost always be found for unanalyzed data; for example, in the classroom. However, the relatively high cost of community studies may not be consistent with such use of data.

Community studies undertaken for the purpose of planning health services are, almost by definition, valuable to the community. By contrast, the direct value to a given community of epidemiological investigations of disease etiology may be limited: these are designed to study diseases, rather than diseased community residents. This distinction assumes importance to the degree that the co-operation and responsiveness of a community is required for a study's successful completion. It suggests a technical criterion for the evaluation of community studies, viz., the nonresponse rate. A related criterion would be the extent to which outmigrants and other nonrespondents are followed in order to secure relevant information about them. As a final, technical criterion of methodological quality we can suggest the extent to which an independent validation is sought of the patients' responses made at personal interview.

The major criteria suggested for the evaluation of community studies may be summarized as follows:

GENERAL CRITERIA
1. Productivity in generating new hypotheses
2. Productivity in testing old hypotheses
3. Direct utility to the community

TECHNICAL CRITERIA
1. Nonresponse rates
2. Follow-up of outmigrants and nonrespondents
3. Independent validation of responses

REALIZING THE POTENTIAL OF COMMUNITY STUDIES

For community studies to fully realize their potential, a number of conditions should be satisfied. The first, and most obvious, is an *appropriate choice of the community*. Administrative convenience is not unimportant, but the methodologic suitability of a specific community for a specific study must not be ignored. To accomplish this, all available information on the medical, environmental, and socioeconomic attributes of the community should be examined. Community studies sometimes disregard the distinguishing features of the communities per se as variables of importance. To remedy this, close collaboration between epidemiologists and sociologists is suggested, in order that due consideration be accorded all relevant community characteristics in future studies.

A second condition concerns the *objectives of the study*. These should be specified in advance and as precisely as possible. If large amounts of descriptive data are to be collected in order to confirm the results of other studies, this can often be efficiently and economically combined with the statistical testing of specific etiologic hypotheses.

The *use of control communities* is also suggested. One type of control community, in which outcome is measured but in which no manipulation by interview or examination takes place, may make it possible to control for the effects of the study procedures independently of the study variables. The effect of a community characteristic (for example, air pollution) may be studied by using another type of control community, one in which the characteristic is lacking.

A high degree of *co-ordination between community laboratories*, especially in regard to methods and operational definitions, is very desirable. This will not only eliminate unnecessary duplications of effort but will also permit meaningful comparisons to be drawn between findings in the various studies.

Collaboration with local public health departments and other sources of data on morbidity, mortality, and demography will often make it possible to obtain an independent validation of questionnaire responses and other study findings. The laboratory, in turn, may be of service to the public health agencies, by conducting evaluations of various ongoing programs, for example.

A final desideratum for community studies should be a mechanism, preferably built-in, for *periodic evaluation* with a view to possible modification or even termination. The procedure should seek to determine whether the objectives are as relevant as they were at the study's inception and whether changes in emphasis or in design are indicated by new advances in knowledge.

It is difficult to evaluate the degree to which the community studies discussed here have fulfilled their objectives. In their collection of descriptive data on disease, all the studies may said to have been successful, although this is true almost by definition. In regard to analytical investigation and hypothesis testing, it is not easy to generalize. A number of previously observed associations were replicated or confirmed and some new hypotheses were generated, but the expected number of such hypotheses was small in any event. Nevertheless, community studies should probably be held to a higher standard of scientific excellence, if only because of their large size, great expense, and long duration.

EDITORIAL COMMENTS

The salient features of the community studies in this casebook, together with some critical comments, are presented in Table 1–1, which should help the reader to identify the essential similarities and differences between them and, perhaps, to suggest modifications that might be incorporated into future surveys. More detailed editorial comments on various aspects of the community studies are presented at the end of each text chapter. While the comments are directed to particular studies they are often applicable to others as well. They are intended to offer a critical but objective examination of the concept of the population laboratory, its shortcomings, its achievements, and its potential. The reader should bear in mind that the viewpoint of the editors was that of medicine and epidemiology rather than of social science. While these fields are complementary, there are important distinctions in their philosophy and scientific orientation.

We do not believe, nor do we hope, that our editorial comments will remain unchallenged. Many of them were, in fact, intended to stimulate discussion and interchange of ideas among medical and social scientists and their students. To the extent that such a dialogue is stimulated, the objectives of this volume will have been realized.

TABLE 1–1. CHARACTERISTICS OF THE COMMUNITY STUDIES

Community	Tecumseh	Olmsted County	Washington County
Population size	10,000	75,000	100,000
Character	Urban and rural White Middle class	Urban and rural White Middle class	Urban and rural White Middle class
Medical care facilities	1 general hospital	3 general hospitals several other hospitals	1 general hospital 3 other hospitals
Study instruments	Private census Interview survey with annual surveillance follow-up Examination survey Monitoring of local hospital admissions, death certificates, school absence records, newspaper items Mail canvass of out-migrants Interviewer observations Sample surveys Laboratory tests	Existing medical records Death certificates Survival status ascertainment of all patients studied	Private census Existing medical records Death certificates Birth certificates Special sample surveys

TABLE 1–1.   (Continued)

Community	Tecumseh	Olmsted County	Washington County
Study interests	Cardiovascular diseases Diabetes Mellitus Rheumatic diseases Respiratory diseases Etc.	Neurological diseases Cancer Etc.	Cervical cancer Tuberculosis Chronic diseases Etc.
Comments	1. Outmigrants generally excluded 2. Adults number about 6,000 3. 34% nonresponse to 1st exam	1. Only 100 records out of 3,000,000 have been lost 2. Multiphasic screening of community sample planned 3. Self-administered patient inventory questionnaire in preparation	1. Commercial source supplied addresses for mailed census 2. Most institutionalized persons excluded 3. Census not updated in 6 years

Community	Evans County	Charleston County	North Carolina
Population size	7,000	216,000	4,500,000
Character	Rural White and nonwhite Agricultural	Urban, partly rural White and nonwhite All social classes	Urban and rural White and nonwhite All social classes
Medical care facilities	Very few	Many and varied	Many and varied

Study instruments	Private census
	Total survey, persons 40–74:
	50% sample survey, persons 15–39:
	   Personal interview
	   Physical examination
	   Laboratory tests
	Monitoring of deaths:
	   Obituaries
	   Morticians
	   Ministers
	   State vital records
	Repeat census
	Repeat survey
		Stratified sample survey persons over 34:
		   Personal interview
		   Physical examination
		   Laboratory tests
			Medical records of selected hospitals
			Monitoring of death certificates
			Federal census data

Study interests	Cardiovascular diseases	Cardiovascular diseases	Cardiovascular diseases

Comments	1. 92% initial response
	2. Large outmigration of young adults; follow-up planned
	3. Recent outmigrants excluded from initial prevalence survey
		1. Response:
		   whites = 85.3%
		   nonwhites = 81.5%
			1. Half of State's hospitals are excluded
			2. Epidemiologic surveillance by nurses being set up in 12 hospitals
			3. Co-ordination with regional medical program planned

TABLE 1–1. (Continued)

Community	Framingham	Alameda County	Washington Heights
Population size Character	50,000 Suburban White Middle class	1,000,000 Urban, metropolitan White and nonwhite All social classes	270,000 Urban, metropolitan White and nonwhite Lower and lower middle class
Medical care facilities	1 local hospital, many others nearby	Many and varied	Many and varied
Study instruments	Sample of adults, age 30–59, for panel cohort study: Interviews Physical examinations Laboratory tests Death certificates (every 2 years)	Area probability sample for household survey: Self-administered questionnaires for adults Re-survey planned	Stratified, clustered sample for household survey: Interviews Selective re-interviews Re-sample and re-survey
Study interests	Cardiovascular diseases	Socioeconomic factors, stress, and health	Socioeconomic status, ethnic background, and health behavior Social pathology Survey methodology
Comments	1. Initial nonresponse: 31.2% 2. Sample supplemented by volunteers 3. Nonrespondents not traced 4. Initial sampling frame based on town list which differed from U.S. census list by 11%	1. Initial nonresponse: 14% 2. Health evaluation based solely on responses to mailed questionnaire	1. Nonresponse: 21.4% 2. Planned sample size reduced by 25% for reasons of time and money

Community	Rhode Island	Stirling County	New York City
Population size	890,000	20,000	8,000,000
Character	Urban White and nonwhite All social classes	Rural White, French, English Lower and lower middle class	Urban, metropolitan Multiracial (whites studied) All social classes
Medical care facilities	Many and varied	Few	Many and varied

TABLE 1–1. (Continued)

Community	Rhode Island	Stirling County	New York City
Study instru- ments	Stratified, clustered sample, cumulative over 5 years, for household surveys: Interviews Vital records Hospital records Physician records Physician inter- views	Area probability sample Questionnaire inter- view Interviewer observa- tions Physician records Hospital records Psychiatric assess- ment from records	Stratified sample from 8 census tracts: Interview Interviewer ob- servations Medical records Psychiatric as- sessment from records
Study interests	Health Health behavior Fertility behavior Etc.	Sociocultural deter- minants of psychi- atric symptoms and symptom clusters	Sociocultural deter- minants of psychi- atric symptoms and symptom clusters
Comments	1. Initial nonresponse: 19.2% 2. Close collaboration with state health and vital statistics departments	1. Nonresponse: 7% 2. Interpsychiatrist re- liability: 65–72% 3. Questionnaire not independently validated	1. Nonresponse: 15% 2. Interpsychiatrist re- liability: 40–90% 3. Questionnaire not independently validated

Community	University Hospital
Population size	745 beds
Character	Large teaching hospi- tal, patients of all races and social classes

Medical care facilities	Same

Study instru- ments	5% random sample of white married pa- tients living with spouse: Personal interviews and observations over 2-year period of: Patients Spouses Physicians Nurses Other hospital personnel Assessment by physi- cian and sociologist

TABLE 1–1.   (Continued)

Community	University Hospital
Study interests	Perceptions of and re- actions to illness among patients and their spouses
Comments	1. 25% of patients died before com- pletion of fieldwork 2. Psychiatric and physical impacts of illness confounded

Community	United States	Puerto Rico	Colombia
Population size	200,000,000	2,300,000	18,000,000
Character	Largely urban All races All social classes	Half rural, half urban Whites and nonwhites All social classes (mainly lower and lower middle)	Largely rural Multiracial All social classes (mainly lower)
Medical care facilities	Many and varied	Many and varied	Varied; lacking in some areas

Study instru- ments	Decennial census
	Vital statistics regis- tration
	Stratified clustered samples for:
	  Household inter- views
	  Physical exami- nations
	  Screening surveys
	  Institutionalized population sur- veys
		Area probability sam- ple for household surveys:
		  Questionnaire interviews
			Area probability sam- ple for household surveys:
			  Questionnaire interviews
			  Physical exami- nations
			  Screening surveys

Study interests	Comprehensive	Comprehensive	Comprehensive
Comments	1. Hypothesis testing studies rare 2. Slowness of data collection a prob- lem 3. Survey samples too small to yield esti- mates for individual states	1. Sample includes survivors from 2 earlier surveys as well as newly se- lected persons. 2. Original cohort ap- proach discarded in favor of annual new samples.	1. Over 75% of re- spondents had a primary education or less. 2. Unequal recall peri- ods for some health questions. 3. Unusual adminis- trative problems en- countered in con- ducting survey and analyzing results.

References

Addams, Jane and other residents of Hull House. 1895. *Hull House Maps and Papers: A Presentation of Nationalities and Wages in a Congested District of Chicago.* Library of Economics and Politics, no. 5. New York: Thomas Y. Crowell Co.

Booth, C. 1892–97. *Life and Labour of the People of London.* 17 vols. London: Macmillan & Co., Ltd.

Chadwick, Sir Edwin. 1843. *Report on the Sanitary Condition of the Labouring Population of Great Britain.* London: Clowes and Sons.

Farr, W. 1885. *Vital Statistics: A Memorial Volume of Selections from the Reports and Writings of W. Farr.* Edited by Humphreys, N.A. London: The Sanitary Institute of Great Britain.

Fisher, Sir Ronald A. 1958. *Statistical Methods for Research Workers.* 13th ed. Edinburgh: Oliver and Boyd.

Galton, Sir Francis. 1889. *Natural Inheritance.* London: Macmillan and Co., Ltd.

Garnet, J. D. 1958. Constitutional stigmas associated with endometrial carcinoma. *Am. J. Obstet. Gynec.* 76:11–19.

Graunt, J. 1939. *Natural and Political Observations Made Upon the Bills of Mortality.* Edited by Willcox, W. F. Baltimore: The Johns Hopkins Press.

Homans, G. C. 1941. The Western Electric Researches. In *Fatigue of Workers: Its Relation to Industrial Production by the Committee on Work in Industry of the National Research Council.* New York: Reinhold Publishing Co.

Howard, J. 1784. *The State of the Prisons in England and Wales, with Preliminary Observations and an Account of Some Foreign Prisons and Hospitals.* 3d ed. Warrington: Wm. Eyres.

Karunas, T. 1969. Department of Epidemiology, University of Michigan School of Public Health, personal communication.

Kellogg, P. U., ed. 1909–14. *The Pittsburgh Survey.* 6 vols., New York: Russell Sage Foundation.

Le Play, P. G. F. 1877–79. *Les Ouvries Européens.* 2d ed., 6 vols. Paris: Imprimeries Impériales.

Lilienfeld, A. M., Pedersen, E., and Dowd, J. E. 1967. *Cancer Epidemiology: Methods of Study.* Baltimore: The Johns Hopkins Press.

MacMahon, B., Pugh, T. F., and Ipsen, J. 1960. *Epidemiologic Methods.* Boston: Little, Brown and Company.

Panum, P. L. 1940. *Observations Made During the Epidemic of Measles on the Faroe Islands in the Year 1846.* Translated from the Danish by A. Sommerville Hatcher, 1940. New York: Delta Omega Society.

Pearl, R. 1929. Cancer and tuberculosis. *Am. J. Hyg.* 9:97–159.

Pearson, E. S. 1938. *Karl Pearson: An Appreciation of Some Aspects of His Life and Work.* Cambridge: The Univ. Press.

Rowntree, B. S. 1902. *Poverty: A Study of Town Life.* London: Macmillan & Co., Ltd.

Shattuck, L. 1850 (Comm.). Massachusetts Sanitary Commission 1850. *Report of a General Plan for the Promotion of Public and Personal Health, Devised, Prepared and Recommended by the Commissioners Appointed Under a Resolve of the Legislature of Massachusetts, Relating to a Sanitary Survey of the State.* Boston: Dutton & Wentworth.

Smith, T. V. and White, L. D. 1929. Chicago: *An Experiment in Social Science Research.* Chicago: University of Chicago Press.

Snow. J. 1885. *On the Mode of Communication of Cholera.* 2d ed. London: John Churchill.

Way, S. 1954. The aetiology of carcinoma of the body of the uterus. *J. Obstet. Gynaec. Brit. Emp.* 61:46–59.

Woods, R. A. 1923. *The Neighborhood in Nation-building: A Running Commentary of Thirty Years at the South End House.* Boston: Houghton, Mifflin.

PART I

COMPREHENSIVE STUDIES OF DISEASE IN
TOTAL COMMUNITIES

The Tecumseh project is a classical example of the community as an epidemiologic laboratory. Data is collected longitudinally from interviews, medical examinations, laboratory tests, hospitals, and vital records. All residents of Tecumseh are studied, but it has been necessary to draw population samples for certain purposes even here. The methods, problems, and potentials of the Tecumseh project are of considerable relevance to the planning of community studies everywhere.

THE TECUMSEH, MICHIGAN COMMUNITY HEALTH STUDY

John A. Napier, Benjamin C. Johnson, and Frederick H. Epstein

INTRODUCTION

The purpose of the Tecumseh Community Health Study has been to develop and to maintain a study of the origins, course, and distribution of disease and disability and of their biological and social determinants in a total community. Major emphasis is placed on investigation into the etiology of chronic diseases, with special efforts directed at the early detection of high-risk groups and of diseases in their preclinical stages. The ultimate goal is prevention. The Tecumseh studies comprise integrated investigations in the community, laboratory, and clinic in the search for causative mechanisms and ecological interrelations. The target diseases are primarily the cardiovascular disorders, especially atherosclerosis and its consequences, diabetes, chronic respiratory disease, and the rheumatic disorders. The field studies are based in Tecumseh, Michigan, a total, defined community of about 10,000 inhabitants.

Since its beginning in 1957, the Tecumseh Community Health Study has proceeded on the basic assumption that a disease develops and becomes manifest in a community within a general ecological setting in which previous disease experience, environmental exposures, and genetic predisposition all play important roles. For this reason the total community approach has an important potential for the clarification of the interrelationships between these factors.

Coronary heart disease is the prime concern of the investigative effort, although other diseases are also under study. More is known about the distribution of and factors of relevance to coronary disease than perhaps about any other major chronic disease. Risk factors of considerable predictive power have been identified. A great deal has also been learned about the underlying lesion, atherosclerosis. Indeed, in the view of some authorities, if the knowledge now at hand were applied to preventive measures the premature toll of the disease might be appreciably reduced.

When persons enrolled in a prospective study develop manifest illness, one can look back and observe how these persons differ from those who remain healthy. The identification of such differences may provide clues to etiology. It is also known that apparently susceptible persons sometimes remain healthy, while apparently low-risk individuals become ill. Within this web of predisposition and resistance, the factors which protect in the face of increased risk or which seemingly override immune mechanisms remain to be elucidated.

The search for these factors is traditionally directed toward specific diseases. However, it is our clinical impression and tentative epidemiological judgment, from studies in Tecumseh and elsewhere, that diseases are not randomly distributed in populations but that some people are prone to a multiplicity of disorders while others are spared. If this is true, then the simultaneous investigation of multiple diseases in the same general study has patent advantages. For each disease, data can be collected and analyzed with regard to etiological factors specific to that disease, and at the same time, a search can be made for clusters of diseases among the same individuals, which would suggest common etiological factors that might otherwise be overlooked or wrongly considered to be specific for one disease alone. A further step would consist of looking at predisposing factors in an attempt to determine which diseases have common precursors. In a total community setting, the study of multiple conditions requires little more effort or expense than the study of a single condition. However, the total inferential information gained may well exceed that to be expected from the several individual studies. Even if this does not prove to be true, the community study will probably be more economical, because several categorical studies have been done at a total cost not much above that of a single disease study. In fact, it might be difficult to justify the investigation of only one categorical disease in a total community, because such a study could probably be done more easily on an appropriately stratified population sample.

Having argued against limiting community studies to a single disease category, we must add that the Tecumseh program does not attempt to study everything in everybody. Such an all-encompassing approach, even if it were desirable, would not be feasible. The greater the scope of a study the greater the methodological problems and the more difficult it is to control the quality of the data. The Tecumseh study attempts to avoid the extremes of inclusiveness and exclusiveness. As stated above, priority is given to cardiovascular and related disorders and to certain other diseases.

THE COMMUNITY

The Tecumseh Community Health Study is being conducted in a defined community consisting of the city of Tecumseh, Michigan and the rural area immediately surrounding it. The study area comprises about 56 square miles; approximately one-third of the community residents live outside the town limits. Geographically Tecumseh is 27 miles southwest of Ann Arbor in Lenawee County, Michigan, approximately 55 miles southwest of Detroit and 35 miles northwest of Toledo, Ohio. Adrian, the county seat of Lenawee County, is located 12 miles southwest of Tecumseh and about 7 miles from the southern boundary of the study area, which is entirely within Lenawee County.

Selection of the Community

Tecumseh was selected after criteria were developed and applied to all cities, towns, and villages located within a 50-mile radius of the University of Michigan in Ann Arbor. The criteria included proximity to the study center in Ann Arbor and to neighboring communities, as well as size, population characteristics, health facilities, community organizations, and degree of interest in participation. Of all the communities considered, Tecumseh appeared to be the most suitable, and initial contacts with community leaders were favorably received.

Three types of information were used to determine the Tecumseh community: (1) fixed boundaries such as political subdivisions, school and postal districts, utility service areas, etc., (2) opinions of well-informed persons living in the area, and (3) information on the shopping habits and the patterns of local organizational membership of rural residents. The boundaries were fixed so that almost all persons living within them were members of the Tecumseh "community."

Nature of the Community

Tecumseh was formerly quite rural in character but, like many midwestern communities, has been undergoing a fairly rapid industrialization. Its largest industry, Tecumseh Products, is the largest manufacturer of refrigeration compressors in the world. In 1966 General Motors opened an upholstery plant within the study area, and the Anderson Division of the Stauffer Chemical Company opened a plastics plant adjacent to it. About 40 per cent of the labor force hold white-collar jobs, such as clerical, sales, managerial, and professional positions. Of the 60 per cent in blue-collar activities, over two-thirds hold skilled or semi-skilled jobs in manufacturing. Approximately one-third of these industrial workers are employed by Tecumseh Products, while the remaining two-thirds are distributed over a wide variety of other enterprises. In all, Tecumseh has about 150 private businesses dealing in a wide range of goods and services.

According to the U.S. Bureau of the Census, the city of Tecumseh had a population of 4,020 in 1950 and 7,045 in 1960. The size of the entire study community was not known until the completion of a private census in the fall of 1957. At that time the study community had a population of 8,787, of whom 6,246 were residents of Tecumseh City and 2,541 were living in the rural fringe. By 1967 the population had grown to approximately 9,800, made up almost entirely of Caucasians, mostly of northern and central European extraction. There is only one Negro family and there are about 30 families of Spanish or Mexican descent.

From 1830 to 1930 the population of Tecumseh Village grew very slowly—from 1,727 to 2,456 persons. Since the establishment of its major industry in 1934, the rate of population increase has doubled during each census period: 19 per cent from 1930 to 1940, 38 per cent from 1940 to 1950, and 76 per cent from 1950 to 1960. Since 1930 Tecumseh's population has nearly tripled in size, a growth rate considerably higher than the national average. In recent years there has been an influx of workers from larger urban centers seeking employment opportunities.

Compared with places of similar size in Michigan and in the United States as a whole, the population of Tecumseh has a slightly lower median age, a smaller proportion of men and women who are widowed, a distinctly lower unemployment rate among males, a slightly higher median level of education, a higher percentage of employed persons in manufacturing industries, and a higher median family income.

The community has little air pollution; levels of solid particulate matter, airborne lead, and carbon monoxide are well below those found in large metropolitan areas. Drinking water, the municipal supply as well as private rural wells, contains high concentrations of calcium, magnesium, and iron and would be classified as "hard" or "very hard" by the usual standards.

Study Facilities

When field work was begun in 1957, a small office in downtown Tecumseh was leased and occupied as headquarters for the field staff. Before the first round of medical examinations, in 1959, the basement of the Herrick Memorial Hospital in Tecumseh was leased and extensively renovated to provide space for the clinic where the first two rounds of examinations were conducted. In 1966 a separate building, located on the city outskirts, was leased and extensively renovated to house the examination clinic, the exercise physiology laboratory, and the field staff.

The research staff currently has office space in the main building of the University of Michigan School of Public Health and in a separate building in Ann Arbor, which also houses the record files and the clerical staff. By 1970 new construction is planned to provide for the consolidation of all Ann Arbor-based activities at one location within the School of Public Health–Medical Center complex.

Two laboratories at the School of Public Health are used for the immunologic-serologic studies and for the processing of the sera and other specimens from the field examinations in the Tecumseh clinic. Another laboratory at the University is used for various biochemical studies. Tests for genetic markers are carried out in the University's Department of Human Genetics.

METHODS

The Tecumseh studies are directed toward the entire population of the defined community, but the operating procedures also allow for special studies among identified subgroups. Initial contacts with subjects are made by trained lay interviewers who visit each dwelling unit in a prescribed order. These units are allocated to one of ten samples randomly selected from five geographic strata. The ten samples are kept current by random allocation of new dwelling units created by construction or conversion. Each cycle of interviewer visits begins with sample I and continues with the other samples in sequence. Dwelling units within each sample are assigned randomly to the interviewers, and each interviewer is assigned a random order of visits. In this way the impact of any bias due to interviewer variability is randomly distributed.

For analytic purposes all members of the Tecumseh community are identified as individuals, as members of family units, as members of households, and as members of kindreds or bloodlines. They are grouped in sibships as well as in parent-child and husband-wife combinations.

The study instruments include carefully designed questionnaires administered by interviewers, self-administered interval histories, medical examinations, clinical tests, and laboratory tests.

Two rounds of medical examinations have now been completed. In the first round (during 1959–60) 8,641 persons were examined; this number comprised 88 per cent of all persons contacted. In the second round, completed in June 1965, 9,226 persons, including 2,499 new residents, were examined. A third round was begun in 1967.

The purpose of the medical examination cycles have been, first, to obtain, as baseline information, the lifetime disease experience of all persons in the community; second, to assess changes in health status and in potentially disease-related risk factors over time; third, to uncover new relationships between risk factors and target diseases; and, finally, to develop new etiological hypotheses.

In the third examination cycle, a sequence different from that of the first two cycles was followed in order to permit earlier and more frequent observation of certain specified individuals. The latter include the following, listed in the order of their study priority:

1. Relatives of all persons identified in the first cycle as having coronary heart disease or diabetes mellitus (case kindreds) and relatives of controls without these diseases who are of similar age and sex to the cases (control kindreds).

2. All other persons over age 35 who had previously been examined.

3. Propositi identified as having chronic pulmonary disease, matched controls, and their immediate families.

Basic Health Evaluation Methods

History and Physical Examinations. During the first two cycles of examinations, exhaustive medical history questionnaires were administered by the interviewers. This provided general information in a standard manner as well as the basis for the more probing questions of the examining physician. In the third cycle, emphasis upon internal health changes necessitated the use of an abbreviated self-administered health questionnaire and a simplified physician's history. A special effort was made to determine the approximate date of onset of all reported symptoms.

The physical examinations were as complete as possible within the time limitation. However, no rectal or pelvic examinations were done. The examiners were drawn primarily from the departments of internal medicine and pediatrics of the University of Michigan Medical School.

Clinic and Laboratory Procedures

Clinic and laboratory tests have been modified with the passage of time, although the basic procedures have been retained in order that comparisons of findings between examinations might be made. The procedures include:

1. Electrocardiography: A 12-lead electrocardiogram was taken in all three examination cycles. This included a modified exercise test in the second cycle and tape recorded tracings for computer analysis, as well as the determination of normalized orthogonal leads, in the third cycle.

2. Pulmonary function measurements: The simple pulmonary function measurements taken in the first cycle were augmented in subsequent examinations to provide for the assessment of pulmonary adequacy and the effects of aging.

3. Anthropometric measurements: Various measures of body build, including estimates of body fatness, skeletal dimensions, and strength tests were made in order to provide indices which might be related to various chronic disease states.

4. Blood pressure determinations: Various methods of blood pressure determinations have been employed, including a standard measurement by the physician, as well as two different semi-automated measurements designed to minimize observer error.

5. X-rays: Standard chest films, 14 x 17 inches, were taken in each cycle, as well as special hand and spine films during the second cycle.

6. Special skin tests: Tuberculin and histoplasmin sensitivity tests were done during the second cycle and five common inhalant allergens were similarly evaluated in the third examination round.

7. Blood tests: A one-hour blood glucose measurement after glucose challenge has been administered in all three cycles in all adults and older children. A hemoglobin determination in cycle I was replaced by a microhematocrit reading in cycle III. Blood tests include determinations of uric acid, as well as various rheumatoid factors. Fasting levels of serum triglycerides were estimated in cycle III by centrifugation of the random bloods, since it has not been feasible to collect fasting specimens. Several 2-milliliter aliquots of serum for each person were also stored for future use such as, for example, immunologic studies related to acute and chronic respiratory disease.

8. Urine tests: The urine tests include measurements of glucose, protein, acetone, occult blood, and acidity, done by a dipstick method. A microscopic examination is done if albumin is noted. If an elevated urinary sugar is noted on examination, a dipstick determination of blood sugar is done on the whole blood.

Surveillance of Health Status between Examination Cycles

The long time interval between the regular cycles of clinical examination probably creates a memory-gap for the recall of certain events relevant to health. Therefore, annual surveillance visits to each dwelling unit have been included among the study procedures. These visits consist of interviews with a household respondent at each dwelling unit and the collection of self-administered health reports on each household member. The household interview serves to identify changes in the composition of the population due to births, deaths, marriages, divorces, or movement away from or into the Tecumseh community. The annual health reports serve to update the medical histories of the study subjects and to suggest areas for further probing by the examining physician at subsequent clinic visits.

Supplemental Sources of Information

In collaboration with the local hospital, the study center has established a system for monitoring the admission of patients with conditions of particular interest to the project, especially myocardial infarction (definite or suspected), pulmonary diseases, and diabetes mellitus. These data can be used to validate the interview responses; they may also yield new information, as well as help to define high-risk groups for special study.

Tecumseh residents over age thirty who move away are canvassed annually by mail and permission is requested for obtaining updated information from hospitals and physicians visited. To date the response rate among former residents has approximated 70 per cent.

The mailed questionnaire seeks to ascertain at regular intervals the live or dead status of the individual and to determine the occurrence of major illnesses or the cause of death. This information is taken into account in the analysis of data based on the experience of the total, original cohort of the Tecumseh community. In addition to this, information is also gathered about people outside Tecumseh, who have never been part of the study, when this is required for the interpretation of data pertaining to kindreds.

A small pilot study has indicated that family members living outside the community are often willing to have their private physician report on their health, obtain an electrocardiogram, and mail in a blood specimen. This approach may be useful in special studies involving nonresident family members. Other sources of surveillance data include:

1. Absence records from the Tecumseh schools, collected rou-

tinely at the end of each six weeks' marking period and, at times, on a weekly basis in special studies of acute upper respiratory disease.

2. Death notices matched against the master files and copies of death certificates which are obtained for all study subjects who have died in Tecumseh or elsewhere.

3. Local (weekly) newspaper and daily newspaper items which pertain to Tecumseh in general or to the community study in particular.

4. Information about local events obtained by the field interviewers who maintain day-to-day contact with the community. This source of information is particularly useful because the interviewer assignments are geographically stratified throughout the community.

Special Study Methods

Acute Respiratory Study. In 1965 special studies of the epidemiology of acute respiratory illness were begun. The subjects were young families with children, with samples studied intensively for one year and then replaced with other sampled families. Blood specimens for serologic study are obtained from each family member at enrollment, at six months, and at year's end. Weekly reports of illness are obtained by telephone interview throughout the year. When acute respiratory illness occurs, specimens are obtained for viral and bacteriological study.

Chronic Respiratory Disease Study. In an effort to assess the relationship of acute infection to emphysema and related chronic pulmonary disorders, a special subgroup of families has been under investigation. Persons already known to have chronic respiratory disease (emphysema, asthma, or chronic bronchitis) were designated as index cases and age-sex matched controls were chosen from nonafflicted persons. The families of both groups are also included in the investigation. After baseline studies of pulmonary and cardiac function, families are kept under weekly telephone surveillance for the detection of illness, as in the acute respiratory study. Specimens are collected for viral and bacterial identification and changes in antibody titers are assessed. During the course of this study, pulmonary function tests are repeated to determine changes, especially among those family members in whom early symptoms or signs may be more likely to develop.

Exercise Physiology Laboratory. A special adjunct of the third examination cycle is the study of the metabolic work capacity of males aged ten to seventy years. Maximum oxygen uptake during a multi-stage treadmill exercise is measured, while the electrocardiogram, respiratory rate, pulse rate, ventilation, blood pressure, and concentration of expired gases are monitored continuously.

These data are of special relevance to cardiovascular diseases, including hypertension, and to pulmonary and certain other diseases. The baseline data will be analyzed and longitudinal changes over time observed. It is also intended to correlate the medical history information with physical and laboratory findings in individuals as well as in family aggregates.

Dietary Studies. Nutritional variables as possible factors in atherogenesis and diabetogenesis came under study in cycle III. Two methods are used: (1) a card-sorting procedure which elicits the respondent's judgment as to the frequency of his use of 110 foods and food groups, and (2) a dietary interview which seeks detailed information regarding food intake during the 24 hours prior to interview.

Sociologic Studies. Studies of social factors that may be associated with chronic disease are also being undertaken in Tecumseh. These are aimed at identifying stresses impinging on individuals which may evoke maladaptive responses and thus contribute to the development of coronary heart disease and other chronic diseases. Also taken into consideration are the individual's verbal descriptions of his subjective reactions to potentially stressful situations.

In the third cycle of interviews, data are obtained from all men and women aged thirty-five to sixty-nine years regarding their current activities and attitudes. Details are elicited regarding the respondent's current occupation, the types of physical activity engaged in on the job, and attitudes toward a variety of aspects of the job. Information is also sought on the formal organizations of which the respondent is a member and his degree of participation in each, the frequency with which he engages in a variety of leisure time activities, and the degree of satisfaction obtained therefrom. Additional questions are concerned with current worries or problems, the extent to which they may interfere with the individual's life, and the degree to which he feels his life goals have been fulfilled.

In order to examine certain long-term sources of stress, including residential mobility, data have been collected on what may loosely be termed the social life history of approximately 1,000 men and women aged thirty-five to sixty-nine from four of the ten samples of the Tecumseh population. The data comprise the following:

1. A detailed occupational history, including job descriptions, remuneration, hours worked, supervisory responsibilities, and over-all job satisfaction.

2. A complete residential history.

3. Family composition during both childhood and adulthood.

4. Nativity, education, religious preference, and occupation of parents.

Genetic Studies. Areas of particular interest in the Tecumseh studies are the familial aggregation of disease and the risk factors of disease. Blood type and salivary secretor status have been studied in the entire population (cycle III). The observed findings will be used:

1. To search for evidence of deviation in the segregation of these polymorphic traits which might indicate differential survival of specific genotypes.

2. To determine whether there are associations between specific genotypes or genetic mating types and levels of fertility.

3. To determine whether specific genotypes are associated with specific diseases (cardiovascular, diabetes, etc.) or with specific laboratory findings (cholesterol levels, uric acid, glucose tolerance, etc.).

4. To obtain data useful in subsequent genetic investigations, e.g., analyses of linkage, gene frequencies, phenotype frequencies, and levels of heterozygosity in the population.

Serological and Biochemical Studies. A principal aim of the serological and biochemical studies is to develop tests which will detect not only the presence of arteriosclerotic heart disease but a susceptibility to it as well. In a study of an inhibitor of lipid hemagglutinins (vaccinial hemagglutinin and cardiolipin) an apparent chemical similarity between the hemagglutinins and a lipid component of the arterial wall suggests that the inhibitor is formed in the blood vessel and released into the plasma. Mechanisms of cholesterol transport are also being investigated.

A Lipid Research Laboratory was established to serve the needs of the Cardiovascular Research Center. Analyses of serum lipids and glucose are carried out here. An investigation of fatty acid metabolism in rats maintained on various dietary régimes has been completed. A series of studies on the separation, identification, and quantification of lipoproteins by chromatographic and other techniques has been undertaken, with the hope of developing relatively simple methods which could be used in the analysis of sera from selected groups of persons in the Tecumseh community. Attempts have also been made to develop a method of serum triglyceride analysis which would obviate the need for fasting specimens. Work has also been done on serological tests for collagen as related to atherosclerosis and on immunological differences as related to the hyperlipemias.

Environmental Studies. Studies of the total ecology of a community require a thorough investigation of all significant aspects of the physical and biological environment. Some progress has already been made with respect to several components of the Tecumseh environment. A thorough review of existing data, augmented by on-the-scene observations, has made it possible to map the community in detail, according to the various types of vegetation and land use. A listing has been prepared of all native vertebrate fauna likely to be found in the area, as well as an estimate of their relative abundance. One study, conducted at a farm site, demonstrated an association of radioactivity in the air and soil with the metabolic pathways of the local plants and farm animals through the food chain. Airborne solid particulate matter was collected and measured daily for 14 months, and less frequently thereafter for four years. During this time the atmosphere was also evaluated for contamination by lead and by carbon monoxide. Although little air pollution was detected, it is planned to continue monitoring in order to detect any changes resulting from the establishment of new industries in the community.

During a 14-month period, in 1964–65, the mineral content of drinking water was analyzed, utilizing monthly samples obtained from 29 locations. The dependent variables included trace elements, hardness, pH, specific conductance, and selected nonmetallic ions. Twenty-five of the 29 sampled locations had high concentrations of calcium, magnesium, and iron and would be classified as very hard water.

PROBLEMS

Representativeness of the Community

Valid extrapolation from studies of sampled or total communities is said to depend upon the representativeness of the population studied. In fact, no community in any geographic area can be representative of all other communities. While Tecumseh is rather similar to other midwestern United States communities of its size, extrapolations to other populations must take into account differences in environmental influences, racial and ethnic composition, and mode of life. This limitation exists in all intercommunity comparisons. The Tecumseh studies were undertaken primarily in order to study the patterns of disease and their possible determinants within this community, rather than for the acquisition of data directly applicable to other communities.

Size of Population

The number of people required for the study of any particular condition depends, in part, upon the prevalence of that condition in the population. It is recognized that Tecumseh's population of 10,000 is not sufficient to study rare diseases in detail, although some inferences may be made about them. Instead, the studies are directed mainly toward those diseases which are sufficiently prevalent to provide adequate numbers of cases for study and for comparison with other groups.

Nonresponse

Longitudinal studies in a total community are dependent upon adequate response rates. About 88 per cent of the identified residents completed their examinations in cycle I, and many of the remainder were interviewed for their medical histories. In the subsequent examination cycles the nonresponse rate has shown no evidence of increasing. It has been highest among older people, persons who are seriously ill, and those who are about to move from or have just moved into the community.

Residential Mobility

In longitudinal studies, selective losses due to changes of residence are unavoidable. The possible effects of such losses in Tecumseh have been examined in some detail. Selected attributes of 6,563 persons who were examined in both cycle I and cycle II were compared with the same characteristics of 1,040 persons who moved from Tecumseh between the two examination rounds. Among the males who moved, the young adults tended to have higher serum uric acid levels, and those over age forty years tended to have higher blood glucose levels than stationary males. Women who moved tended to have normal uric acid levels, lower weight under age forty years and a tendency to higher blood sugars above age forty years. Moving was more common among persons in higher educational and occupational classes and among those who had not been born in Tecumseh or in Michigan. The observed differences between movers and nonmovers have not been of sufficient magnitude to significantly affect the distribution of these parameters in the Tecumseh population, but with the passage of time, the cumulative effect of losses due to moving may become more important. This type of problem can be serious in prospective studies of single cohorts, but the Tecumseh study has admitted new cohorts of inmigrants who, in some respects at least, replace the movers. These new cohorts serve as additional comparison groups within the total community and help to maintain the adequacy of the population's size.

Follow-up of Movers

The extent to which movers should be followed may be estimated by weighing the relative costs in effort and money against the expected yield of information. In the Tecumseh studies, all persons aged thirty years or older are requested to mail in a self-administered health report annually and death certificates are obtained for persons who die after moving away. Except for special groups of particular interest, follow-up of movers is limited to these annual reports and death certificates.

Data Collection and Analysis

A physician of the central staff is responsible for the supervision of clinic activities and for the recording and initial processing of data. His responsibilities include checking the examining physician's records for completeness, and preparing a diagnostic summary of all known conditions as well as any which have developed or recurred in the interval between examinations. Conditions are classified according to standardized diagnostic criteria which minimize variability of diagnoses among the various physicians. After the diagnostic summary is prepared, a letter is mailed to each respondent, indicating whether or not he should consult his physician about the findings of the examination. A letter is also sent to each respondent's physician with pertinent history, physical findings, and laboratory test results. Care is taken to avoid interfering in the physicians' private practice, and no medical advice or treatment is given. Perhaps as a result of this policy, the local physicians remain cordial and co-operative with the study.

A characteristic of large-scale longitudinal studies is that planning, data collection, and analysis proceed simultaneously and usually in the hands of the same study personnel. The competing demands upon the time of the staff physicians are especially critical. Older methods of data processing are not suitable and the computer has become an increasingly indispensable tool.

The major problem with regard to concurrent data analysis is that new data are being generated while earlier data are being analyzed. The complexity of the data and its sheer magnitude have made standard methods of data handling unworkable. Most of the data is coded soon after collection and is otherwise prepared for electronic processing.

Recruitment and Maintenance of Staff

Staff maintenance was made more difficult because of two features of the study, first, the clinic hours (afternoon and evening) made necessary by the voluntary nature of participation and the need to minimize inconvenience to the respondents, and, second, the self-imposed restriction that staff not be hired from within the community. The latter proscription was felt necessary in order to avoid unnecessary involvement in community affairs and to ensure confidentiality of the recorded data. However, this made travel expenses greater, since all field and clinic staff must live outside the study area.

FINDINGS AND POTENTIALS

The uniqueness of the underlying concept of the Tecumseh study explains its appeal, although its success must ultimately be judged by the results. Baseline and follow-up information on most of the areas of interest has already been collected (Figure 2–1). With regard to coronary heart disease, the study represents the first systematic attempt to investigate familial predisposition prospectively in an unselected population. The importance of hyperglycemia as a risk factor has been demonstrated, thereby stimulating a new area of research. The electrocardiographic data have been extensively studied by others. So, too, have the immunologic approaches to the elucidation of various pathogenetic mechanisms. Some of the analytical designs and data have served as models for parallel studies elsewhere. The studies on hyperglycemia-diabetes, chronic respiratory disease, and arthritis have also provided useful baseline data. Specific references to studies in the various areas of interest are found in the references following this chapter.

An important potential of the Tecumseh project lies in its elucidation of risk factors in the health of a population studied in its natural setting. A major effort will be made to identify maximally predictive risk factors incorporating multiple variables which are closely related to the biological determinants of disease. As an example, intensive study of the interrelationships between hyperglycemia, hypertriglyceridemia, and lipoprotein and carbohydrate metabolism in general may yield predictive indices for coronary disease which are more sensitive and more specific than those derived from serum cholesterol measurements alone.

The long-term storage of serially collected sera from a large number of genetically related and unrelated persons in a total community represents a unique resource. This serum bank will permit the testing of new hypotheses as they are formulated in the future. It will also make possible a retrospective study of serological factors in persons who subsequently develop disease.

The Tecumseh population is being studied individually and in family units or kindreds. Analysis in terms of individuals has the major aim of identifying the various risk factors of disease in various subgroups of the population. Analysis in terms of family units is oriented toward the study of the environmental and genetic determinants of disease.

The entire Tecumseh population will continue to be surveyed, although less intensively than previously. In addition, more intensive studies of special kindreds and other subsets of the population will be undertaken. Within these subgroups, clinical investigative methods previously employed only in selected patient groups will be implemented.

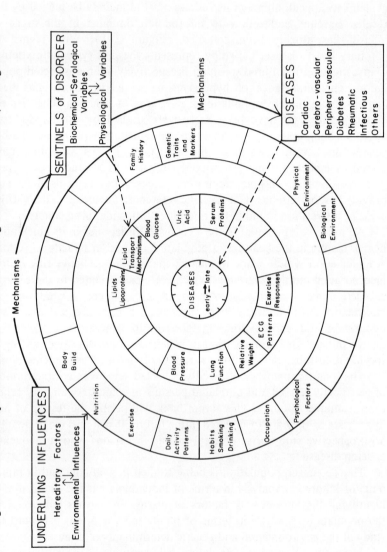

Figure 2-1—Relationships of interest for which data is being collected in Tecumseh, Michigan.

UNDERLYING INFLUENCES

Hereditary Factors
Environmental Influences

SENTINELS of DISORDER

Biochemical-Serological Variables
Physiological Variables

DISEASES

Cardiac
Cerebro-vascular
Peripheral-vascular
Diabetes
Rheumatic
Infectious
Others

Mechanisms

Nutrition
Body Build
Family History
Genetic Traits and Markers
Physical Environment
Biological Environment
Psychological Factors
Occupation
Habits Smoking Drinking
Daily Activity Patterns
Exercise

Lipids Lipoproteins
Lipid Transport Mechanisms
Blood Glucose
Uric Acid
Serum Proteins
Exercise Responses
ECG Patterns
Relative Weight
Lung Function
Blood Pressure

DISEASES

early ⇄ late

The major task of the Tecumseh Community Health Study has been to observe, to measure, and thereby to gain insight into the chains of causation. It is also within the broader scope of the work to envision the possibility, in coming years, of clinical trials of preventive regimens, since a population of this type would offer many advantages for this kind of investigation. Such clinical trials, however, would be secondary to the primary investigative goal of the longitudinal study of a total community.

Acknowledgments

The Tecumseh study was initiated and has been directed by Dr. Thomas Francis, Jr. It was supported by the Cardiovascular Research Center, University of Michigan, under Program Project Grant HE-6378 from the National Heart Institute, National Institutes of Health, U.S. Public Health Service and a Research Career Award (HE-K6-6748) to Dr. Epstein from the National Heart Institute, National Institutes of Health, U.S. Public Health Service.

The present report also includes contributions by other senior participants in the project, particularly Drs. R. A. Beldin, W. D. Block, S. Deutscher, H. J. Dodge, N. S. Hayner, M. P. Higgins, R. U. Marks, A. S. Monto, H. J. Montoye, and L. D. Ostrander, Jr

References

Deutscher, S., Epstein, F. H., and Kjelsberg, M. O. 1966. Familial aggregations of factors associated with coronary heart disease. *Circulation* 38:911–24.

Deutscher, S., Kjelsberg, M. O., and Epstein, F. H. 1967. Relationships between toxemia of pregnancy and essential hypertension in a total community. *Am. J. Epidem.* 85:72–83.

Dodge, H. J., Payne, M. W., Whitehouse, W. M., and Bauman, K. A. 1965. Estimates of the prevalence of tuberculous and histoplasmal infections in a sample of the population of Tecumseh, Michigan, 1960. *Am. Rev. Resp. Dis.* 92:459–69.

Epstein, F. H. 1964. Epidemiological research in total communities: settings and perspectives. *Meth. Inform. Med.* 3:18–22.

———. 1967a. Some uses of prospective observations in the Tecumseh Community Health Study. *Proc. Roy. Soc. Med.* 60:56–60.

———. 1967b. Risk factors in coronary heart disease-environmental and genetic influences. *Israel J. Med. Sci.* 3:594–607.

Epstein, F. H., Francis, T., Jr., Hayner, N. S., Johnson, B. C, Kjelsberg, M. O., Napier, J. A., Ostrander, L. D., Jr., Payne, M. W., and Dodge, H. J. 1965. Prevalence of chronic diseases and distribution of selected physiologic variables in a total community, Tecumseh, Michigan. *Am. J. Epidem.* 81:307–22.

Epstein, F. H., Ostrander, L. D., Johnson, B. C., Payne, M. W., Hayner, N. S., Keller, J. B., and Francis, T., Jr. 1965. Epidemiological studies of cardiovascular disease in a total community—Tecumseh, Michigan. *Ann. Intern. Med.* 62:1170–87.

Evans, J. G. and Ostrander, L. D., Jr. 1967. Fasting serum-triglycerides concentration and distribution of subcutaneous fat. *Lancet* 1:761–62.

Francis, T., Jr. 1961. Aspects of the Tecumseh Study. *Public Health Rep.* 76:963–65.

————. 1967. Epidemiological aspects of coronary heart disease. *Path. Microbiol.* 30:752–65.

Francis, T., Jr. and Epstein, F. H. 1965. Survey methods in general populations. Studies of a total community. Tecumseh, Michigan. *Milbank Mem. Fund Quart.* 43:333–42.

Francis, T., Jr., Ling, N. S., and Krasteff, T. 1965. Transcholesterin, a cholesterol-binding globulin: serological demonstration of a specific interaction between cholesterol and serum globulin. *Proc. Nat. Acad. Sci.* 53:1061–69.

French, J. G., Dodge, H. J., Kjelsberg, M. O., Mikkelsen, W. M., and Schull, W. J. 1967. A study of familial aggregation of serum uric acid levels in the population of Tecumseh, Michigan, 1959–1960. *Am. J. Epidem.* 86:214–24.

Hayner, N. S., Kjelsberg, M. O., Epstein, F. H., and Francis, T., Jr. 1965. Carbohydrate tolerance and diabetes in a total community, Tecumseh, Michigan. I. Effects of age, sex and test conditions on one-hour glucose tolerance in adults. *Diabetes* 14:413–23.

Hennessy, A. V., Davenport, F. M., Horton, R. J. M., Napier, J. A., and Francis, T., Jr. 1964. Asian influenza: occurrence and recurrence, a community and family study. *Milit. Med.* 129:38–50.

Higgins, M. W. and Kjelsberg, M. O. 1966. Characteristics of smokers and non-smokers in Tecumseh, Michigan. II. The distribution of selected physical measurements and physiologic variables and the prevalence of certain diseases in smokers and non-smokers. *Am. J. Epidem.* 86:60–77.

Higgins, M. W., Kjelsberg, M. O., and Metzner, H. L. 1967. Characteristics of smokers and non-smokers in Tecumseh, Michigan. I. The distribution of smoking habits in persons and families and their relationship to social characteristics. *Am. J. Epidem.* 86:45–59.

Johnson, B. C., Epstein, F. H., and Kjelsberg, M. O. 1965. Distributions and familial studies of blood pressure and serum cholesterol levels in a total community—Tecumseh, Michigan. *J. Chronic Dis.* 18:147–60.

Marks, R. U. 1967. Factors involving social and demographic characteristics: A review of empirical findings. *Milbank Mem. Fund Quart.* 45:51–108.

Matovinovic, J., Hayner, N. S., Epstein, F. H., and Kjelsberg, M. O. 1965. Goiter and other thyroid diseases in Tecumseh, Michigan: Studies in a total community. *J.A.M.A.,* 192:234–40.

Mikkelsen, W. M., Dodge, H. J., Duff, I. F., and Kato, H. 1967. Estimates of the prevalence of rheumatic diseases in the population of Tecumseh, Michigan, 1959–60. *J. Chronic Dis.* 20:351–69.

Mikkelsen, W. M., Dodge, H. J., and Valkenburg, H. 1965. The distribution of serum uric acid values in a population unselected as to gout or hyperuricemia. *Am. J. Med.* 39:242–51.

Montoye, H. J. and Epstein, F. H. 1965. Tecumseh Community Health Study: An investigation of health and disease in an entire community. *J. Sports Med.* 5:127–31.

Montoye, H. J., Epstein, F. H., and Kjelsberg, M. O. 1966. Relationship between serum cholesterol and body fatness: An epidemiologic study. *Am. J. Clin. Nutr.* 18:397–406.

Montoye, H. J., Faulkner, J. A., Dodge, H. J., Mikkelsen, W. M., Willis, P. M., III, and Block, W. D. 1967. Serum uric acid concentration among business executives: With observations on other coronary heart disease risk factors. *Ann. Intern. Med.* 66:838–50.

Morton, W. E. and Dodge, H. J. 1963. Modifications of the agar double diffusion precipitin test for tuberculosis. *Am. Rev. Resp. Dis.* 88:264–66.

Napier, J. A. 1962. Field methods and response rates in the Tecumseh Community Health Study. *Am. J. Public Health* 52:208–16.

Neff, B. J., Ackermann, W. W., Epstein, F. H., and Francis, T., Jr. 1962. Inhibition of vaccinial hemmagglutinins by sera of patients with coronary heart disease and other chronic illnesses. *Circulation Res.* 10:836–45.

Neff, B. J., Ackermann, W. W., and Preston, R. E. 1965. Studies of vaccinia hemagglutinin obtained from various vaccinia infected tissues: Density gradient centrifugation and electron microscopy. *Proc. Soc. Exp. Biol. Med.* 118:664–71.

Neff, B. J., Brody, G. L., Epstein, F. H., and Francis, T., Jr. 1962. Serologic and pathologic changes in rats on atherogenic diets. *J. Atheroscler. Res.* 2:306–13.

Ostrander, L. D., Jr. 1966. Serial electrocardiographic findings in a prospective epidemiological study. *Circulation* 34:1069–80.

Ostrander, L. D., Jr., Brandt, R. L., Kjelsberg, M. O., and Epstein, F. H. 1965. Electrocardiographic findings among the adult population of a total natural community, Tecumseh, Michigan. *Circulation* 31:888–98.

Ostrander, L. D., Jr., Francis, T., Jr. Hayner, N. S., Kjelsberg, M. O., and Epstein F. H. 1965. The relationship of cardiovascular disease to hyperglycemia. *Ann. Intern. Med.* 62:1188–98.

Ostrander, L. D., Jr., Neff, B. J., Block, W. D., Francis, T., Jr., and Epstein, F. H. 1967. Hyperglycemia and hypertriglyceridemia among persons with coronary heart disease. *Ann. Intern. Med.* 67:34–41.

Payne, M. W. and Kjelsberg, M. O. 1964. Respiratory symptoms, lung function and smoking habits in an adult population. *Am. J. Public Health* 54:261–77.

Reiff, G. C., Montoye, H. J., Remington, R. D., Napier, J. A., Metzner, H. L., and Epstein, F. H. 1967. Assessment of physical activity by questionnaire and interview. In *Physical Activity and the Heart*, proceedings of a symposium, Helsinki, Finland. Edited by Karvonen, M. J. and Barry, A. J., pp. 336–71. Springfield: C. C Thomas.

Schuman, S. H. and Miller, L. J. 1966. Febrile convulsions in families:

Findings in an epidemiological survey. *Clin. Pediat. (Phila.)* 5:604:08.
Wilcox, K. R., Jr. 1965. A trial of methods for collecting household morbidity data. In *Genetics and the Epidemiology of Chronic Diseases.* Edited by Neel, J. V., Shaw, M. W., and Schull, W. J., pp. 185–205. P.H.S. Pub. No. 1163. Washington: U.S. Government Printing Office.

EDITORIAL COMMENTS

1. The small and relatively homogeneous population of Tecumseh has now (1969) been subjected to surveillance and examination for more than a dozen years. One may ask whether the intensity of the study procedures and the "microscope" under which the residents find themselves have influenced the findings in any way. The Hawthorne effect was discussed in chapter 1, as was the possible merit of selecting an otherwise comparable control community in which outcomes are ascertained but in which the population is not manipulated.

2. The Tecumseh experience emphasizes the need to consider the demographic characteristics of communities which are selected for study. With only about 6,000 adult residents, a majority being young adults without chronic disease, the detailed epidemiologic investigation of relatively infrequent diseases is not feasible in Tecumseh. The unique advantages of the total community approach may, consequently, not be fully realizable there.

3. After several years of total community studies, an increasing number of investigations in Tecumseh are now being performed on specific subgroups. This suggests a shifting of interest to cohort studies of persons at special risk or with special attributes. Of course, it is likely that inadequate sample size will pose an even greater problem in these studies than in the community-wide investigations.

4. The authors suggest that in a total community setting, the study of multiple conditions requires little more effort or expense than the study of a single condition. This advantage would seem to apply to prospective studies in general, rather than to community studies in particular.

5. The authors believe that total community studies tend to be more economical because several investigations can be done at a total cost not much above that of a single retrospective study. This is an impressive argument which would benefit from the presentation of figures comparing the actual costs of data collection and hypothesis-testing in population laboratories with those incurred by more conventional approaches.

6. The authors note that the Tecumseh program does not attempt to study everything in everybody. This is particularly relevant to com-

prehensive community studies of the Tecumseh type, in which the testing of specific hypotheses is not of paramount importance. Where study objectives are not precisely formulated, there may, in fact, be no logical place to draw the line.

7. The nonresponse rate in Tecumseh has been highest among the aged, the seriously ill, and the migrants. The latter group differed from nonmigrants in having higher blood glucose levels and (among young adult males) higher serum uric acid levels. Yet, follow-up of migrants from Tecumseh is presently limited to the collection of death certificates and voluntarily submitted annual reports. This raises the question of whether it might be worth while to allocate additional funds for the intensive tracing of nonrespondents, even at the expense of one or more new studies.

8. The authors state that "the Tecumseh studies were undertaken primarily in order to study the patterns of disease and their possible determinants within this community rather than for the acquisition of data applicable to other communities." If, indeed, there was no intention to generalize the results of the Tecumseh studies, then this community has undergone a remarkably elaborate and costly health surveillance program. A project designed to acquire data for a single community with no prospect of application to other communities is really a public health service rather than a research program. We would hope that many of the findings in Tecumseh will prove of value elsewhere.

9. In regard to the authors' remark that "clinical trials of preventive regimens, especially in the field of coronary heart disease, will be given increasing attention," two reservations come to mind: first, the possible inadequacy of sample sizes in the selected age and sex groups; and, second, the possible difficulty in obtaining an untreated control group in a small town where cases, controls, and physicians probably all know one another.

10. Tecumseh appears to lack any special characteristics which would make its study uniquely appropriate. It has no especially high or low disease prevalences, characteristic dietary patterns, stress factors, or the like. As already noted, it is likely that convenience played a major role in its selection. This is true of most population laboratories, but it raises the question of whether even more appropriate choices could be made if closer attention were paid to the medical, environmental, and other characteristics of communities before their selection. A goal might be the identification of those communities which are best suited for studying specific diseases, environmental agents, or risk factors. To accomplish this would require either the active co-operation of such agencies as the National Center for Health Statistics and the Census Bureau or the establishment of a new national center to collate and

disseminate medical, social, and demographic data on communities. Since the center would utilize only existing data, costs would be moderate, but the potential benefits would be great. On the other hand, the research staff and technical facilities of the Tecumseh Community Health Study are so outstanding that the choice of community may well be of secondary importance.

CHAPTER 3

A renowned medical center with broad research interests and an ingeniously designed central record-keeping system fostered the development of an epidemiologic laboratory in a relatively isolated midwestern community. The advantages of near-complete case ascertainment and valid diagnosis of disease must be weighed against the relatively small sample sizes to be expected here. A question for consideration is whether Rochester might serve as a model for the development of population laboratories in other, larger communities.

POPULATION STUDIES IN ROCHESTER AND OLMSTED COUNTY, MINNESOTA, 1900–1968

Leonard T. Kurland, Lila R. Elveback, and Fred T. Nobrega

INTRODUCTION

At a national meeting on neurological disease 20 years ago, MacLean et al. (1948) described the first population survey of multiple sclerosis in North America. Morbidity rates for the previous 20 years in Rochester, Minnesota, were presented: the prevalence was more than twice as high as that reported elsewhere, and the medical prognosis was far more favorable than in the prevailing view, derived largely from the experience of hospitalized patients. MacLean's description of Rochester anticipated its unique advantages as an epidemiologic laboratory:

Rochester, Minnesota, is a small city of 33,000 inhabitants, the medical facilities of which are to a large extent concentrated within the organization of the Mayo Clinic. Approximately 15,000 residents of the city are at present examined each year in this institution. Data derived from this clinical scrutiny of roughly a half of the population annually, over a long period of years, have been preserved in the available medical records of the institution. A unique opportunity appears to present itself here for the study of disease states in a defined delimited community. We have attempted such a study of multiple sclerosis, in an effort to learn something of the incidence and prevalence of this disorder in our city and to evaluate its social implications. . . .

Although the small number of cases involved prompts one to be cautious in suggesting that the prevalence rate obtained in the present study is definitive, yet the very fact of the small size of the community involved, considering its exceptionally close relation to the Mayo Clinic, makes it quite plausible to believe that we have been able here to locate existing cases more completely than usual. In fact since there is no question as respects the cases we did find, the rates given are minimal estimates of the actual prevalence of multiple sclerosis in Rochester, Minnesota in 1948.

Despite the obvious merits of Rochester for community study, the findings on multiple sclerosis were largely discounted because of the discrepancy between these results and earlier reports and because of the city's small size. During the succeeding decade, however, extensive surveys of other communities in the northern United States and Canada corroborated the high prevalence of multiple sclerosis which had been reported from Rochester (Siedler, Nicholl, and Kurland 1958; White and Wheelan 1959). As the potential value of Rochester as a data resource became increasingly apparent, a series of descriptive epidemiologic studies of other neurologic diseases was conducted (Kurland 1957; 1958 a, b, c; 1959–60). The results offered convincing evidence that other diseases might be explored in similar fashion and led to the development of a research program which is now supported by the National Institutes of Health.

THE COMMUNITY

Historical Perspective

In 1964 Rochester, Minnesota, celebrated the hundredth anniversary of the birth of the Mayo brothers, the seventy-fifth anniversary of St. Mary's Hospital, and the fiftieth anniversary of the Mayo Foundation. The history of these institutions (Clapesattle 1941) reveals a complex mixture of "happenstance, catastrophe, idealism, foresight, and the impact of opportunity upon men prepared" (Schuster 1966). The Mayo Clinic happens to be in Rochester because Dr. William W. Mayo, the father of the Mayo brothers, migrated from England and was appointed by the federal government during the Civil War as Medical Provost Marshall in Rochester. He settled there permanently with his family after the war.

A catastrophe in the form of a tornado which struck Rochester in 1883, leaving 150 persons dead or injured, led to the construction of St. Mary's Hospital by a local order of Franciscan nuns. Doctor W. W. Mayo and his sons William J. and Charles H. practiced there and developed a new concept of group practice. The Mayo Clinic itself began in 1903 as an association of physicians joined together in an integrated and co-ordinated practice of medicine and surgery. Today the Clinic registers nearly 200,000 patients each year, about 15 per cent from Olmsted County and the remainder from the 50 states and many foreign countries.

Closely affiliated with the Mayo Clinic is the Mayo Foundation, a charitable and educational corporation which supports medical education and research. The Clinic and Foundation together have a permanent staff of 450 physicians and medical scientists and the Mayo Graduate School of Medicine, conducted by the Foundation, has an enrollment of nearly 700 in residency training.

The research potentials of Rochester owe their conception and realization, in part, to the relative isolation of this community but, in the main, to the vision and talent of two physicians, Henry Plummer and Joseph Berkson. In 1907 Henry Plummer developed a medical diagnostic index. Rather than a fanciful or theoretical nosology, this was a remarkably practical system for classifying the diagnoses recorded by physicians at the patient's discharge. Plummer also designed a unit record system, perhaps one of the earliest working examples of record linkage. For each patient a single record file is kept for the medical charts, pathological and laboratory reports, and correspondence relating to clinic visits, home visits, and treatments in all affiliated hospitals. Birth records and death certificates are also kept as part of this record.

Joseph Berkson, well known for his contributions to medical statistics, expanded Plummer's diagnostic index and, in 1935, initiated the use of Hollerith punch cards. This broadened the scope of the index so that many additional characteristics of the patient population would be ascertainable. Numerous other indexing procedures introduced by Plummer and Berkson have worked so well that, in spite of the recent technologic advances in data processing, it has not yet become necessary to alter the record system in Rochester appreciably.

The primary purpose of the unit record system is to facilitate the diagnosis and treatment of the patient. However, the ease with which records can be retrieved by diagnostic category has also affected the clinical research activities to the extent that between 500 and 800 diagnostic sets are now assembled each year for a variety of studies. Among these are epidemiological studies which require a clear identification of patients, a complete record of diagnoses and treatments, and longitudinal follow-up as to outcome. These conditions are especially applicable to the records of patients from Rochester and Olmsted County.

The growth of the Mayo Clinic and its two associated general hospitals was accompanied by the gradual disappearance of unaffiliated private medical practitioners in the community. By the end of World War II there were only three or four independent physicians remaining in Olmsted County.

To facilitate the medical care of the local population, the Rochester Section of Internal Medicine and the Newborn, the Well Child, Acute Illness, and Employees Health Services of the Mayo Clinic were organized after 1945. Despite this, the need for additional independent medical resources became acute and, in 1955, with support from members of the Mayo Clinic, the Olmsted Community Hospital was organized. Staffed by local independent physicians, especially those in the newly formed Olmsted Medical Group, the hospital has adopted the unit record system and diagnostic indexing procedures of the Mayo Clinic. In addition, members of the Olmsted Medical Group, as well as other unassociated physicians, participate with the Clinic staff in various community studies. It should be evident that, at least since 1935, most of the diagnosed cases of chronic progressive disease in Olmsted County residents can be identified from existing records of the Mayo Clinic, the Olmsted Community Hospital, the Olmsted Medical Group, the Rochester State Hospital (the local mental institution), and county death certificates. It is likely that the few remaining cases could also be identified from our central file which contains diagnostic summaries of the records of county residents who have been patients at the University and Veterans Administration Hospitals in Minneapolis, the county tuberculosis sanitorium, and several state hospitals for the mentally ill. Present plans also call for indexing the records of all other institutionalized residents of Olmsted County, viz., the blind, the mentally retarded, and the deaf, although most of these individuals have already established records in the existing master file.

Rochester Today

Rochester, the seat of Olmsted County, is 85 miles southeast of Minneapolis. The county is approximately square in shape, with boundaries about 12 miles on a side. About two-thirds of its population reside within the city and 10 per cent are employed by, or in training at, the clinic or the affiliated hospitals. IBM has been a major employer in Rochester since the opening of a computer component assembly plant and the establishment of a Medical Applications Department in 1957. Other local industries include electronics, food processing, and manufacturing of medical and allied equipment. There is no heavy industry and essentially no industrial air pollution. The population of Rochester and of the county (including Rochester) has more than doubled since 1930 (Table 3–1). Ninety-nine per cent of the population is white and primarily of northern European extraction. Rochester's growth rate parallels that of the rest of Olmsted County, which exceeds that of Minnesota as well as of the United States as a whole. The city's population growth reflects not only its natural increase but also the continued expansion of the Mayo Clinic, the establishment of diversified industries, and the periodic annexation of populous suburbs.

METHODS

A first step in the expansion of community studies in Rochester was the consolidation of the central record file. This has already been accomplished for the 200,000 persons who are now, or have been, Olmsted County residents since 1935. Their 372,000 medical and death records from a variety of sources have been abstracted and diagnostic punch cards prepared (Table 3–2). The death records include the death certificates of Olmsted residents dying in any part of Minnesota since 1935 and anywhere in the United States since about 1949.

The initial studies were designed to provide experience in the utilization of the master file and were limited to diseases for which this data source was considered to be especially appropriate. The projects included delineation of long-term trends in leukemia, lymphoma, myeloma, and cancers of the lung and thyroid.

TABLE 3–1. POPULATION OF ROCHESTER AND OLMSTED COUNTY[a] (1930–65)

Place	1930[b]	1940[b]	1950[b]	1960[b]	1965[c]
Rochester	20,621	26,312	29,885	40,663	47,797
Olmsted County[a]	35,426	42,658	48,228	65,332	75,217

[a] Including Rochester.
[b] From U.S. Census, 1930 to 1960.
[c] Estimated from special census of Rochester.

TABLE 3–2. SUMMARY OF RECORDS CATALOGED IN CENTRAL FILE (JANUARY 1, 1969)

Source	Number of Olmsted County records abstracted and coded by diagnosis
Mayo Clinic[a]	200,000
Death certificates	14,500
Autopsies	10,000
Olmsted Community Hospital	50,000
Olmsted Medical Group	90,000
Rochester State Hospital	4,000
University and V.A. Hospitals	4,000
Total	372,500

[a] In existing Mayo Clinic medical and surgical diagnostic file.

As was expected, nearly all cases seen prior to 1955 were identified through the diagnostic file of the Mayo Clinic. For example, of 137 cases of lung cancer, 124 were found in Mayo Clinic records (Table 3–3). The comparable figures for leukemia were 125 and 116, respectively. It is likely that the relative contribution of cases from other sources, especially the Olmsted Medical Group, will increase over time.

Project teams usually consist of a clinical specialist from the Mayo Clinic or a collaborating institution, a pathologist, and an epidemiologist or statistician. A medical resident, working under the supervision of the clinical consultant, may also be the principal investigator for a particular project to be published as a scientific paper or a doctoral thesis (Michel, Olsen, and Dockerty 1967). In co-operation with the pathologist, the clinician usually establishes the diagnostic criteria for the disease in question and designs and pretests those sections of the study abstract concerned with the clinical and pathological data. In addition, he attempts to estimate the stage of the disease and to identify antecedent or associated conditions. The pathologist identifies potential cases from the tissue registry, autopsy files, and death certificates and classifies the cases according to current concepts in pathology. The epidemiologists and statisticians, in turn, provide guidance in study design and execution, from the planning of abstract forms to final analysis of the data. The assistance of a well-trained paramedical staff is essential for such aspects of data collection as the determination of residence eligibility, current status, time and cause of death, and (if required) person years of observation, not to mention the coding of the data for card punching.

PROBLEMS

Use of Death Certificates

Death certificates afford an independent check on the completeness of case ascertainment from the master file. An effort was, therefore, made to determine: (1) the proportion of cases identified from death certificates, and (2) the proportion of certificates which failed to mention the disease under study.

In the leukemia study, 113 patients were known to have died and the death certificates of 112, including 2 who died outside of Minnesota, were located (Kyle et al. 1968). Leukemia was given as the underlying cause of death in 98 of these and as a contributory cause or complication in 7. Of the remaining seven cases in which leukemia was not mentioned, the diagnosis had been made before death in five and at autopsy in two instances.

TABLE 3-3. CASES OF BRONCHOGENIC CARCINOMA IN OLMSTED COUNTY, BY DECADE AND SOURCE OF DATA ON INITIAL DIAGNOSIS (1935-64)

Source of data	1935-44	1945-54	1955-64	Total
Mayo Clinic	11	41	72	124
Olmsted Community Hospital	—	—	2	2
Rochester State Hospital	—	1	3	4
Veterans Administration Hospital	—	—	5	5
University of Minnesota Hospital	—	—	1	1
Other	—	—	1	1
Total	11	42	84	137

The examination of death certificates revealed that 13 deaths had been ascribed to leukemia which could not be substantiated by subsequent review of all available clinical data. Two cases were certified as agnogenic myeloid metaplasia and one each as idiopathic monocytosis, Hodgkin's disease, lymphoproliferative disease, leukemoid reaction from a peritonsillar abscess, and refractory anemia. Two other cases showed a clinical pattern consistent with acute leukemia, but the peripheral blood smears were not diagnostic and the cases were excluded from study. Two cases were identified after an extensive histopathologic review as lymphocytic lymphosarcoma and in the remaining two cases no information other than that on the death certificate could be obtained.

Of the 137 patients with lung cancer, 128 have died and death certificates have been obtained for all (Byrd et al.). Bronchogenic carcinoma was recorded as the underlying cause of death in 116 cases (91 per cent). Among the other 12, death was attributed to other primary malignant disease in 4, to coronary artery disease in 5, and to peritonitis, bronchopneumonia, and cerebrovascular disease in the remaining 3. In addition to these 128 patients, 10 other county residents had their causes of death certified as bronchogenic carcinoma from 1935 to 1964. Medical records, including a few autopsy protocols, gave no evidence of lung cancer in six of these, while clinical data were unavailable for review in the other four. However, the inclusion of these four cases in the calculation of incidence rates would not have altered them appreciably.

For some diseases, particularly those of elderly patients dying at home, there were death certificates for which no clinical reports could be located. In the study of cerebrovascular disease for the period 1945–54, 649 cases were identified through clinical and pathological sources and 30 from death certificates alone (Fitzgibbons et al. 1968). Most of the latter had died at home, attended or seen after death by an unassociated general practitioner. In comparison with the decedents who had clinical records, those without them were more likely to have their deaths certified to cerebral hemorrhage (50 per cent vs. 10 per cent) or ill-defined conditions (apoplexy, stroke, etc.).

In a study of stomach cancer, from 1935 to 1964, it was noted that of the 143 case reports, only 3 before 1954 and 6 thereafter came from sources other than the Mayo Clinic (Smith et al.). The age-adjusted annual incidence rates, based on cases with medical records and histological confirmation, were 18, 14, and 12 per 100,000 in the 3 successive decades. The numbers of death-certificate-only cases in each decade were 13, 3, and 1, respectively, and their addition to the other cases would have exaggerated the downward trend in stomach cancer markedly. It has been suggested that the term "cancer of the stomach" may have been employed, especially in the 1935–44 period, for indeterminate abdominal malignancy or cachectic disease in which attempts at specific diagnosis were considered unnecessary or undesirable in view of the age and general health of the patients.

Histologic Confirmation of Diagnosis

Histologic confirmation of the diagnosis was made in 122 of the 125 leukemias and in 131 of the 137 pulmonary cancers. As would be expected, the proportion was somewhat lower for stomach cancer (120 of 143 cases confirmed), where X-ray and clinical findings more often provided the basis for diagnosis.

The extent of diagnosis at autopsy varied with the disease, the patients' age, and, to a slight extent, the time period—being somewhat more frequent from 1948 to 1958. The over-all autopsy rate in Rochester during this time was about 70 per cent. In a special study of infant deaths from 1946 to 1965, 75 per cent were autopsied; but among those with sudden, unexplained deaths 90 per cent were autopsied (Ludwig et al. 1969). About 55 per cent of elderly decedents with cerebrovascular disease were autopsied, the proportion being somewhat higher among those dying within 30 days of an acute episode which, presumably, increased their likelihood of dying in a hospital. Less than 2 per cent of clinically diagnosed strokes could not be confirmed at post-mortem; however, 10 per cent of the strokes found at autopsy had not been diagnosed previously (Fitzgibbons et al. 1968). The latter tended to occur in clinically silent regions and the patients were usually elderly persons treated (if at all) at home. Of 13 clinically diagnosed cases of multiple sclerosis which came to autopsy, 12 were histologically confirmed (Percy et al.). This is a somewhat higher rate than reported in other studies (Stazio et al. 1964).

Completeness of Follow-up

Most of the diseases studied in Rochester were serious and progressive, terminating in death or in disability requiring continued medical management. Consequently, the follow-up of most patients to establish live or dead status required only a search for the latest entries in the file or retrieval of the death certificate and autopsy report, if any. Follow-up is more difficult if the patient has not been seen in recent years or if the death was not noted in the clinical record. In these cases the history is reviewed for possible clues and the city directory is checked to determine dates of residence and to identify relatives or neighbors who might have some useful information. Additional inquiries are made by telephone and, when possible, patients are traced through the post office or the Retail Credit Bureau. If there is reason to believe the patient has died, death certificates for the years after the date last known alive are searched in Minnesota and, if necessary, in other states.

These extensive procedures do not have to be employed for most patients with rapidly progressive disease, including some of the malignancies, since the medical record alone suffices in 85 to 90 per cent of such cases. One of the studies which did require such follow-up was that of stroke diagnosed in Rochester residents between 1945 and 1954 (Fitzgibbons et al. 1968). Of 649 patients, 646 were known to have died (and their death certificates were obtained) or were known to be alive on January 1, 1968. This high percentage of follow-up was attained only after considerable difficulty due, in part, to the necessity for tracing patients 13 to 23 years after their stroke and, in part, because of the many residential changes made by elderly patients surviving their first stroke. Some of these had residual neurologic disability and were transferred from relative to relative, sometimes out of the county or even out of the state, or from one nursing home to another. The extensive follow-up procedures had to be instituted in about 150 of the approximately 500 stroke patients who survived the acute episode.

For the rapidly fatal diseases such as amyotrophic lateral sclerosis or for diseases requiring frequent medical attention, such as systemic lupus erythematosus or multiple sclerosis, there was relatively little difficulty in achieving complete follow-up (Kurland, Choi, and Sayre 1969; Nobrega et al. 1966; Percy et al.). Parkinsonism, with its slowly progressive course, was less of a problem in follow-up than stroke, since most of the patients remained ambulatory and could generally attend to their personal needs better than those who had suffered strokes (Kurland et al. 1969).

It is likely that this degree of success in follow-up will not be attained in studies of less progressive or fatal diseases, especially if cases occurring prior to 1945 are included.

FINDINGS

The measurement of time-trends in disease incidence is important because such trends may reflect changes in exposure to etiologic factors, if variations in case ascertainment can be excluded. Most studies of time-trends have been based on hospital admissions, autopsied cases, or death certificates—data sources with well-recognized potential biases. The Rochester project, in which the degree of case ascertainment and the accuracy of clinical diagnosis are both unusually high, is relatively free of such selective factors. Other problems remain, however: the population may be too small to permit the detection of any but large deviations in the incidence of rare diseases; changes in diagnostic procedures may supervene; and the medical records may fail to mention exposure to a suspected etiologic agent.

Multiple Sclerosis

Some investigators have suggested that multiple sclerosis has been increasing in frequency over time. There is no evidence of an increase in the average annual incidence of this disease over a 60 year period in Rochester (Table 3–4). The rates in Rochester are, on the whole, somewhat higher than those reported for other cities in the northern United States and Canada, perhaps because of more complete case ascertainment. To our knowledge, the only other long-term studies of annual incidence, those from New Orleans and Winnipeg, also show no increase in rates (Stazio, Paddison, and Kurland 1967).

TABLE 3–4. NUMBER OF CASES AND AVERAGE INCIDENCE RATES OF MULTIPLE SCLEROSIS IN RESIDENTS OF ROCHESTER, MINNESOTA (1905–64) BY SEX AND DECADE

| Years | Number of cases | | | |
	Male	Female	Total	Incidence /100,000
1905–14	0	4	4	5.1
1915–24	2	3	5	3.6
1925–34	0	11	11	5.3
1935–44	2	4	6	2.3
1945–54	3	5	8	2.7
1955–64	7	6	13	3.2
Total	14	33	47	3.2[a]

[a] Weighted average.

The survivorship for multiple sclerosis in Rochester is appreciably better than that reported from other sources, with almost 75 per cent surviving 25 years after the onset of disease (Percy et al.). These survivorship data suggest that the essentially complete case ascertainment in this community results in the identification of a higher proportion of mild cases than do most studies of clinic or hospital patients.

Amyotrophic Lateral Sclerosis

The mean age of onset in amyotrophic lateral sclerosis has been reported in several clinical studies as being about fifty-two years (Mulder 1957; Friedman and Freedman 1950). Since the mean duration of this fatal disease is three to four years, these data are hard to reconcile with U.S. mortality statistics showing a mean age at death of 64.4 years. All cases diagnosed in Rochester over a 40-year period were identified and the mean age at onset was calculated to be sixty-four years. This suggests that the other clinical studies may have been biased toward the selection of younger patients who were more likely to have been seen by specialists capable of diagnosing rare neurological conditions. Therefore, the mean age at onset may be closer to sixty years than to the fifty-two years generally reported (Kurland, Choi, and Sayre 1969).

Parkinsonism

During the period 1945–54 the age-specific rates for parkinsonism increased continuously with age (Kurland et al. 1969). During the decades just prior to 1945 and immediately after 1955, the rate increased up to seventy-five years of age but declined slightly thereafter. It is believed that the most complete case ascertainment for parkinsonism was achieved during the 1945–54 period and that the true rate increases continuously over the life span.

The mean age at onset in five-year intervals after 1934 (line 3 in Figure 3–1) tends to parallel the mean age of the Rochester population thirty-five years and older (line 2). At the same time it contrasts with the steeply increasing trend of age at onset (line 1) reported by Poskanzer and Schwab (1963) from their study of patients at the Massachusetts General Hospital. Poskanzer and Schwab noted a "steady upward progression in age of onset" and stated that these data "suggest the presence of a cohort, a group in the population aging together. Between 1920–1924 and 1955–1959, a period of 35 years, the mean age at onset of our population with Parkinson's syndrome has increased 27 years." This analysis and other arguments cited with it were used by

Figure 3–1. Age at onset of parkinsonism: Massachusetts General Hospital and Rochester–Olmsted County. *Source*: Nobrega et al. 1969.

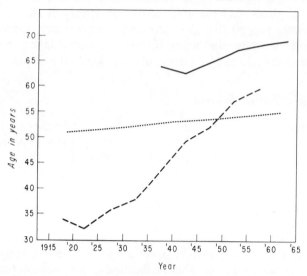

------Age at onset, Massachusetts General Hospital
----------Mean age (over thirty-four years), Rochester–Olmsted County
————Age at onset, Rochester–Olmsted County

Poskanzer and Schwab as the basis for predicting a "precipitous drop" in the incidence of parkinsonism in the United States within about ten years. The Rochester data, however, do not substantiate these findings, and when our analysis is extended to include all Mayo Clinic patients with parkinsonism, or another neurologic disease—herpes zoster—since 1935, a similar pattern of increasing age over time is noted.

The findings in the Boston study may be attributable to an artifact related to changing patterns of medical care, rather than to a shift in the age distribution of the disease. The Rochester material, consisting of patients seen by general practitioners as well as specialists, probably reflects the actual characteristics of the disease, including its age distribution, with greater accuracy.

There are indications that in the United States increasing numbers of older parkinsonism patients, who had formerly remained at home without treatment, are now seeking the care of family physicians and specialists. Such a change in the acceptance of medical care by the aged seems to offer a reasonable explanation for the increase in mean age at disease onset among the hospitalized patients seen at the Massachusetts General Hospital. The stability in mean age of onset among the Rochester patients during the past three decades is probably a reflection of the general acceptance by the elderly in Rochester of medical care at the Mayo Clinic and its affiliates (Nobrega, et al. 1969).

In our opinion, the shift in age distribution of parkinsonism patients at the Massachusetts General Hospital is not necessarily due to the cohort effect of common exposure to the encephalitis lethargica epidemic as postulated by Poskanzer and Schwab. Such a shift can be explained equally well, and perhaps better, as a reflection of changes in medical practice, and particularly in specialty services sought and received with increasing frequency by elderly persons in recent years. The highly specialized medical institutions in the United States are being called on to attend to an increasing proportion of the chronic and progressive illnesses among elderly patients which previously have largely been the responsibility of the general practitioner.

Cerebrovascular Disease

In a study of strokes occurring prior to the era of anticoagulants and antihypertensive drugs Fitzgibbons et al. (1968) measured survivorship and residual deficits at given intervals. Case fatality within one month after the acute episode was 27 per cent for cerebral infarction, 83 per cent for cerebral hemorrhage, and 64 per cent for subarachnoid hemorrhage. The latter is a higher percentage than is generally reported from other studies, and it may be related to the unusual promptness of hospitalization in Rochester, which could permit such patients to survive long enough to be diagnosed.

Systemic Lupus Erythematosus

The average annual incidence rates of systemic lupus erythematosus in Rochester were calculated for the periods 1950–59 and 1960–65. Among males the rates increased from about 1 to 6 per 100,000 and among females, from 4 to 7 per 100,000 (Nobrega et al. 1966). A study in New York has also demonstrated an increase in rates with time, but it is generally believed that diagnostic improvements rather than true increases have taken place (Siegel et al. 1962). It is of interest that in New York the reported incidence was higher among Negroes and Puerto Ricans than among whites, whereas in predominantly white Rochester the rate exceeded that of all groups in New York. It is possible that case ascertainment was not equal for each of the population subgroups in the New York study (Siegel et al. 1962).

In both New York and Rochester prior to 1960, females with systemic lupus predominated over males seven to one (Siegel et al. 1964). Since 1960, however, the sex ratio among Rochester cases has changed so that it is now about two to one in favor of females. The explanation of this is still lacking.

The development and growing utilization of the LE cell test since 1950 has resulted in an increasing recognition of this disease. The sharp increase in its reported incidence may be due to the inclusion of less advanced, earlier diagnosed cases in recent years. If this is true, then the long-range trends should show increases in incidence and prevalence and decreases in case fatality rates. Case fatality in Rochester has, in fact, decreased from 33 per cent in 1950–59 to 17 per cent more recently.

Leukemia

During the past 30 years, leukemia mortality rates per 100,000 U.S. whites have shown a threefold rise from about 2.4 in 1930 to 7.5 in 1963 (U.S. Bureau of the Census 1934; U.S.P.H.S. 1965). Incidence figures from state tumor registries in New York and Connecticut demonstrate a similar upward trend (Bailar, King, and Mason 1964; Griswold et al. 1955).

In Olmsted County, the average annual leukemia incidence rates for the three decades from 1935 to 1964 were 7.7, 6.8, and 9.0 respectively (Kyle et al. 1968). The rates are not appreciably affected by age and sex adjustment to the 1950 Olmsted County population. Although the rate increased slightly during the most recent decade, there is no obvious trend or significant difference in these rates over the entire period. The incidence rates by cell type have also not changed significantly over time. The age distribution has remained stable except for persons seventy-five years old and more, among whom there was an increase in the most recent decade. Males showed a consistent and slightly higher incidence than females over the entire period.

Other studies in the United States and abroad have suggested that leukemia is more common in urban than in rural areas. In Olmsted County the urban rate exceeded the rural except from 1945 to 1954, but these differences were not significant.

Reports of the onset of leukemia symptoms by season have shown no consistent pattern (Hayes 1961; Lee 1964). In Olmsted County there was a tendency for the disease to appear in the fall and winter, although in an appreciable number of cases the date of onset was uncertain. There was no seasonal pattern by date of diagnosis for acute lymphocytic leukemia, acute leukemia in general, or for all types combined. Because of the relatively small number of cases in Rochester, however, one would not expect to detect a seasonal variation unless it was quite sizable.

The question of whether leukemia occurs in geographical clusters has been of interest since the first reports of such clustering in Buffalo, New York, and Niles, Illinois (Pinkel and Nefzger 1959; Heath and Hasterlik 1963). There was no obvious spatial clustering in Olmsted County.

In contrast to the reported rise in leukemia mortality over the past 30 years in the United States, the incidence of leukemia has not changed significantly during this time in Olmsted County (Kyle et al. 1968). In fact, the average annual incidence rate for males and females from 1935 through 1944 in Olmsted County was identical to the incidence rates reported in Norway and Sweden in 1959 and to the mortality rate among U.S. whites (Court-Brown, Doll, and Hill 1964; U.S.P.H.S. 1963). Furthermore, there has been no major change during these 30 years in leukemia incidence by sex, cell type, or urban-rural residence.

In the last decade or two in the United States, bone-marrow examinations and other improved diagnostic techniques have been increasingly utilized. In addition, supportive therapy now enables some patients who might otherwise have died from associated septicemia or cerebrovascular accidents to survive long enough for an underlying leukemic process to be recognized. Because of the nature of the Rochester data, it is our impression that the findings there reflect the secular trend in leukemia incidence more accurately than do the U.S. mortality data.

Bronchogenic Carcinoma

The average annual incidence of lung cancer increased markedly among males—from 3 per 100,000 in 1935–44 to 24 per 100,000 in 1955–64 (Byrd et al.). There was no increase over time in females. Especially large, temporal increases were observed for squamous-cell, small-cell, and large-cell carcinoma, while adenocarcinoma increased moderately among males and not at all among females (Figures 3–2 and 3–3). The observed increases were much greater in the urban as compared with the rural males, the incidence rising fifteenfold among the former and only threefold among the latter. To some extent these differences may reflect differential rates of case ascertainment.

The age-specific incidence of bronchogenic carcinoma rose fairly steadily between forty-five and seventy-five years of age; beyond seventy-five years it continued to increase from 1945 to 1954 but declined during the other two decades studied. Other observers of a rate decrease among the elderly have suggested that the rapid increase in lung cancer incidence is coming to an end and that the death rate will become stabilized within the next 15 years (Ravenholt and Foege 1963).

Figure 3–2. Lung cancer in Olmstead County males: 1935–64. *Source:* Byrd et al.

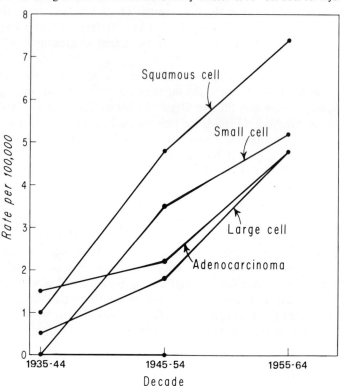

Incidence rates of disease are very much affected by competing risks of death from other causes. This is especially true of the elderly, who are subject to high risks of many diseases. It is doubtful, however, whether the secular trends for lung cancer among the elderly Rochester males can be explained on this basis. A more probable explanation is that case ascertainment among the elderly had improved in 1945–54 over the earlier period but that it declined somewhat in the third decade, as less comprehensive data sources than the Mayo Clinic were beginning to be utilized.

Thyroid Cancer

Although United States death rates for thyroid cancer have remained essentially unchanged in 30 years, there have been recent reports of an increase in incidence (Goldman et al. 1967). Through an examination of medical records, death certificates, and other data sources, 59 cases of thyroid cancer among Olmsted County residents from 1935 to 1965

Figure 3–3. Lung cancer in Olmstead County females: 1935–64. *Source:* Byrd
   et al.

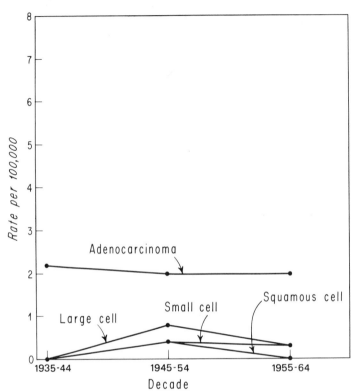

were identified (Verby et al. 1969). The average annual incidence rose
only slightly during each of the last two decades, suggesting that there
has been little increase in the incidence of thyroid cancer in Olmsted
County since 1935. The study confirmed that there had been improvements in case ascertainment, particularly in autopsies performed since
about 1950. The occult, grade I papillary carcinoma is still of question-
able malignancy, however, and it would appear that the inclusion of
such cases in recent years, as well as a more intensive search for thyroid
tumors in general, has been responsible for the apparent secular increase in incidence which others have reported.

Primary Brain Neoplasms

The findings on primary brain neoplasms in Rochester differed
from those reported in a number of other studies (Figure 3–4). The
average annual age-specific incidence in these other studies decreased
among persons sixty-five years of age and above. In Rochester, by

Figure 3–4. Average annual incidence of primary neoplasms of the brain, by age: Rochester–Olmsted County and three other populations. *Source*: Kurland 1958*a*.

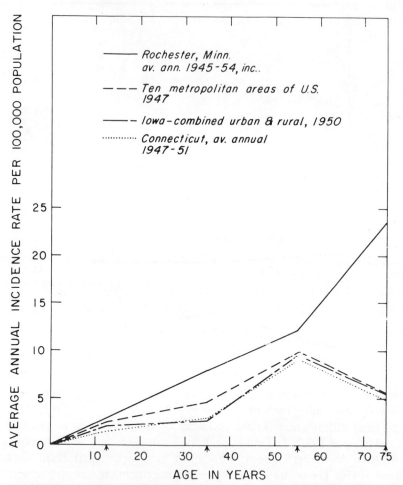

contrast, the rate increased continuously with age. The explanation may lie in the relatively more complete and accurate diagnoses of brain neoplasms among the elderly in Rochester as compared with the other areas (Kurland 1958*a*).

Multiple Myeloma

The incidence of multiple myeloma from 1945 to 1964 in both sexes combined was 3.1 per 100,000, a rate approximating that recorded in Malmo, Sweden, but higher than both white and Negro rates reported in an earlier study in Brooklyn, N.Y. (Kyle, Nobrega, and Kurland

1969; Waldenström 1960; MacMahon and Clark 1956). Clinical reports have suggested that the age-specific incidence increases up to sixty or sixty-five years of age and then decreases. In Olmsted County the average annual incidence rates in males and in both sexes combined increased with age and were highest for persons over eighty.

POTENTIALS

The epidemiologic laboratory in Rochester is well adapted for both retrospective and prospective approaches to the study of disease. An especially valuable feature of the central record file is that it permits the identification of numerous categories of diseased patients with little more effort than is required for a single disease. For these reasons, among others, we are studying not only the common diseases but also the uncommon or relatively rare conditions such as pheochromocytoma and pancreatic islet cell tumors. Other epidemiologic studies in progress or being planned include investigations of chronic ulcerative colitis, sudden death in infancy, Bell's palsy (Annis et al.), childhood epilepsy, and various connective tissue disorders.

In other study centers, the data sources on such diseases are often inadequate, either because of the sophisticated diagnostic techniques which are necessary or because it is not considered worth while to code infrequent events. With its ready access to information on both mild and severe cases of identifiable conditions, the Rochester Community Study may constitute one of the few reliable sources of incidence data on many of the uncommon diseases. That such data can serve for comparison with experience in other populations has already been demonstrated by our studies on multiple sclerosis, amyotrophic lateral sclerosis, and epilepsy.

The completeness of the medical histories in Rochester makes possible the study of relationships between existing clinical or physiologic abnormalities and the subsequent risk of specific diseases. The spurious statistical associations often found in data derived from selectively admitted hospital patients should be absent from our studies of a total population (Berkson 1946). We also anticipate that the additional advantages of accuracy and completeness in case ascertainment will outweigh the disadvantage of Rochester's small population size.

The Rochester project is well suited to evaluate time-trend data based on mortality statistics with their inherent errors and inconsistencies. For example, Yates (1966) has reported that in England and Wales over the past 30 years there has been an appreciable drop in the death rate for cerebral hemorrhage and a concomitant rise in that for cerebral infarction. A similar trend has been noted in the United

States, where the death rate from hypertension has also been falling. With our resources in Rochester we may be able to determine whether these trends reflect changing fashions in death certification or true changes in disease incidence.

The follow-up procedures in use at the Mayo Clinic have made possible the conduct of many survivorship studies (Berkson and Gage 1950; Elveback 1958). Application of these methods to the entire Olmsted County population may improve the calculated survivorship estimates by reflecting the totality of diagnosed cases, mild and severe, occurring in a population. This would contrast with studies based only on cases (presumably the more severe) which were treated at a particular hospital or clinic. Such survivorship statistics would be especially useful in evaluating new methods of treatment (e.g., for hypertension) or of early diagnosis (e.g., for cervical cancer).

The recorded prior medical history is usually well-documented in our records. Family histories are often inadequate but could be improved if a program for linkage of family records proves to be feasible. The descriptions of occupational and other environmental exposures are not generally satisfactory; case-control studies with specific questioning on such exposures, therefore, continues to be the method of choice.

To strengthen our data resources and to extend the usefulness of the Rochester-Olmsted project even further, two new instruments are being considered for use in our long-range plans. In conjunction with current efforts at the Mayo Clinic to develop an automated self-administered patient-inventory questionnaire, we intend to explore the use of an even more detailed questionnaire for Olmsted County residents. In future studies, this should provide us with appreciably more information than is now available on prior medical history, family history, and environmental exposures. It should make possible the validation of those aspects of personal and family history which have been entered in both the questionnaire and the existing medical records of the patient and his family in the central file.

The other instrument under consideration is a multi-phasic screening examination which would be extended to a large sample (perhaps 25 per cent) of the local population. A major function of this examination would be the early detection of disease. Because of our highly efficient follow-up of Rochester patients after their hospitalization it should be possible to compare the extent of early disease detection among those who have been screened and those who have not.

Acknowledgments

This investigation was supported in part by Research Grant GM-14231 from the National Institutes of Health, United States Public Health Service.

References

Annis, J. P., Mulder, D., Sayre, G. P., and Kurland, L. T. Incidence of Bell's palsy in the Olmsted County population, 1955–1967, inclusive. (Unpublished data.)

Bailar, J. C., III, King, H., and Mason, M. J. 1964. *Cancer Rates and Risks.* P.H.S. Pub. No. 1148. Washington: U.S. Government Printing Office.

Berkson, J. 1946. Limitations of the application of fourfold table analysis to hospital data. *Biometrics* 2:47–57.

Berkson, J. and Gage, R. P. 1950. Calculation of survival rates for cancer. *Mayo Clin. Proc.* 25:270–86.

Byrd, R., Nobrega, F. T., Divertie, M. B., Carr, D. T., Woolner, L. B., and Kurland, L. T. The 30-year trend in carcinoma of the bronchus in Olmsted County, Minnesota, 1935–64. (Unpublished data.)

Clapesattle, H. 1941. *The Doctors Mayo.* Minneapolis: University of Minnesota Press.

Court Brown, W. M., Doll, R., and Hill, I. D. 1964. Leukaemia in Britain and Scandinavia. *Path. Microbiol.* 27:644–54.

Elveback, L. 1958. Estimation of survivorship in chronic disease: The "actuarial" method. *J. Am. Statist. Ass.* 53:420–40.

Fitzgibbons, J. P., Jr., Sayre, G. P., Whisnant, J. P., and Kurland, L. T. Incidence and outcome of stroke in Rochester, Minnesota, Phase I, 1945–1954. Presented at the meeting of the American Heart Association, Bal Harbour, Florida, 24 November 1968.

Friedman, A. P. and Freedman, D. 1950. Amyotrophic lateral sclerosis. *J. Nerv. Ment. Dis.* 111:1–18.

Goldman, L., Greenspan, F. S., McCorkle, H. J., and Lindsay, S. 1967. Thyroid cancer climbing sharply. *Med. World News* 8:35.

Griswold, M. H., Wilder, C. S., Cutler, S. J., and Pollack, E. S. 1955. *Cancer in Connecticut, 1935–1951.* Hartford: Connecticut State Department of Health.

Hayes, D. M. 1961. The seasonal incidence of acute leukemia: A contribution to the epidemiology of the disease. *Cancer* 14:1301–05.

Heath, C. W., Jr., and Hasterlik, R. J. 1963. Leukemia among children in a suburban community. *Am. J. Med.* 34:796–812.

Kurland, L. T. 1957. Definitions of cerebral palsy and their role in epidemiologic research. *Neurology* 7:641–54.

———. 1958*a*. The frequency of intracranial and intraspinal neoplasms in the resident population of Rochester, Minnesota. *J. Neurosurg.* 15:627–41.

———. 1958*b*. Descriptive epidemiology of selected neurologic and myopathic disorders with particular reference to a survey in Rochester, Minnesota. *J. Chronic Dis.* 8:378–418.

———. 1958*c*. Epidemiology: Incidence, geographic distribution and genetic considerations. In *Pathogenesis and Treatment of Parkinsonism.* Edited by Fields, W. S. pp. 5–49. Springfield: C. C. Thomas.

————. 1959–60. The incidence and prevalence of convulsive disorders in a small urban community. *Epilepsia* 1:143–61.

Kurland, L. T., Choi, N. W., and Sayre, G. P. 1969. Implications of incidence and geographic patterns on the classification of amyotrophic lateral sclerosis. In *Motor Neuron Diseases: Research on Amyotrophic Lateral Sclerosis and Related Disorders*. Edited by Norris, F. H., Jr., and Kurland, L. T. New York: Grune & Stratton, in press.

Kurland, L. T., Hauser, W. A., Okazaki, H., and Nobrega, F. T. 1969. Epidemiologic studies of parkinsonism with special reference to the cohort hypothesis. In *Proc. Symposium on Parkinsonism*, in press.

Kyle, R. A., Nobrega, F. T., Kurland, L. T., and Elveback, L. R. 1968. The 30-year trend of leukemia in Olmsted County, Minnesota, 1935 through 1964. *Mayo Clin. Proc.* 43:342–53.

Kyle, R. A., Nobrega, F. T., and Kurland, L. T. 1969. Multiple myeloma in Olmsted County, Minnesota, 1945–1964. *Blood* 33:739–45.

Lee, J. A. H. 1964. Seasonal variations in the incidence of the clinical onset of leukemia. *Path. Microbiol.* 27:772–76.

Ludwig, J., Fitzgibbons, J. P., Jr., and Nobrega, F. T. 1969. Sudden unexpected unexplained death in infants: a comparative clinicopathologic study. *Virchow Arch. Path. Anat.* 346:287–301.

MacLean, A. R., Berkson, J., Woltman, H. W., and Schionneman, L. 1948. Multiple sclerosis in a rural community. *Ass. Res. Nerv. Ment. Dis.* 28:25–27.

MacMahon, B. and Clark, D. W. 1956. The incidence of multiple myeloma. *J. Chronic Dis.* 4:508–15.

Michel, J. O., Olsen, A. M., and Dockerty, M. B. 1967. The association of diaphragmatic hiatal hernia and gastroesophageal carcinoma. *Surg. Gynec. Obstet.* 124:583–89.

Mulder, D. W. 1957. The clinical syndrome of amyotrophic lateral sclerosis. *Mayo Clin. Proc.* 32:427–36.

Nobrega, F. T., Ferguson, R. H., Kurland, L. T., and Hargraves, M. M. 1966. Lupus erythematosus in Rochester, Minnesota 1950–1965: A preliminary study. In *Proc. of the 3d International Symposium on Population Studies of the Rheumatic Diseases, 1966*. Edited by Bennett, P. H. and Wood, P. H. N., pp. 259–66. International Congress Series, no. 148. Amsterdam: Excerpta Medica Foundation.

Nobrega, F. T., Glattre, E., Kurland, L. T., and Okazaki, H. 1969. Comments on the epidemiology of parkinsonism including prevalence and incidence statistics for Rochester, Minnesota, 1935–1966. In *Progress in Neuro-Genetics*. Edited by Barbeau, A. and Brunette, J. R., pp. 474–85. Amsterdam: Excerpta Medica Foundation.

Percy, A., Nobrega, F. T., Glattre, E., and Okazaki, H. Multiple sclerosis in a rural community: A reevaluation. (Unpublished data.)

Pinkel, D. and Nefzger, D. 1959. Some epidemiological features of childhood leukemia in the Buffalo, N.Y. area. *Cancer* 12:351–58.

Poskanzer, D. C. and Schwab, R. S. 1963. Cohort analysis of Parkinson's syndrome: Evidence for a single etiology related to subclinical infection about 1920. *J. Chronic Dis.* 16:961–73.

Ravenholt, R. T. and Foege, W. H. 1963. Epidemiology and treatment of lung cancer in Seattle. *Dis. Chest* 44:174–85.

Schuster, G. S. 1966. Speech presented to the American Association for the History of Medicine, 13 May 1966. (Unpublished data.)

Siedler, H. D., Nicholl, W., and Kurland, L. T. 1958. The prevalence and incidence of multiple sclerosis in Missoula County, Montana. *J. Lancet* 78:358–60.

Siegel, M., Lee, S. L., Widelock, D., Reilly, E. B., Wise, G. J., Zingale, S. B., and Fuerst, H. T. 1962. The epidemiology of systemic lupus erythematosus: Preliminary results in New York City. *J. Chronic Dis.* 15:131–40.

Siegel, M., Reilly, E. B., Lee, S. L., Fuerst, H. T., and Seelenfreund, M. 1964. Epidemiology of systemic lupus erythematosus: Time trend and racial differences. *Am. J. Public Health* 54:33–43.

Smith, L. A., Nobrega, F. T., Cain, J. C., Dockerty, M. B., and ReMine, W. H. Carcinoma of the stomach in Olmsted County, Minnesota, 1935–1964. (Unpublished data.)

Stazio, A., Kurland, L. T., Bell, L. G., Saunders, M.G., and Rogot, E. 1964. Multiple sclerosis in Winnipeg, Manitoba: Methodological considerations of epidemiologic survey: Ten year follow-up of a community wide study, and population re-survey. *J. Chronic Dis.* 17:415–38.

Stazio, A., Paddison, R. M., and Kurland, L. T. 1967. Multiple sclerosis in New Orleans, Louisiana, and Winnipeg, Manitoba, Canada: Follow-up of a previous survey in New Orleans, and comparisons between the patient populations in the two communities. *J. Chronic Dis.* 20:311–32.

U.S. Bureau of the Census. 1934. Mortality Statistics, 1930. Washington: U.S. Government Printing Office.

U.S. Public Health Service. 1963. Vital Statistics of the United States, 1960, vol. II: Mortality, parts A and B. Washington: U.S. Government Printing Office.

U.S. Public Health Service. 1965. Vital Statistics of the United States, 1963, vol. II: Mortality, parts A and B. Washington: U.S. Government Printing Office.

Verby, J. E., Woolner, L. B., Nobrega, F. T., Kurland, L. T., and McConahey, W. M. 1969. Thyroid cancer in Olmsted County, 1935–1965. (Unpublished data.)

Waldenström, J. 1960. Diseases associated with abnormal plasma proteins. *Proc. Roy. Soc. Med.* 53:789–92.

White, D. N. and Wheelan, L. 1959. Disseminated sclerosis: A survey of patients in the Kingston, Ontario area. *Neurology* 9:256–72.

Yates, P. O. 1966. The changing pattern of cerebrovascular disease in the United Kingdom. In *Cerebral Vascular Diseases: Transactions of the 5th Conference.* Edited by Millikan, C. H., Siekert, R. G., and Whisnant, J. P., pp. 67–82. New York: Grune & Stratton.

EDITORIAL COMMENTS

1. The near-total population coverage of the Rochester studies is not usually achieved in hospital-based surveys of disease. The centripetal pattern of health services for Olmsted County residents and the rather unique system of record linkage between their medical institutions have made this possible in Rochester. Important contributing factors are, first, the near-absence of physicians who are unaffiliated with these institutions, and, second, the phenomenally low number of missing records at the Mayo Clinic: about 100 lost out of a total of 3 million.

2. Despite the unusually complete hospital records in Rochester, some persons with such diseases of interest as leukemia, lung cancer, and stroke are known to have eluded detection. The extent of these losses is uncertain, but this suggests the desirability of supplementing the existing methods of case ascertainment with periodic community surveys. The planned multi-phasic screening program and the self-administered health inventory questionnaire now in preparation may make possible the development of a survey-based community laboratory in Rochester.

3. There would seem to be a number of advantages in developing a community survey mechanism for Rochester, including the existence of a large medical staff and ample laboratory facilities. Thus, problems of recruitment and capital expenditures would be minimal. The incorporation of a Tecumseh-like survey mechanism into a community with the comprehensive and outstanding medical diagnostic services of Rochester is an intriguing notion.

4. Some of the advantages and disadvantages of hospital-based studies are well exemplified in Rochester. Rare diseases such as multiple sclerosis, amyotrophic lateral sclerosis, thyroid cancer, or multiple myeloma are best studied retrospectively, from existing medical records. The high degree of diagnostic validity which is of paramount importance in such studies is undoubtedly achieved in the Mayo-affiliated institutions. On the other hand, valid survivorship studies in diseases for which patients are not usually hospitalized, cannot be made solely on hospital-based populations.

5. The authors point to the relative inadequacy of family and social data in the existing records. An attempt is being made to remedy this by improving the record linkage system. However, it would seem that the ultimate solution lies in the collection of information in a standardized fashion. The development of the self-administered inventory questionnaire, already mentioned, may go far toward resolving this problem.

PART II

EPIDEMIOLOGIC SURVEYS OF SPECIFIC DISEASES

For a community to serve as an epidemiologic laboratory, there must exist a system for the registration of denominator data (population figures) and numerator data (vital events). A total community census, conducted under private auspices, represents one approach to community studies. The Washington County, Maryland, census exemplifies the advantages and disadvantages inherent in this approach. Also of relevance are the considerations which entered into the choice of Washington County as the community for study.

THE NONOFFICIAL CENSUS AS A BASIC TOOL FOR EPIDEMIOLOGIC OBSERVATIONS IN WASHINGTON COUNTY, MARYLAND

George W. Comstock, Helen Abbey, and Frank E. Lundin, Jr.

INTRODUCTION

The currently popular application of the word "laboratory" to a human community seems somewhat inappropriate, even apart from its disquieting association with guinea pigs. A laboratory suggests a place where experiments are conducted, and experiments imply deliberate manipulation and controls. Controlled manipulations are probably never instigated by nature, and when performed by man, they are rarely conducted on a community-wide basis. "Observation" is a more inclusive and felicitous term than "experiment," and encompasses most community-based epidemiologic research. Unfortunately, an accurate and catchy substitute for "laboratory" does not come to mind.

Valid epidemiologic observations demand knowledge of the characteristics of both the diseased and the population at risk, in this instance the population of an entire community. Although information about the population base may be estimated from various sampling techniques, a more generally useful procedure, particularly when epidemiologic studies of many diseases are envisioned, is the complete enumeration or census.

73

The official decennial censuses in the United States collect tremendous amounts of information about individuals in every community in the country. Tabulations are published in considerable detail for a wide variety of population units, from states and regions down to individual city blocks. Additional tabulations may be obtained by special arrangement, and this vast assemblage of information may be supplemented or brought up to date by special censuses and sampling procedures conducted between the census years.

In spite of their obvious utility, official census data have serious limitations from the epidemiologist's point of view. For one thing, the information is oriented more toward economics than health. But much more important is the inviolate confidentiality of census data. Because information on individuals is not released, case records cannot be matched to the population base, except by special arrangement with the Bureau of the Census to do the matching for the investigator. Only statistical tabulations will be returned to him, and the questions and problems that arise during matching can be made known only in a general way. In the future, computer matching may make this procedure less cumbersome, but the basic difficulties imposed by confidentiality will remain. For most of us, the best solution is to conduct our own enumeration, a nonofficial census.

To the best of our knowledge, the first censuses for health purposes were taken in the period 1912–16, when house-to-house canvasses of six cotton-mill villages in South Carolina were made for studies of pellagra (Siler, Garrison, and MacNeal 1914; Goldberger, Wheeler, and Sydenstricker 1920). However, both groups of investigators appear to have deliberately omitted certain classes of households and thus failed to study the entire community. Enumerations more nearly approaching community-wide coverage comprised the series of health-related censuses of the Eastern Health District of Baltimore. These were stimulated by Frost, Reed, and Sydenstricker, and were carried out periodically from 1933 to 1947 (Fales 1951; Cochran 1952). What may well have been the first census for general health research on a county-wide basis was initiated as recently as 1946 in Muscogee County, Georgia, by Yerushalmy and Palmer (Burke, Schenck, and Thrash 1949; Comstock 1964).

The present discussion will be based in part on the censuses of the Eastern Health District and of Muscogee County, but mostly on a more recent nonofficial census of Washington County, Maryland. The latter was conducted, in large part, to provide a major resource for the Training Center for Public Health Research, an investigational facility of the Johns Hopkins School of Hygiene and Public Health. The Training Center is operated in co-operation with the Washington County Department of Health and the Maryland State Health Department with the dual purposes of providing population data and a geographic area for student research.

In selecting a study community, the county should be given primary consideration over other geographic entities. Counties throughout most of the United States are the official units for collecting and storing legal records, including birth and death certificates and marriage and divorce records, all of which have obvious uses in public health studies. County tax records are useful in locating rural homes. Records of health department services, too, are still largely kept on a county basis. Of course, no record is useful that is not readily available. Obviously, then, if a county is selected as a study area in order to take advantage of the available information in legal records, an important consideration is the existence of a good record system.

Size of population is another important consideration. The community should be large enough to provide adequate numbers of subjects with important health conditions and to support a wide range of medical, paramedical, and social services. On the other hand, the population should be small enough to make a census financially feasible. Informing the public about proposed studies and maintaining long-term follow-up observations are also easier in a small community. In our opinion, for the epidemiologic study of many diseases the best balance between the respective advantages of largeness and smallness is struck in a community of approximately 100,000 persons.

Stability of the population is also desirable, both to maintain the usefulness of census data after it is collected and for long-term studies which may be developed from the census findings. Losses due to emigration are, of course, more serious than dilution of the original population by immigration.

Perhaps the major criterion in the selection of a community is the degree of its self-sufficiency. A single centralized location for medical, social, and economic activities not only simplifies communication with the population but ensures that peripheral areas of the county are attracted to their own center rather than to other counties. It matters little if outsiders are also drawn to the county center, for the effect of this, like that of immigration, is merely dilution of the study population. What does matter is that pertinent health information on county residents is collected inside the county to the greatest extent possible. Consequently, the county should be far enough from major metropolitan centers to minimize their attraction, especially as regards medical facilities and specialists. Suburban counties can be difficult areas in which to mount many types of health studies, because the major communications media are aimed at the entire metropolitan area rather than being focused on the study community, and because health and medical information on suburban residents can be scattered among many institutions.

THE COMMUNITY

For all of the above reasons Washington County, Maryland, was attractive as a community for study. As can be seen in Figure 4–1, it is located about 70 miles west of both Baltimore and Washington, D.C., sufficiently distant so that the problems of suburbia are still remote. Its population remained at about 92,000 from 1960 to 1963 and has recently increased to over 100,000. A single central city, Hagerstown, is the economic, cultural, and medical center for the county and for much of the adjacent area as well. An excellent county record system makes public records readily available.

Figure 4–1. Map of Maryland showing location of Washington County.

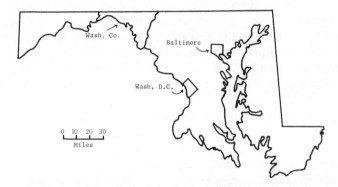

An additional important feature was the existence of public health research activities in Washington County over the past several decades (Turner 1952). In the early 1920's, Sydenstricker of the U.S. Public Health Service initiated a morbidity survey in Hagerstown, the first of a series which eventually culminated in the National Health Survey of the present. Dental surveys, also started at that time, came into full flower in the 1930's, with the work of Klein and Palmer leading them, among other accomplishments, to the development of the DMF index— a widely used epidemiologic index of dental deterioration based upon the number of decayed, missing, and filled teeth (Klein, Palmer, and Knutson 1938). Major contributions to knowledge of childhood growth and development and to familial aggregation of disease were also made at this time (Palmer and Reed 1935; Ciocco 1941). Although largely unpublicized, Washington County also played a key role in the history of tuberculosis investigation. In 1938 a meeting was held in Hagerstown to bring together tuberculosis experts from many areas to investigate two puzzling observations. The first was that pulmonary calcification, then thought to be pathognomonic of tuberculosis, was often not associated with tuberculin sensitivity; the second was the distinctive geographic distributions of sensitivity to large and small doses of tuberculin. Palmer left this meeting with the seeds of future discovery already planted— seeds that were to culminate in demonstrations that pulmonary calcifications were often the result of histoplasmosis and that tuberculin sensitivity was often caused by a variety of nontuberculous, mycobacterial infections (Palmer 1946; Palmer and Edwards 1967). More recently, extensive studies by the National Cancer Institute have left a legacy of survey information about the rural areas of the county, including detailed maps, and a cancer registry dating back to 1948. The basic records of all of these studies are still on file in Washington County and are available to qualified investigators, including graduate students.

Along with the advantages of Washington County as a site for community-oriented research, there are also drawbacks, the most important of which is its relatively long distance from potential investigators. The institutions most likely to be interested in conducting community studies there have been the Johns Hopkins University and the University of Maryland in Baltimore, and the National Institutes of Health in Bethesda, Maryland. The same distance that keeps Washington County residents from seeking medical care in the metropolitan centers also acts as a deterrent to travel by metropolitan investigators.

Population movement is a problem in Washington County, as elsewhere, although, fortunately, immigration has been greater than emigration. The mobility of Washington County residents, as measured by the 1960 census, was less than the average for Maryland counties. The only more stable areas were either small counties on the Eastern Shore or counties located much farther from Baltimore and Bethesda than Washington County. The local population is homogenous, being mostly white Protestant of English and German extraction. For this reason racial and ethnic differences cannot be investigated there, but by the same token, one need not adjust for these factors in the analysis of study findings.

Most of Washington County lies in the great limestone valley between the Blue Ridge on the east and the rest of the Appalachian mountains to the west. The distribution of the population in 1963, according to major political subdivisions, is shown in Figure 4–2. Slightly more than half of the 92,000 residents lived in Hagerstown or its suburbs, the remainder being distributed with some unevenness across the rest of the county. The largest industries are the manufacture of airplanes, truck engines and transmissions, and dust control equipment. Dairy farming in the valley and orchards on the mountain slopes are the major agricultural pursuits.

The county is served by a single general hospital which is sufficiently well-equipped and staffed so that it draws patients from the surrounding areas. A private mental hospital with strong community orientation, a state chronic disease hospital, and a Veterans Administration hospital only a few miles outside the county comprise the remaining local hospital facilities. In 1960, 90 per cent of the births to county residents, and 84 per cent of the discharges of county residents from general hospitals occurred within the county (Maryland State Planning Commission 1963). In the period 1963–66, 86 per cent of all deaths of residents occurred within the county; of those dying in a general hospital, 93 per cent occurred in Washington County Hospital. This concentration of events within the county facilitates the identification of cases in the study of various diseases.

Figure 4–2. Map of Washington County showing boundaries and populations for Hagerstown and election districts outside of Hagerstown, with other incorporated places indicated.

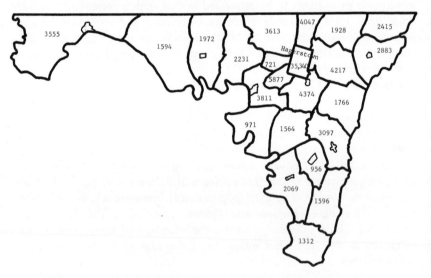

METHODS

To provide baseline information about the population of Washington County, Maryland, for use in health-related studies, a nonofficial census was taken in 1963 under the sponsorship of the National Cancer Institute, the Johns Hopkins School of Hygiene and Public Health, the Washington County Health Department, and the Maryland State Department of Health. The basic plan was to obtain information of possible relevance to health and to do record linkage studies of various diseases, both prospectively and retrospectively, among survivors of an earlier diagnosis. Characteristics associated with participation in public health programs would also be studied by record linkage. The existence of a total census has the advantage of facilitating the random sampling of a population or any of its subgroups. Such sampling might be used for gathering additional data or for selection of controls. For example, questionnaires or screening kits might be sent to members of the sampled population.

The format and content of the census questionnaire is shown in the Appendix to this chapter. The typed entries represent information which was requested from all residents by mail, with a follow-up visit by an enumerator to collect or complete the questionnaires. Handwritten entries indicate information or coding recorded in the local study center. The questions were largely copied from those used by the Bureau of the Census or from earlier surveys in Washington County by the National Cancer Institute.

Just above the list of household names is a six digit number which, together with the two digits preceding each name, is an identifying census number for each individual. The first two digits indicate the enumeration district in which the household was located, and, together with the middle four digits, identify the household. Houses without numbered street addresses could be located accurately on detailed maps of rural enumeration districts. Identification of individuals was further facilitated by the registration of complete birth dates and the maiden names of married women.

Questions relating to house construction and to the date of moving into present domicile were originally inserted to permit comparison with studies done by the National Cancer Institute, but these have proved useful for other studies as well. Crowding, in terms of persons per room, was calculated by computer from information in the questionnaire. Source of drinking water, aside from its relation to sanitation, was of interest because of the wide range of water hardness in Washington County. The rural water supplies are divided between the very hard water of most deep wells and the very soft water of cisterns which collect rainwater. The municipal water supplies also vary in their hardness but tend to be neither very hard nor very soft. The number of complete bathrooms in a house has obvious sanitary implications but, in addition, has proved to be a useful indicator of socioeconomic status. Heating and cooking facilities have not yet proven their utility as questionnaire entries. The presence of animals on the premises has been an item of interest in studies of histoplasmosis, mycobacterial infections, and the possible relationship of epilepsy to animal parasites.

The personal characteristics requested in the census were those having some relevance for investigational purposes. Marital history was desired primarily for studies on cancer of the cervix. Smoking is associated in some way with so many aspects of health that information on this habit was deemed essential. Attendance at religious services was included largely because this touches on an important aspect of social life hitherto omitted from health studies, a notable exception to this being its reported association with hypertension (Scotch 1963). Its inclusion in the census has been vindicated by our observation that the frequency of religious attendance is related to health with a consistency approaching that of cigarette smoking.

It was not possible to obtain all the census information that might have been desired. Each additional question costs money by lengthening the questionnaire, by increasing the time needed for interviewing and data processing, and, finally, by adding to the complexity of the analysis. Among the many bits of information that had to be omitted, three items seem to represent losses of some importance. Full middle names would have helped with identification problems, but recording them would have required much space on the questionnaire, and an additional deck of punched cards. Occupation and income would have been most useful additions as indicators of socioeconomic status. Their omission resulted largely from the number of questions which would have to be asked in order to obtain a reasonably accurate classification of these variables.

Following a trial of the questionnaire in about 50 households, 24,000 forms were mailed by a direct mail advertising company to all known residential addresses in Washington County. The cost for printing, addressing, and mailing was approximately five cents per questionnaire. From this point on, the general procedures of the U.S. Census Bureau were followed. In each of the 91 enumeration districts, an enumerator went from door-to-door to collect the questionnaires or to fill one out if the original form had not been received or had been mislaid. About 36,000 questionnaires were needed for the 27,000 households in the county.

Personnel for the census included a director, associate director, two supervisors (office and field), bookkeeper, secretary, 10 crew leaders, and 91 enumerators. Much of the enumeration was done within three weeks; the census was virtually completed in six. As the enumerators completed their own assignments they were sent to help in other districts or were brought into the office as coders and editors.

Completeness of enumeration was checked in a number of ways. Addresses of enumerated households were compared with those in the City Directory to make certain that all known addresses in Hagerstown, its suburbs, and the small towns had been included. Similar checking was done against lists prepared for most of the rural areas of the county in previous surveys by the National Cancer Institute. To estimate the completeness of coverage a stratified area sample of the county was selected. In the nonrural areas this consisted of a 10 per cent sample of blocks, selected with the help of a table of random numbers. In the rural areas the county was divided into small squares, approximately one mile on a side, and then sampled.

Incomplete rural squares around the periphery were considered in groups, the area of each group approximating that of a complete square. A 5 per cent sample of the grouped areas was then selected. The rural sampling unit was defined as houses along all roads and lanes within each selected square and along their extensions into other areas to their end or to the next intersection. This procedure was simple, accurate, and practicable; it yielded a sample of approximately 10 per cent of the population. Enumerators who revisited the sampled areas to check on completeness of coverage were able to secure only limited additional information because the questionnaire respondents tended to resent having the same questions asked again. In these circumstances, the returning enumerators merely ascertained the location of all households, the names of the household heads, and the total number of persons in each unit. Analysis of the findings indicated that over 98 per cent of the households had been enumerated in the original census.

The data from the 1963 census is available in a number of forms. The original questionnaires and maps are filed by census number, and the findings are recorded on punched cards and magnetic tape. A considerable number of basic tabulations have already been prepared, including a useful listing of all persons and households surveyed. Also recorded are the personal characteristics of the enumerated population, listed alphabetically by last name and maiden name. Households are grouped together by census number, as are housing characteristics.

PROBLEMS

A community census is not inexpensive. The total cost will be influenced by a number of factors, primarily the size of the community and the amount and quality of information that is desired. The census of Washington County cost about $100,000, or slightly more than one dollar per person enumerated. However, this expense should be prorated over all of the studies which make use of the census data. At present, six such studies have been published (Naguib, Comstock, and Davis 1966; Naguib, Lundin, and Davis 1966; Comstock and Lundin 1967; Kuemmerer and Comstock 1967; Whatley, Comstock, Garber, and Sanchez 1968; Comstock et al. 1968). Seven other papers, ranging from a sample survey of immunization status to a doctoral thesis, are in various stages of preparation. Three Johns Hopkins School of Hygiene classroom problems, one in biostatistics and two in epidemiology, have also drawn on census-related studies. In addition to these, six student research projects have been completed. With several other studies now being initiated, the prorated cost of the census continues to decline.

The degree to which an *enumerated* population represents the *actual* population of a community is a matter of great importance. Fortunately, the initial coverage of the Washington County census was highly complete, an estimated 98.4 per cent of the households having been enumerated. Information obtained on some subjects was more complete than on others, but even the questions yielding the poorest response— those relating to religious attendance—were answered by more than 90 per cent of the subjects.

Persons in institutions were not as well enumerated as persons at home. County and state medical and penal institutions furnished lists of their Washington County residents, including name, age, race, sex, and nearest relative. Of the 1,197 county residents reported as being in these institutions, only 32 per cent were listed on census forms by their families; the information on the remaining 68 per cent is consequently limited to that furnished by the institutions. Persons in the armed services or in federal institutions were enumerated only if their families listed them on the census form, and there is no direct way to estimate the number who were not enumerated. Because the census was conducted in the summer, failures to count college students appear to have been minimal.

Though a community may be completely enumerated in a census, all populations change with time, as death and emigration take their toll, and births and immigrants dilute the survivors. Without continuous registration of residents there appears to be no feasible way to keep census data up to date. In the Baltimore Eastern Health District, censuses were repeated at intervals of three to eight years in order to maintain a reasonably current population list (Fales 1951; Cochran 1952). In Muscogee County an attempt was made to add births and newly arrived residents as they received various health department services and to remove decedents from the rolls (Comstock 1949). The rewards of this effort were not sufficient to justify the cost, and the attempt to maintain a current population register has been discontinued.

The demographic changes that occur over time in a community may not pose as serious a methodologic problem as they might appear to at first glance. In exploratory studies, correcting for population losses is usually not necessary. In most other studies the primary interest is not in determining absolute rates but rather in a comparison of rates among persons with and without particular attributes. Losses are certain to occur in both population groups, but only rarely will the attrition of one group be so different from that of the other that the two rates being measured are not comparable. The significance of this problem is time-dependent because even a small differential loss, if sustained over a long period, can vitiate comparisons. In the more definitive studies, the groups selected to represent the denominator of the rates (the control groups) can be sampled in order to provide an estimate of losses in the various categories (Comstock and Palmer 1966). Household lists used as sampling frames can be readily brought up to date in many localities by sampling building permits or tax records for dwelling units built after the date of the census.

The most commonly voiced criticism of community studies is that they are not representative. This allegation cannot be categorically denied, for the fact of the matter is that the population of one county is not likely to be completely representative of any other population. But it is also a fact that almost none of the epidemiologic knowledge we now possess was derived from a totally "representative" population. For most investigative purposes there is no such thing.

The criticism stems in part from two different meanings of the word "representative" as applied to populations. There is the statistical or sampling sense of the word, indicating that the study population is similar to its parent population or universe in all pertinent respects. This type of study population is essential when the magnitude of a health problem must be precisely measured in order to plan for treatment or control programs.

A broader sense of the word "representative" implies that a population so designated has a wide range of study attributes, thereby assuring that there will be sufficient numbers of subjects in all important categories of the attributes. If an attribute does not exist in a community, its effect cannot be investigated there, nor will studies be fruitful if the attribute has a very limited distribution. For example, it would be difficult to identify the association of a condition with degree of formal education in a population composed entirely of university faculty members. Provided that adequate numbers of subjects are available in all categories, the relative frequency of an attribute is probably not important.

The subject of primary interest in most studies is not likely to be the over-all frequency of a particular condition in a total population— a rate which depends on the composition of the population. The fundamental question is much more likely to be the risk of the condition among persons with a given attribute compared with the risk among persons without it. This relative risk may not be greatly affected by whether the proportion of all persons with the attribute is high or low.

Doubts as to the representativeness of a community may arise because of certain characteristics of its population. To the extent that these affect cases and non-cases and persons with and without the study attributes equally, estimates of relative risks will not be affected. However, selective factors such as employment, hospitalization, membership in special organizations, etc., increase the possibility that various population subgroups will be affected unequally. Intuitively, it seems that the operation of selective factors, which may be very subtle, will be minimized if an entire community is selected for study rather than a more limited population group.

Losses by death and emigration will obviously affect the representativeness of a census population in the statistical sense of this term. However, the population census may continue to serve as a sampling frame for households if it can be supplemented by complete lists of new households. Case-control studies can also continue to be done so long as the procedures assure that the controls represent the surviving population to the same extent as the cases. To the extent that certain attributes are concentrated among persons who die or emigrate, the surviving population will become deficient in persons with these attributes. Such effects, however, are likely to become serious only after the lapse of considerable time.

A final problem concerns the frequency with which community censuses should be repeated. No standard answer is possible. The need for a new population base will increase with the emigration rate and with the importance of residential mobility to the research problem. At the present time, and balancing all considerations, it appears that 8 to 12 years may be the optimum interval between censuses in a relatively stable community.

FINDINGS AND POTENTIALS

Data from a nonofficial community census are sometimes uniquely valuable because they represent information collected from all the individuals in a given population at one time. An illustration of the use of such data, obtained in the Washington County census, is the tabulation of cigarette smoking patterns among whites over the age of sixteen and one-half years by sex, education, residence, and marital status (Table 4–1). Because the table is based on information from nearly 60,000 people, most of the individual cells represent substantial numbers of individuals. In all subcategories more males than females were current cigarette smokers, except among those between the ages of

TABLE 4–1. PERCENTAGE OF PERSONS WHO PRESENTLY SMOKE CIGARETTES AND WHO HAVE STOPPED SMOKING CIGARETTES, BY SEX, AGE, YEARS OF SCHOOLING, RESIDENCE AND MARITAL STATUS (WHITE RESIDENTS OF WASHINGTON COUNTY, MD., 1963)

	Present smokers				Ex-smokers			
	Age group				Age group			
MALES	16–	25–	45–	65+	16–	25–	45–	65+
Years of schooling								
More than high school	41	50	42	23	9	20	30	31
9–12 grades	52	63	54	25	6	15	21	26
0–8 grades	62	62	53	26	4	14	19	23
Residence								
Urban	55	67	57	27	7	14	20	26
Suburban	41	66	48	27	8	19	25	23
Small towns	66	62	54	26	7	14	20	27
Rural	47	56	46	24	6	16	20	22
Marital status								
Married in 1963:								
Married only once	71	59	50	24	11	17	22	26
Married more than once	—ᵃ	73	59	33	—	13	22	28
Widowed	—	—	57	23	—	—	16	22
Divorced or separated	78	78	67	41	2	6	15	26
Never married	46	67	49	30	5	8	17	12

	Present smokers				Ex-smokers			
	Age group				Age group			
FEMALES	16–	25–	45–	65+	16–	25–	45–	65+
Years of schooling								
More than high school	34	42	46	14	9	13	13	7
9–12 grades	29	41	33	8	8	9	8	3
0–8 grades	41	39	22	6	10	8	5	2
Residence								
Urban	38	50	34	9	9	10	8	4
Suburban	27	44	35	6	7	11	10	4
Small towns	33	39	27	7	9	10	7	3
Rural	22	33	22	4	7	9	6	2
Marital status								
Married in 1963:								
Married only once	37	38	26	7	12	10	8	2
Married more than once	56	58	41	16	15	12	9	7
Widowed	—	55	27	7	—	8	7	3
Divorced or separated	57	60	47	13	12	9	7	3
Never married	22	30	26	4	4	5	5	3

ᵃ — signifies that base population was less than 50 persons.

forty-five and sixty-five years who had received more than a high school education. In the latter group, nearly one-third of the males had stopped smoking cigarettes, while this was true for only 13 per cent of the females. Differences in smoking habits by attained educational level were most marked among women over forty-five years, and were almost nonexistent among those twenty-five to forty-four years of age. Among women sixteen to twenty-four years of age, those with the least education comprised the highest proportion of smokers. This suggests a shift from circumstances in the past, when smoking was more common among upper class women, to the present pattern of more frequent smoking among women of lower social class, a situation which parallels that among males today.

Census data can be used to furnish denominators in the estimation of rates. While hardly a sufficient reason for conducting a nonofficial census, judicious interpretation of such estimates may provide useful information which is not otherwise obtainable. Table 4–2 shows estimated tuberculosis case rates for 1960–64 which were developed from data of the Washington County census. Only those cases which could be matched to persons identified in the 1963 census are included; the few who died prior to the census and the appreciable number who moved away are excluded. Although they are not shown in this table, the case rates were nearly equal for urban and rural residents; the apparent urban excess in total case rate resulted from the fact that highly mobile patients tended to be city residents when reported. Most of the findings in Table 4–2 are consistent with generally held beliefs about tuberculosis; namely, that it is more common among males, non-whites, the elderly, and the poorly educated. The findings also suggest that promoting participation in chest X-ray surveys by advertising in church bulletins is likely to be unrewarding.

A nonofficial census, if done at the proper time, permits accurate estimates to be made of the degree of community participation in ongoing public health programs. The primary purpose of the 1946 census of Muscogee County, Georgia, was to determine which segments of the population had been examined and which segments had not been examined in a survey for tuberculosis and syphilis (Burke, Schenck, and Thrash 1949). The Washington County census was conducted immediately after the completion of a cervical cancer screening program utilizing the Davis self-administered cyto-pipette. This made possible a study of factors associated with participation in this program (Naguib, Geiser, and Comstock 1968).

Ad hoc epidemiologic studies can often be greatly facilitated by information previously or subsequently obtained in a community census. In Washington County, a number of projects had already been completed prior to the 1963 census (Abraham and Nordsieck 1960). One that depended extensively on census information was an investigation of the relationship between parental smoking during pregnancy and perinatal mortality (Comstock and Lundin 1967). Neonatal deaths among the 19,000 live births occurring during the ten-year period prior to the census were identified; actually, the number of live births in each study category was estimated from a 3 per cent systematic sample of birth certificates. The neonatal deaths and the sampled records were then matched to the 1963 census listings. The results of the study are summarized in Tables 4–3 and 4–4. Of the 570 sampled live births and 551 deaths, slightly more than 20 percent were excluded because neither parent could be identified in the 1963 census. The few nonwhites were also excluded to achieve greater homogeneity. Another 17–18 per cent were excluded because some other essential information, usually the date when the ex-smokers had stopped smoking, was lacking. Losses from the birth sample and from the deaths were essentially equal, however, and there is no indication that differentially selective factors were operative in the two groups.

TABLE 4–2. CHARACTERISTICS OF CASES OF TUBERCULOSIS REPORTED 1960–64, THAT COULD BE MATCHED AGAINST 1963 CENSUS

Attribute		No. of cases[a]	Estimated rate/ 100,000 in 5 years
Total		56	62
Race and sex	WM	38	88
	WF	11	25
	NM	5	570
	NF	2	210
Age	0–19	4	12
	20–39	17	44
	40–59	16	75
	60+	19	168
Age at first marriage[b]	<20	8	51[d]
	20–29	31	110[d]
	30+	5	140[d]
Years of school[b]	0	2	580
	1–7	9	101
	8–12	35	94
	13+	4	53
Attendance, religious services[c]	At least weekly	14	57
	About once a month	15	84
	Twice a year or less	18	138

[a] Numbers in each category may not add to total because cases with missing information are omitted.

[b] Limited to persons 20+ years of age.

[c] Limited to persons 16½+ years of age.

[d] Adjusted to the age distribution of the total known cases.

TABLE 4-3. STUDY OF PARENTAL SMOKING AND PERINATAL MORTALITY LOSSES DUE TO INELIGIBILITY AND INCOMPLETENESS

	Sample of births		Neonatal deaths	
	No.	%	No.	%
Initial number	570	100.0	551	100.0
Exclusion of ineligible cases[a]				
Neither parent in 1963 census	110	19.3	110	20.0
Nonwhite	14	2.5	20	3.6
Study group, after exclusions	448	78.6	431	78.2
Study group, after exclusion of incomplete cases	376	66.0	337	61.2

[a] Some subjects excluded for more than one reason.

TABLE 4-4. NEONATAL DEATH RATES PER 1000 LIVE BIRTHS ACCORDING TO SMOKING STATUS OF MOTHER AND EDUCATION OF FATHER

	Mother nonsmoker			Mother smoker		
Education of father	Sample of births[a]	Deaths		Sample of births	Deaths	
		No.	Rate		No.	Rate
Total	238	180	22.9	138	157	34.5
0–8 grades	59	56	28.7	23	50	65.9
9+ grades	179	124	21.0	115	107	28.2

[a] 3% systematic sample of births; see text.

Neonatal death rates per 1,000 live births were calculated by dividing the deaths by the total number of births as estimated from the 3 per cent sample. A slight excess in infant mortality was noted for children of smoking mothers, but this was almost entirely limited to the group in which the father was poorly educated. Review of all findings in this study led to the conclusion that infant mortality was not directly associated with maternal smoking but rather with certain other characteristics of smokers. The nonofficial census of Washington County made this study possible without having to wait years for adequate numbers of neonatal deaths to occur. It also made it possible to obtain smoking history independently of the fate of the infant. Another advantage was the fact that the study could be done with little additional financial investment. A significant disadvantage stemmed from the fact that the census questionnaire was not specifically designed for this study and, consequently, losses occurred because the smoking history was not recorded in sufficient detail. Nevertheless, the study was rapidly completed, a useful conclusion was reached, and the groundwork was laid for further studies, now in progress, of etiological factors in the increased infant mortality observed among the offspring of lower socio-economic class mothers who smoke.

Experiences with nonofficial censuses in the Eastern Health District of Baltimore, in Muscogee County, Georgia, and in Washington County have all shown their value in providing sampling frames for community studies. The census has several different applications in sampling. The first is to provide a sample of persons with specified characteristics at the time of the census. This is a survivor population because some persons will have died or emigrated before they can be studied. Illustrative of this type of sample is a study of the association of urban residence with signs of chronic obstructive respiratory disease (Stebbings 1969). The desired study population was to consist of white males who were thirty-five to sixty-four years of age, had never smoked, currently lived in or near Hagerstown, and had previously lived outside the county for at least 20 years. To find such a population in most communities would require extensive field work. With census information on magnetic tape, the desired sample was identified in a very short time.

The community census also provides the basis for an updated sample of the population, provided that the investigator is satisfied to have a sample of households. A list of dwelling units obtained at the time of the census will represent the great majority of these units for years to come, and households currently living in these units can be sampled directly from the list. New housing can be sampled from lists or records at the county tax office. With the excellent record system in Washington County, this supplementation can be achieved simply and rapidly.

The major usefulness of a census is to provide a defined population from which both cases of disease and their controls can be drawn. Two of the fundamental assumptions for determining relative risks in case-control studies are that the cases and controls come from the same population, and that the controls are a representative sample of that population. Without a census it is difficult to be certain that these conditions obtain. Illustrative of this is our study of the association of water hardness and fatal coronary heart disease. Previous investigators have reported an association of cardiovascular death rates with the hardness of local water supplies. If this relationship were one of cause and effect, it would be of great public health significance because of the ease with which the hardness of water can be modified. However, it is not easy to do a definitive study of this association, because many individuals are mobile and few obtain drinking water from a single source. In spite of these difficulties, a preliminary study was undertaken in Washington

County, where the local water supplies show a wide range of water hardness and the older male population tends to have lived in one place for a long time. The cases were white males between the ages of forty-five and sixty-five years in 1963 who died of coronary heart disease in the three-year period following the census. With the help of the census lists it was easy to establish that 185 of these deaths occurred among persons enumerated in the census. It was also easy to select two controls for each death in such a way that the controls comprised a representative sample of the census population stratified by race, sex, and birth year.

Some preliminary findings of this study are shown in Table 4–5. The excess risk associated with not being the head of the household at the time of the census suggests that such persons may have been ill at that time, a point that needs to be investigated further. Infrequent attendance at church and moderate to heavy cigarette smoking are two personal characteristics which suggest that one's way of life is somehow associated with coronary artery disease. The next three attributes— failure to complete high school, owning a dog, and lack of a complete bathroom in the house—are all associated with low socioeconomic status as well as with a slight increased risk of coronary disease. The findings with respect to water supply do not support the maxim, "hard water, soft arteries." Length of residence and degree of crowding within the home were similar for cases and controls. Further studies are planned to examine the association with water hardness in greater detail.

TABLE 4–5. ASSOCIATION OF VARIOUS ATTRIBUTES WITH FATAL CORONARY DISEASE IN THE FIRST THREE YEARS AFTER THE 1963 WASHINGTON COUNTY CENSUS (WHITE MALES, 45–64 YEARS OF AGE IN 1963 AND ENUMERATED IN THE CENSUS)

Attribute	Cases	Controls	Relative risk
Total number	185	370	—
Not head of household in 1963	25	17	3.2
Church attendance less than once weekly	122	193	1.8
1+ packs cigarettes per day	59	81	1.7
Less than 12 years' schooling	143	252	1.6
Dog on premises	89	143	1.4
House without complete bathroom	36	58	1.3
Drinking water source:			
Deep well (mostly hard water)	26	42	1.3
Cistern (mostly soft water)	15	47	0.6
Average number of years in county	43.9	43.3	—
Average persons per room, 1963	0.61	0.56	—

Acknowledgments

Many senior staff members of the U.S. Bureau of the Census gave freely of their time and advice during the planning phases of this private census. They saved us much time and many mistakes.

We are also grateful to Dr. Philip E. Sartwell, professor of epidemiology at the Johns Hopkins School of Hygiene and Public Health, for his encouragement and advice.

Dr. D. Crosby Greene, Washington County Health Officer, at the time worked actively to ensure that the census was accepted wholeheartedly by the entire community. Although it is not possible to thank all of the crew leaders, enumerators, and office workers whose tact and diligence made the enumeration virtually complete, we are particularly indebted to Mr. Jack B. Gunderman and Mr. James E. Hawthorne, Jr., for their effective work as field and office supervisors, respectively.

The Board of County Commissioners of Washington County not only endorsed the census but advanced the funds necessary to initiate it. The major portion of the financial support came from the National Cancer Institute, through Contract PH-43-63-1170. Analysis of the census findings and preparation of this paper were partially supported by Graduate Training Grant CD-00001 and Research Career Award K6-HE-21,670 from the Bureau of Disease Prevention and Environmental Control and the National Heart Institute, respectively, Public Health Service, U.S. Department of Health, Education, and Welfare.

References

Abraham, S. and Nordsieck, M. 1960. Relationship of excess weight in children and adults. *Public Health Rep.* 75:263–73.

Burke, M. H., Schenck, H. C., and Thrash, J. A. 1949. Tuberculosis studies in Muscogee County, Georgia. II. X-ray findings in a community-wide survey and its coverage as determined by a population census. *Public Health Rep.* 64:263–94.

Ciocco, A. 1914. On the mortality in brother-sister and husband-wife pairings. *Hum. Biol.* 13:189–202.

Cochran, W. G. 1952. An appraisal of the repeated population censuses in the Eastern Health District, Baltimore. In *Research in Public Health,* pp. 255–65. New York: Millbank Memorial Fund.

Comstock, G. W. 1949. Tuberculosis studies in Muscogee County, Georgia. I. Community-wide tuberculosis research. *Public Health Rep.* 64:259–63.

———. 1964. Community research in tuberculosis in Muscogee County, Georgia. *Public Health Rep.* 79:1045–56.

Comstock, G. W. and Lundin, F. E., Jr. 1967. Parental smoking and perinatal mortality. *Am. J. Obstet. Gynec.* 98:708–18.

Comstock, G. W. and Palmer, C. E. 1966. Long-term results of BCG vaccination in the southern United States. *Am. Rev. Resp. Dis.* 93:171–83.

Comstock, G. W., Vicens, C. N., Goodman, N. L., and Collins, S. 1968.

Differences in the distribution of sensitivity to histoplasmin and isolations of Histoplasma capsulatum. *Am. J. Epidem.* 88:195–209.

Fales, W. T. 1951. Matched population records in the Eastern Health District, Baltimore, Maryland: A base for epidemiological study of chronic disease. *Am. J. Public Health* 41:91–110.

Goldberger, J., Wheeler, G. A., and Sydenstricker, E. 1920. Pellagra incidence in relation to sex, age, season, occupation, and "disabling sickness" in seven cotton-mill villages of South Carolina during 1916. *Public Health Rep.* 35: 1650–64.

Klein, H., Palmer, C. E., and Knutson, J. W. 1938. Studies on dental caries. I. Dental status and dental needs of elementary school children. *Public Health Rep.* 53:751–65.

Kuemmerer, J. M. and Comstock, G. W. 1967. Sociologic concomitants of tuberculin sensitivity. *Am. Rev. Resp. Dis.* 96:885–92.

Maryland State Planning Commission, Committee on Medical Care, 1963. *Report on Community Health Services.* Pub. No. 123. Baltimore: State Planning Department.

Naguib, S. M., Comstock, G. W., and Davis, H. J. 1966. Epidemiologic study of trichomoniasis in normal women. *Obstet. Gynec.* 27:607–16.

Naguib, S. M., Geiser, P. B., and Comstock, G. W. 1968. Response to a program of screening for cervical cancer. *Public Health Rep.* 83:990–98.

Naguib, S. M., Lundin, F. E., Jr., and Davis, H. J. 1966. Relation of various epidemiologic factors to cervical cancer as determined by a screening program. *Obstet. Gynec.* 28:451–59.

Palmer, C. E. 1946. Geographic differences in sensitivity to histoplasmin among student nurses. *Public Health Rep.* 61:475–87.

Palmer, C. E. and Edwards, L. B. 1967. Tuberculin test in retrospect and prospect. *Arch. Environ. Health* 15:792–808.

Palmer, C. E. and Reed, L. J. 1935. Anthropometric studies of individual growth. I. Age, height, and rate of growth in height, elementary school children. *Hum. Biol.* 7:319–34.

Scotch, N. A. 1963. Sociocultural factors in the epidemiology of Zulu hypertension. *Am. J. Public Health* 53:1205–13.

Siler, J. F., Garrison, P. E., and MacNeal, W. J. 1914. A statistical study of the relation of pellagra to use of certain foods and to location of domicile in six selected communities. *Arch. Int. Med.* 14:293–373.

Stebbings, J. H., Jr. 1969. Respiratory disease in a population of residentially-mobile nonsmokers in Hagerstown, Maryland. Doctor of Science dissertation, the Johns Hopkins University, Baltimore, Md.

Turner, V. B. 1952. *Hagerstown Health Studies. An Annotated Bibliography.* Public Health Bibliography Series no. 6. P.H.S. Pub. No. 148. Washington: U.S. Government Printing Office.

Whatley, T. R., Comstock, G. W., Garber, H. J., and Sanchez, F. S., Jr. 1968. A waterborne outbreak of infectious hepatitis in a small Maryland town. *Am. J. Epidem.* 87:138–47.

APPENDIX: FORMAT OF QUESTIONNAIRE USED IN 1963 CENSUS

WASHINGTON COUNTY HEALTH DEPARTMENT
HAGERSTOWN, MARYLAND

1963 CENSUS OF WASHINGTON COUNTY, MD.

Dear Householder:

Washington County's leadership in public health research
is being continued through cooperative studies with the U. S.
Public Health Service, Maryland Department of Health, and the
Johns Hopkins University. To provide a foundation for future
studies, a complete census of the county is being conducted
this summer.

This report form is for you to fill out before the census
taker calls to complete the census of your household. Please
fill it out carefully and keep it ready for the census taker who
will call for it in the next few weeks.

The census information will be used only for medical and
public health research. It will be kept confidential and will not
be used for purposes of taxation, investigation or regulation.

Thank you for your help in making our county, and the world,
a healthier place in which to live and work.

Sincerely yours,

D. Crosby Greene, M.D.
County Health Officer

BULK RATE
U.S. Postage
PAID
Permit No. 450
Hagerstown, Md.

Sample

PHS- 5-63	WASHINGTON COUNTY HEALTH DEPARTMENT IN COOPERATION WITH U.S. PUBLIC HEALTH SERVICE MARYLAND STATE HEALTH DEPARTMENT JOHNS HOPKINS UNIVERSITY WASHINGTON COUNTY, MARYLAND	SECTION A – IN THIS SECTION LIST: 1. Everyone who usually lives here whether related to you or not. 2. All persons staying here who have no other home. PLEASE NOTE BEFORE YOU START that some people should be listed in Section B.

NAMES OF PERSONS LIVING HERE ON JULY 15, 1963, AND THOSE STAYING HERE WHO HAVE NO OTHER HOME:

Write names in this order
- Head of household
- Wife of head
- Unmarried children, oldest first
- Married children, and their families
- Other relatives
- Others not related to head of household

If there are more than 12 names on your list, use an additional sheet.

What is the relationship of each person to the head of this household?

(For example: Wife, son daughter, grandson, mother-in-law, lodger, lodger's wife)

47-9786 (1)

Line Number	Last name	First name	Middle initial	Maiden name	(2)
01	Doe	John	D		1 Head
02	Doe	Jane	-	Roe	2 Wife
03	Doe	Robert	L		3 Son
04	Doe	June	-		3 Daughter
05					
06					
07					
08					
09					
10					
11					
12					

SECTION B – IN THIS SECTION, PLEASE LIST PERSONS WHO USUALLY LIVE HERE, BUT WHO ARE IN ONE OF THE FOLLOWING GROUPS:

- Persons stationed away from here in the Armed Forces.
- College students who are away at college.
- Persons away in institutions, such as, a sanitarium, home for the aged, nursing home, mental hospital, or other institution.

91	Doe 2	John Jr.	D		3 Son
92					
93					
94					
95					

PHS-T222-1
6-63

Sample___ Budget Bureau No. 68-6334; Approval expires April 30, 1968

PLEASE BE SURE TO LIST IN SECTION A —

●All members of your family living with you, including babies.
●All other relatives living here.
●Lodgers and boarders living here.
●Servants, hired hands, others not related to you who are living here.
●Anyone else staying here but who has no other home.

ALSO LIST:
Persons who usually live here but who are temporarily away on business, on vacation, or in a general hospital.

Male or Female (M or F) (3)	Is this person— White, Negro, Other race? (4)	When was this person born? (5)			Is this person now— Married, Widowed, Divorced, Separated, Single (Never married)? (6)	How many years has this person lived in Washington County? (7)	How many grades of school, including college did this person complete? (8)	Line Number
		Month	Day	Year				
/ M	/ W	0 9	30	908	/ Married	54	16	01
2 F	/ W	01	7	915	/ Married	26	16	02
/ M	/ W	12	23	945	5 Single	17	11	03
2 F	/ W	07	21	948	5 Single	15	09	04
								05
								06
								07
								08
								09
								10
								11
								12

/ M	/ W	01	27	9 43	4 Separated	20	14	91
								92
								93
								94
								95

Sample

SECTION C: Fill out one part of Section C for EVERY PERSON listed in Sections A or B who was
BORN IN 1946 OR BEFORE (persons now more than 16½ years old).

1. NAME OF THIS PERSON

C1   John D. Doe

	MONTH AND YEAR
2. When did this person move into this house or apartment?	*06/63*

	AGE AT FIRST MARRIAGE (Years)
3. MARRIAGE INFORMATION 1 ☐ Never married?	
Has this person .... 2 ☐ Married only once?	*30*
3 ☐ Married more than once?	

4A. What is this person's religion?___ Episcopalian

13   (Baptist, Jewish, Mennonite, Presbyterian, Roman Catholic, etc.)

B. Does this person USUALLY attend religious services?

1 ☐ More than once a week   4 ☒ Two to twelve times a year
2 ☐ About once a week   5 ☐ Less than twice a year
3 ☐ More than once a month   6 ☐ Never

5A. Has this person EVER smoked Cigarettes?   1 ☐ Yes   2 ☒ No
                                    Cigars?   1 ☐ Yes   2 ☒ No
                                    Pipes?   1 ☒ Yes   2 ☐ No

B. Does this person smoke CIGARETTES NOW?   1 ☐ Yes   2 ☒ No
C. What was the greatest number of CIGARETTES this person ever smoked REGULARLY?

9   1 ☐ Smoked once in a while, not every day   4 ☐ 21 to 40 a day (1 to 2 packs)
      2 ☐ Less than 10 a day (less than ½ pack)   5 ☐ More than 40 a day (More than 2 packs)
      3 ☐ 10-20 a day (½ to 1 pack)

	YEARS
D. How old was this person when he first started to smoke REGULARLY?	*20*

SECTION C: Fill out one part of Section C for EVERY PERSON listed in Sections A or B who was
BORN IN 1946 OR BEFORE (persons now more than 16½ years old).

1. NAME OF THIS PERSON

02   Jane Doe

	MONTH AND YEAR
2. When did this person move into this house or apartment?	*06/63*

	AGE AT FIRST MARRIAGE (Years)
1 ☐ Never married?	
3. MARRIAGE INFORMATION 2 ☒ Married only once?	*24*
Has this person .... 3 ☐ Married more than once?	

4A. What is this person's religion?___ Presbyterian

25   (Baptist, Jewish, Mennonite, Presbyterian, Roman Catholic, etc.)

B. Does this person USUALLY attend religious services?

1 ☐ More than once a week   4 ☐ Two to twelve times a year
2 ☐ About once a week   5 ☐ Less than twice a year
3 ☒ More than once a month   6 ☐ Never

5A: Has this person EVER smoked Cigarettes?   1 ☒ Yes   2 ☐ No
                                    Cigars?   1 ☐ Yes   2 ☒ No
                                    Pipes?   1 ☐ Yes   2 ☒ No

B. Does this person smoke CIGARETTES NOW?   1 ☐ Yes   2 ☒ No
C. What was the greatest number of CIGARETTES this person ever smoked REGULARLY?

      1 ☐ Smoked once in a while, not every day   4 ☐ 21 to 40 a day (1 to 2 packs)
      2 ☐ Less than 10 a day (less than ½ pack)   5 ☐ More than 40 a day (More than 2 packs)
Tel. call → 3 ☒ 10-20 a day (½ to 1 pack)

	YEARS
D. How old was this person when he first started to smoke REGULARLY?	*22*

Sample

HOUSEHOLD CENSUS

St. Peter's Rd.   4.

(Street Address)
1 ☒ Md.

2 ☐ W. Va.

Rt. 7, Hagerstown
3 ☐ Pa.

(Town or Post Office Address)

1. ┌─┬─┬─┬─┬─┬─┐
   │4│7│9│7│8│6│
   └─┴─┴─┴─┴─┴─┘
   ┌─┬─┬─┬─┬─┬─┬─┐
   │RT│7│ST│PETERS│RD│ │
   └─┴─┴─┴─┴─┴─┴─┘
   ┌─┬─┬─┬─┬─┬─┬─┐
   │HAGERSTOWN│ │ │
   └─┴─┴─┴─┴─┴─┴─┘

INSTRUCTIONS: Questions 5, 6, 7 and 8 refer to the whole building. The other questions refer to your house
or the part of the house which you occupy, or to the apartment, flat or rooms in which you live.

**5. About when was this house originally built?
IN:**

1 ☒ 1961 to 1963   4 ☐ 1945 to 1954
2 ☐ 1959 to 1960   5 ☐ 1900 to 1944
3 ☐ 1955 to 1958   6 ☐ 1899 or earlier

6. What material covers most of the roof?

1 ☐ Slate   5 ☐ Metal painted
2 ☐ Wood Shingle   6 ☐ Metal Unpainted
3 ☒ Asbestos Shingle   7 ☐ Tile
4 ☐ Asphalt Shingle   8 ☐ Other
  or paper

7. What material is used for most of the outside walls?

1 ☐ Stone   4 ☐ Asbestos Shingle
2 ☒ Brick   5 ☐ Wood
3 ☐ Concrete or   6 ☐ Other
  concrete block

88. Is this house built:

1 ☒ With a basement or cellar with a
  concrete floor?

2 ☐ With a basement or cellar without a
  concrete floor?

3 ☐ On a concrete slab and no basement?

4 ☐ In another way?

9. How many rooms are in your house or apartment?
(Count Kitchen as a room but do not count bathrooms)

Number of rooms ____ *050 7*

**10. Is there hot and cold running water in this
house or building?**

1 ☒ Hot and cold running water inside the
  house or building?

2 ☐ Only cold running water inside

3 ☐ Running water on property but not
  inside building

4 ☐ No running water

11. Where does your drinking water come from?

1 ☐ City water   4 ☐ Cistern
2 ☒ Deep well   5 ☐ Spring
  (over 50 ft.)   6 ☐ Other Source
3 ☐ Shallow well
  (under 50 ft.)

12. How many bathrooms are in your house or apartment?
A **complete** bathroom has **both** flush toilet and
bathing facilities (bathtub or shower). A **partial**
bathroom has a flush toilet **or** bathing facilities
but not both.

1 ☐ No bathroom or only a partial bathroom
2 ☐ 1 complete bathroom
3 ☒ 1 complete bathroom, plus partial
  bathroom(s)
4 ☐ 2 or more complete bathrooms

13. How is your house or apartment heated?

1 ☐ Steam or hot water

2 ☐ Warm air furnace with individual room
  registers

3 ☐ Floor, wall, or pipeless furnace

4 ☒ Built-in electric units

5 ☐ Room heater(s) connected to chimney or
  flue

6 ☐ Room heater(s) **not** connected to chimney or
  flue

7 ☐ Other (specify) _____

8 ☐ Not heated

14. What type of fuel do you use for heating?

1 ☐ Coal, coke or wood

2 ☐ Utility gas from pipes serving the
  neighborhood

3 ☐ Bottled, tank or LP gas

4 ☒ Electricity

5 ☐ Fuel oil or Kerosene

6 ☐ Other fuel

7 ☐ No fuel used

15. What type of fuel do you use for cooking?

1 ☐ Coal, coke or wood

2 ☐ Utility gas from pipes serving the
  neighborhood

3 ☐ Bottled tank, or LP gas

4 ☒ Electricity

5 ☐ Fuel oil or kerosene

6 ☐ Other fuel

7 ☐ No fuel

**16. On the property on which you live, are there any
of the following animals or pets?**

1 ☐ Cattle   5 ☐ Chickens or birds
2 ☐ Horses   6 ☐ Others
3 ☒ Dogs   7 ☐ No animals
4 ☐ Cats

**17. Is there a telephone on which people who live here
can be called?**

☒ YES   ☐ NO

If yes, what is the Telephone NO. **428-2942**

Is the telephone in your house or apartment?

☒ YES   ☐ NO

EDITORIAL COMMENTS

1. The private census of Washington County differed in at least two important respects from the Tecumseh census: First, it was not done by door-to-door enumeration but by a form mailed to residential addresses supplied by a commercial firm. Second, it was intended to collect substantive as well as the usual demographic data with the same instrument.

2. The difficulties experienced with this "two birds with one stone" approach are illustrated by the study of parental smoking and perinatal mortality: the smoking histories pertained to the census date rather than to the time of the relevant pregnancy. Further, as the authors note, "losses occurred because the smoking history was not recorded in sufficient detail."

3. The authors describe the advantages of the private census *cum* survey but then recommend that the enumeration be repeated every "eight to twelve years in a relatively stable community." Since this would coincide approximately with the decennial federal census, it may be that equivalent data could be obtained more easily from official sources supplemented by a sample survey. An additional problem in utilizing infrequently collected private census data for epidemiologic study is that one cannot usually anticipate the pertinent variables long in advance of their investigation. Prior to the 1950's, for example, few would have considered the inclusion in protocols of smoking histories, dietary cholesterol intakes, or exposures to atmospheric pollution. The authors' argument would be more telling if they recommended a more frequent census in a small and relatively stable community.

4. The authors point to the fact that private censuses have been of value in providing sampling frames for community studies. While this is undoubtedly true, one may ask whether other means are available to accomplish this: by using existing demographic data from federal, state, local, or commercial sources, perhaps. A private census would provide more detailed information than these other sources, but it is not easy to agree that the extra information (for example, Stebbing's identification of a sample of white male nonsmokers aged thirty-five to sixty-four who currently resided in Hagerstown but had previously lived outside the county for at least 20 years) justifies a private census. Nevertheless, one can understand the authors' exasperation with some of the confidentiality restrictions of the federal census.

5. A periodic total census combined with substantive data collection may be advantageous in longitudinal studies of very small communities, perhaps the size of Tecumseh. On the other hand, the sample

survey approach would seem to have merit in studies of such relatively large and populous areas as Washington County.

6. Despite these comments on the private census, there remain some very cogent arguments in favor of a community laboratory in Washington County. An important one is the long history of prior community studies there. Because of this, time-trend analyses for selected diseases are facilitated and there is an increased likelihood of favorable community response to the surveys. Other advantages include the relative stability of the local population, a largely centripetal pattern of medical care, and the existence of a cancer registry, to say nothing of the affiliation with an outstanding university medical center.

CHAPTER 5

Some interesting contrasts are evident in the epidemiologic studies of cardiovascular disease in three southeastern communities of high reported prevalence. Evans County, Georgia, was small enough to permit a special census, followed by a survey of all resident adults. Population samples were drawn in the much more populous Charleston County, South Carolina, but all upper class Negroes had to be included in order to provide sufficient numbers for analysis. The studies in North Carolina were largely based on existing records of hospitals and vital statistics registers, but a novel system of epidemiologic surveillance by hospital nurses is being tested. The use of area-adjusted maps to permit visual study of epidemiologic patterns is also illustrated.

EPIDEMIOLOGIC STUDIES OF CARDIOVASCULAR DISEASE IN THREE COMMUNITIES OF THE SOUTHEASTERN UNITED STATES

Herman A. Tyroler

INTRODUCTION

During the past few decades a large body of information relating to the empirical risk of cardiovascular disease in adults has been collected by application of epidemiologic methods. The same period has also seen unparalleled growth in our understanding of the biomedical bases of these diseases and in clinical and technical developments related to their treatment. These advances in epidemiologic knowledge and clinical modalities must now be supplemented with evaluations of the extent to which the increased knowledge has led to increased primary or secondary prevention of heart disease. Such research might, ideally, be accomplished in four steps:

1. Identification of subsegments of a given community which experience different risks of heart disease.
2. Characterization of the environment, life style, and existing patterns of medical services in the community.

3. Experimental modification in an aspect of the existing medical services which is thought to affect the expression of heart disease in the community.
4. Assessment of the biological outcome over time.

The type of research program suggested above has been undertaken, in one form or another, by various investigators, although the four levels of study have not usually been pursued in the same reference population. The development of the Regional Medical Program should make possible such comprehensive studies in individual communities. The main purpose of this chapter is to illustrate some of the uses and limitations of the epidemiologic approach to the study of cardiovascular disease in communities, with examples from the Evans County Cardiovascular Survey, the Charleston County Heart Study, and the North Carolina Regional Medical Program. In addition, some problems of general interest in epidemiologic studies of etiology in a community-based setting will be discussed.

THE COMMUNITIES

The community-based epidemiologic studies in Georgia, South Carolina, and North Carolina were conducted in very contrasting circumstances. Evans County, Georgia, was small enough (population 6,952) to permit an intensive surveillance, over time, of all adult residents according to household and first decree genetic relationship. The studies in Charleston County, South Carolina (population 216,383), required sampling of residents for comprehensive examination. North Carolina (population 4,556,155) was large and complex enough to suggest the need for exploring multiple methods of study. The three states represented in these studies are contiguous, southeastern, coastal states. They resemble each other in having reported death rates attributed to coronary heart disease which are among the highest in the United States (Figure 5–1).

In Evans County approximately half of the population resides on farms; the other half lives in a few small villages and the town of Claxton (population 2,000). The county is only 19 miles in greatest diameter. In contrast, Charleston County measures some 140 miles in length, and extends 35 miles inland from the coast. Although approximately 75 per cent of the population reside in urban areas, there are also many small rural communities. These are notable for their social and geographic isolation which will be discussed below. For the purposes of this exposition, the significant attributes of North Carolina are its large size and its heterogeneity.

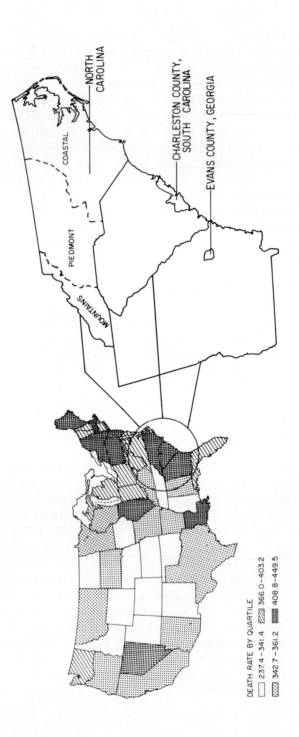

Figure 5–1. Average annual age-adjusted arteriosclerotic heart disease death rates (ISC 420), per 100,000 population, for white males, by state (1959–61).

Methods

Evans County

The Evans County Cardiovascular Field Study was initiated by, and has remained under the direction of, Dr. Curtis G. Hames, a medical practitioner and county health officer in Evans County. Dr. Hames was prompted to undertake a community study when he observed that coronary disease seemed to occur less commonly among Negroes than whites in his clinical practice.

The apparent protection of the Negro from coronary heart disease contrasted sharply with his greater risk of hypertension. However, clinical observations in a private medical practice do not necessarily reflect community levels of disease incidence or prevalence, and an epidemiologic survey was undertaken to test the observation. The research design was developed through the collaborative effort of a number of institutions and individual scientists (McDonough et al. 1963). At present the analysis is primarily the responsibility of the Department of Epidemiology at the University of North Carolina School of Public Health. There is a point worth emphasizing here in the context of community studies: an effective relationship between a highly motivated practitioner of clinical medicine and public health and a University staff can lead to productive research in which community participation and interest remain high.

Prior to an initial survey of coronary heart disease, synthetic estimates of its prevalence were derived by relating the prevalence observed in other reported studies to the population structure of Evans County. From these estimates it was judged that the Negro population would not generate an adequate number of cases for analysis in the contemplated survey. In order to augment the number of Negroes, a portion of adjoining Bulloch County was, therefore, added to Evans County for survey purposes. Before the survey itself, a special census of the area was conducted by five specially trained enumerators and a supervisor. The enumerators were paid $.50 per completed household census and the supervisor received $15 per day. Total cost of the county census, including transportation and printing expenses, was $1,900.

The target population for the survey consisted of the entire Evans County population (Negro and white) aged forty to seventy-four years, the Bulloch County population aged forty to seventy-four (Negro only), and a randomly selected 50 per cent sample of the Evans County population aged fifteen to thirty-nine years. The older group was chosen for prevalence studies of manifest disease, while the younger population served as a base for longitudinal studies of disease incidence, risk factors, familial associations, and other studies. Over a two year period, examinations were made on ten sub-samples in randomized sequence, in order to minimize the possible biasing effects of seasonal or secular morbidity trends. Participation in the prevalence survey of 1958–60 was 92 per cent (3,107 out of 3,377 eligible subjects). This high response rate was due to a combination of factors, including:

1. Ready acceptance of the study by residents of the county, due largely to the efforts of Dr. Hames.
2. Relative ease of locating all subjects on a specially prepared spot map of the county, laid out at the time of the census.
3. Provision for examining in their homes any subjects who were unable or unwilling to come to the study center.
4. A sampling system that made possible an earlier and more systematic approach to nonresponse.
5. Persistent re-visits to persons who refused examination or who were not found at home.

Detailed social, occupational, and behavioral information was collected through interview. In addition, comprehensive medical histories were taken, physical examinations performed, and laboratory procedures completed.

After the prevalence survey in 1960, an ongoing mechanism was set up to monitor deaths among community residents. This involved review of local obituaries, contacts with morticians and ministers, and name checks with the State Office of Vital Records. A recensus of the population and a re-examination cycle was begun in 1967 and is currently nearing completion.

Charleston County

The Charleston Heart Study was initiated by Dr. Edwin Boyle, Jr., while director of the lipid metabolism laboratory of the Medical College of South Carolina. Dr. Boyle was prompted to study the epidemiology of coronary heart disease and hypertension in that community as a result of observations based on an analysis of mortality statistics: he noted that death rates attributed to arteriosclerotic heart disease, cerebral vascular disease, and hypertensive disease were consistently higher in Charleston County than in the United States among persons aged thirty-five to sixty-four years of each race and sex.

In addition, age-adjusted mortality ratios showed striking differences between the races in Charleston County: expressed in sequence of white male to white female to Negro male to Negro female, the ratios were 5:1:3:2 for arteriosclerotic heart disease; 2:1:10:11 for cerebro-vascular disease; and 1:1:7:8 for hypertensive disease. The pattern of an excess mortality from coronary disease in white males and a marked excess of hypertensive disease mortality in Negroes had also been observed in Evans County.

To confirm these apparent racial differences in cardiovascular disease, a community study was undertaken. As described by Boyle et al. (1967):

A population sample based on the 1950 census was drawn by Dr. Alva Finkner of the Research Triangle Institute of Durham, North Carolina. The expected yield was 2,500 men and women over the age of 35 years. The average sampling rate was 3.825 per cent.

The county was divided into the city proper, the urban fringe, the open country and rural places. These areas were subdivided into units of 12 households each. One hundred and sixty units were selected, visited and all adults 35 years of age and over approached for examination. Prior to the drawing of the sample, a preliminary practice area was set aside containing 129 individuals and excluded subsequently from the population sample.

Community acceptance of the study was encouraged by newspaper, radio, and television publicity and letters soliciting aid from ministers and school principals. Repeated attempts were made to obtain cooperation from reluctant subjects.

A mobile trailer containing its own power supply was utilized to examine the study subjects at their place of residence by a staff consisting of a registered nurse, public health advisor, and supervising physician.

The examination procedure consisted of a brief medical history and interview regarding personal habits plus history of residence; a supine and seated blood pressure (fifth phase) utilizing repeatedly standardized aneroid manometer and standard cuff, 99 per cent of all pressures being taken by the same registered nurse (repeated audiometric examinations were performed on this observer); an eight lead electrocardiogram; bilateral recording ankle oscillometrics; height; weight; skin pigmentation reflectance by Photovolt Corp. Model 610; serum cholesterol; K-agar test; and blood type. Rh phenotypes and hemoglobin electrophoresis were also obtained.

In the subsequent analysis of the data it became obvious that social status was an important variable of study in this setting. Unfortunately, the occupational structure and the racial distribution of Charleston County were such that the sampled population contained very few Negroes in either nonmanual or upper social class occupations. For this reason, Dr. Boyle attempted to augment the sample with all upper social class Negroes of Charleston, i.e., all professional and managerial personnel, and owners of large businesses. The necessary information was obtained from previously identified upper social class Negro informants and by peer group nominations. A total of 103 upper social class Negro males was ascertained by this method. The over-all survey participation rates were 85.3 per cent among the whites and 81.5 per cent among the nonwhites of the random sample, including 82.4 per cent of the upper social class nonwhites.

North Carolina

The only data on heart disease which is currently available on all residents of North Carolina is that provided by census-based vital statistics. Death certificates are received from the North Carolina State Board of Health and the number of deaths attributed to each disease is determined. Cross tabulations are then generated which permit the study of decedent groups by variables of interest, such as date and place of death, residence, hospital, etc. From those data, tables, graphs, and maps are prepared which document the mortality attributed to each categorical disease.

Hospital data are currently available through a standardized reporting system for approximately half the hospitals of North Carolina. Statistics on morbidity and case fatality for conditions such as acute myocardial infarction are generated therefrom. Epidemiologic studies have been facilitated by the development of computer programs to select cases with given diagnoses and to select samples matched by age, race, sex, and date of admission. A mechanism for the ascertainment of death after discharge from the hospital has been established through the state office of vital statistics. The latter has made possible an analysis of the effect of diagnostic "fashion" in the medical certification of deaths attributed to coronary heart disease in urban and rural hospitals.

The problems of reliability and validity in the reporting of disease are many. A number of attempts are being made to overcome them. One is an experiment in which medical practitioners are being trained in methods of standardizing data collection. Another is an attempt to develop an epidemiologic surveillance system as part of a training program for supervisory nurses in coronary care units. After completing the program, the nurses are now functioning as supervisors of coronary care units in 12 community hospitals throughout the state. Each is assisting in the development of a uniform method for the collection and recording of demographic, medical, and outcome data. If this approach succeeds, a valuable new source of epidemiologic information will become available to describe the outcome of treatment of coronary heart disease in widely different types of medical care facilities in North Carolina.

FINDINGS

Evans County

In common with the other southeastern communities discussed in this chapter, Evans County is characterized by an excessive mortality from cardiovascular disease. Various studies conducted here have documented the relationship of various physiologic factors (blood pressure and serum cholesterol), genetic factors (family and population), and psychological factors to coronary disease. There is additional interest in studies relating behavioral and social attributes of changing life styles to coronary heart disease.

McDonough et al. (1965) and Skinner et al. (1966) found that coronary heart disease was more prevalent in whites than nonwhites, (despite the "epidemic" hypertension among the latter) and that, among white males, it was increased among those in the upper social class. These observations led them to propose that differences in physical activity at work may explain most of the observed social class differences in coronary heart disease. Although the specific mechanism underlying this relationship is not yet known, the implications for communities in the southeastern United States seem clear: as they are transformed from a rural, predominantly agrarian economy to an urban, industrialized one, the problem of coronary heart disease, particularly in the middle-aged white male, can be predicted to increase.

The familial aggregation of coronary disease and its risk factors is not only theoretically interesting but it is relevant to program planning. This is exemplified by a study of blood pressure levels among family members in Evans County (Hayes et al. 1967). Pearson product-moment correlation coefficients were computed for each examinee, based on standard blood pressure scores. Means and standard deviations were computed for each of the race-sex categories in ten-year age groupings. The standard score was derived as the algebraic difference between the observed value and the mean for that age-race-sex group, divided by the standard deviation for the same grouping. The correlation coefficients for systolic blood pressure among first-degree relatives ranged from 0.13 to 0.26 (Table 5–1). These values differ significantly from zero, and they compare with coefficients reported in other populations (Johnson, Epstein, and Kjelsberg 1965). With the exception of parent-offspring correlations of 0.26 for systolic blood pressure among Negroes and 0.13 among whites, the various kin relationships show no sizable differences between the races. Correlation coefficients for height were also calculated (Table 5–1). These ranged in value from 0.34 to 0.44 for the first-degree relatives residing in Evans County. This is consistent with findings in

TABLE 5–1. FAMILIAL AGGREGATION OF BLOOD PRESSURE LEVELS—EVANS COUNTY PREVALENCE SURVEY

	Number of pairs	Correlation coefficients[a]		
		Diastolic blood pressure	Systolic blood pressure	Height
Spouse pairs				
White	669	0.08[b]	0.13[c]	0.13[c]
Negro	308	−0.05	−0.03	0.11[b]
Sib pairs				
White	545	0.17[c]	0.20[c]	0.41[c]
Negro	191	0.19[c]	0.14[b]	0.34[c]
Parent-offspring pairs				
White	635	0.14[c]	0.13[c]	0.44[c]
Negro	263	0.17[b]	0.26[c]	0.40[c]

[a] Computation of the product moment correlation coefficients was based upon standard scores, specific for race, sex, and ten-year age group.
[b] $P < 0.05$.
[c] $P < 0.01$.

other populations and adds to our confidence in the values obtained for blood pressure. Recently, however, some doubt has been cast on the validity of this conclusion (Acheson and Fowler 1967).

White spouse pairs showed a significant similarity in blood pressure values, with correlation coefficients of 0.08 for diastolic and 0.13 for systolic blood pressure. This was not found among Negro couples and has not been reported in other studies to date.

The aggregation of elevated blood pressure levels in white spouse pairs was examined in greater detail by comparing the observed number of hypertensive pairs with expected numbers calculated under the null hypothesis (Table 5–2). No excessive concordance was observed among spouse pairs in which the wife's age was under forty years. For wives aged forty to sixty years there was an excess of concordant pairs with diastolic hypertension which was maximal at wife's age of fifty to fifty-nine years. In the oldest age group concordance approximated expectation. For systolic hypertension a slight excess of concordant pairs was observed only when the wife's age was fifty years or older.

The results of this study in Evans County have, in general, been consistent with other population-based studies of the familial aggregation of blood pressure levels. Of special interest is the finding that first-degree relatives of both races are about equally concordant, despite the much higher prevalence of hypertension in Negroes.

The concordance measures in this study were based entirely upon casual blood pressure readings. No attempt was made to exclude sec-

TABLE 5–2. NUMBER OF SPOUSE PAIRS CONCORDANT FOR ELEVATED BLOOD PRESSURE BY AGE OF WIFE—EVANS COUNTY PREVALENCE SURVEY

Wife's age	Diastolic BP ⩾ 95 White: Number of concordant pairs			Systolic BP ⩾ 150 White: Number of concordant pairs		
	Observed	Expected[a]	O/E × 100	Observed	Expected[a]	O/E × 100
15–29	0	0.19	—	0	0.04	—
30–39	2	2.33	86	3	1.95	(154)
40–49	26	18.98	137	15	14.92	101
50–59	27	19.28	140	37	32.97	112
60+	18	17.46	103	45	40.35	112
All ages	73	58.24	125	101	90.23	111

[a] The expected number of pairs was computed under the assumption of independence between the pair, given the prevalence of elevated blood pressure specific for age, race, and sex.

ondary hypertension or to adjust for time of examination or antecedent activity. In view of the intra-individual variability of blood pressure and the well-recognized differential responses to environmental, biological, and psychological stimuli, one must be impressed with the observed concordances. However, no light has been shed here on the Negro-white differences in population levels of blood pressure. The similarity in degree of blood pressure concordance among genetic relatives of both races residing in Evans County suggests that the factors influencing aggregation act with equal force on the two populations whose mean blood pressures are, in effect, set at different levels.

The findings on aggregation of hypertension in spouse pairs also deserve comment. Winkelstein et al. (1966) reported that this was a function of length of marriage. Data from Tecumseh suggest the possibility of an association in those marital pairs where female age is fifty years or above, although the investigators questioned the significance of this (Johnson, Epstein, and Kjelsberg 1965).

If chance associations or systematic biases in measurement can be ruled out, shared life experiences as a function of length of marriage emerge as possible determinants of spouse concordance. While shared experience appears to be a reasonable explanation for aggregation in the middle aged, the disappearance of such aggregation at the older ages may seem surprising. An explanation becomes apparent if one considers the selective factors which might cause a differentially greater number of withdrawals from observation of elderly couples who are concordantly hypertensive than of discordant couples. The major selective force operating on hypertensives over the age of fifty years is death, and death rates from hypertension are known to be higher in males than females. Furthermore, all of the concordantly hypertensive pairs must contain a male, while among the discordant pairs there will be an excess of hypertensive females, since the prevalence of hypertension is higher in females than in males over age fifty. Thus, in the middle aged, there will be a higher proportion of hypertensive males in concordant than in discordant couples. By age sixty-five or seventy years it can be expected that there will have been a greater number of withdrawals (due to death) from the concordant than from the discordant couples, thus leading to a reduction in the proportion of concordant couples.

This age effect on spouse concordance (a result of the combined effects of shared experience and selective withdrawal) may explain the contradictory results that have been obtained in other studies of spouse aggregation. According to our explanation the degree of such aggregation will be greatly influenced by the age distribution of the population, and the analysis should in all cases take account of this.

The failure to demonstrate aggregation of hypertension in Negro spouse pairs in the Evans County study is noteworthy. One possible explanation is that different environmental mechanisms may be operative in the two races, both in producing high blood pressure and in producing its familial aggregation. An alternative explanation is that the higher rates of mortality, divorce, and separation in Negroes result in shorter average durations of shared experience and selective withdrawal of spouse pairs which reduces the possibility of concordance. There will be an opportunity to test some of these hypotheses in a follow-up study of the Evans County cohort of 1960–62.

Charleston County

The excess of hypertension among Negroes which had been observed clinically and evaluated in death certificate studies was confirmed in the prevalence survey of Charleston County (Boyle et al. 1967). Studies of associated characteristics which might help to explain this finding are now under way. One study, concerning the possible relationship between sickle cell trait and hypertension, is of particular relevance in the context of this chapter, as it demonstrates the need for a community-based, multi-variable approach. The possibility of a direct relationship between sickle cell trait and hypertension has been suggested by the high values of each in American Negro populations, and by evidence of altered renal functioning (Cochran 1963) and renal pathologic changes in individuals with sickle cell trait (Femi-Pearse and Odungo 1968).

Sickle cell trait, as determined by paper electrophoresis, was found in 113 out of the 775 Negro adults in the random sample of Charleston County. This proportion (14.6 per cent) is one of the highest reported in the United States and is one of very few values which have been derived from randomly sampled residents of a community. The trait was almost equally prevalent in males and females, and there was little or no evidence of variation with age (Boyle et al. 1968).

The latter finding is at variance with the results of other studies in the United States which have reported less sickling among older patients (Rucknagel and Neel 1961). These earlier studies also provided some indication of an increased death rate among adult sicklers as compared with normal adults in a nontropical environment. Our data, based on a random sample of Charleston residents, do not support the suggestion that adults with sickle cell trait experience a significantly increased death rate.

The observed relationship of sickle cell trait to diastolic blood pressure among Charleston Negroes is set out in Table 5–3. The mean diastolic blood pressure for sampled males with the trait was 92.0 and for those without it 90.1. Among sampled females the values were 91.8 and 92.1, respectively. There are no significant differences between these values. However, blood pressures in the younger males with sickle cell trait were somewhat higher than in males without it—a pattern which is reversed after age fifty-four. This pattern is consistent with the hypothesized association of the trait with hypertension in earlier adulthood and selective mortality in the older ages. It is not consistent with the findings observed in females (Table 5–3).

The prevalence of sickle cell trait in Charleston County varied significantly in subpopulations stratified by occupation and place of

TABLE 5–3. MEAN DIASTOLIC BLOOD PRESSURE IN NEGROES WITH AND WITHOUT SICKLE CELL TRAIT—CHARLESTON COUNTY

Age (Years)	With trait			Without trait		
	Sample size	M.D.B. pressure	Standard deviation	Sample size	M.D.B. pressure	Standard deviation
	MALES					
35–44	22	91.5	13.4	120	85.8	11.6
45–54	8	96.0	17.2	71	93.0	14.4
55–64	11	92.9	12.2	53	94.5	15.6
65+	7	88.0	16.0	35	92.8	16.0
All ages	48	92.0	13.9	279	90.1	14.2
	FEMALES					
35–44	27	86.4	13.0	166	87.0	12.6
45–54	16	91.6	11.7	88	95.9	13.0
55–64	11	98.0	11.5	65	97.0	14.0
65+	11	99.5	7.3	64	95.5	13.6
All ages	65	91.8	12.6	383	92.1	13.8

Figure 5–2. Prevalence of the sickle cell trait in geographic subdivisions of Charleston County, South Carolina. Reproduced with permission from *Arch. Env. Health* 17:6, 891–98. Dec., 1968, E. Boyle, MD., et al.

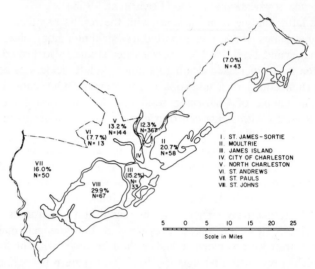

residence (Figure 5–2). It was highest (29.9 per cent) in the lowest socioeconomic stratum of rural St. John's Island and lowest (5.5 per cent) in the upper stratum of the city.

This differential distribution of a genetically determined trait within a region as small as Charleston County is particularly interesting in view of the relative genetic purity of the local Negro population, the "Gullah." Although many of them have emigrated, there has been minimal Negro immigration and minimal white gene diffusion. Thus the Gullah have preserved the biological and cultural traits their ancestors possessed when they first came to the United States (Pollitzer 1968; Pollitzer et al. 1964).

North Carolina

The geographic distribution of deaths attributed to cerebrovascular disease among persons forty-five to sixty-four years of age in North Carolina was examined by plotting on a map the average annual number of such deaths from 1959 to 1961 by county of residence (Figure 5–3). The distribution is grossly heterogenous: there are dense clusters of deaths in the thickly populated, industrialized counties of the Piedmont and also in the Upper Coastal Plain where the state's Negroes are relatively concentrated. On the other hand, very few deaths occurred in the sparsely populated counties of the western mountain area.

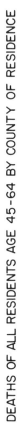

Figure 5–3. The distribution of deaths attributed to cerebrovascular disease (1959–60–61), by county of residence in North Carolina. Reproduced with permission from *Am. J. Public Health*. Tyroler, H. A. and Smith, H. L., 1968. Epidemiology and planning for the North Carolina Regional Medical Program. 58:1058–67. No. 6.

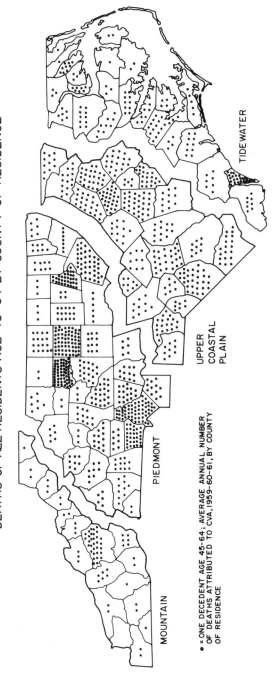

DEATHS OF ALL RESIDENTS AGE 45-64 BY COUNTY OF RESIDENCE

MOUNTAIN

PIEDMONT

UPPER COASTAL PLAIN

TIDEWATER

• = ONE DECEDENT AGE 45-64; AVERAGE ANNUAL NUMBER OF DEATHS ATTRIBUTED TO CVA, 1959-60-61, BY COUNTY OF RESIDENCE

To assist in the interpretation of this geographic distribution, epi-demiologic area-adjusted maps were constructed. In this technique, the counties are redrawn with their dimensions proportionate to population rather than to area, although the general spatial relations (county borders, north-south and east-west orientation, etc.) are preserved (Levison and Haddon 1965). Such area-adjusted maps were constructed for white and nonwhite cerebrovascular deaths in North Carolina (Figures 5–4 and 5–5). The previously noted clustering of deaths in the Piedmont and Upper Coastal Plain is no longer apparent as these more densely popu-lated areas are now in scale. By the same token, the higher stroke mortality of Negroes as compared with whites is plainly evident.

Figure 5–4. Epidemiologic area-adjusted map. Deaths of white residents age forty-five to sixty-four by county of residence.

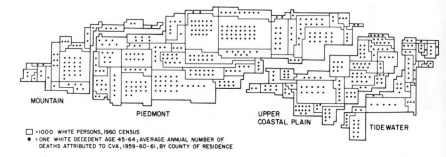

☐ =1000 WHITE PERSONS, 1960 CENSUS
● = ONE WHITE DECEDENT AGE 45-64 ; AVERAGE ANNUAL NUMBER OF
DEATHS ATTRIBUTED TO CVA, 1959-60-61, BY COUNTY OF RESIDENCE

Figure 5–5. Epidemiologic area-adjusted map. Deaths of nonwhite residents age forty-five to sixty-four by county of residence.

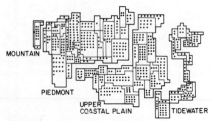

☐ = 1000 NON-WHITE PERSONS, 1960 CENSUS
● = ONE NON-WHITE DECEDENT AGE 45-64 ; AVERAGE ANNUAL NUMBER OF DEATHS ATTRIBUTED
TO CVA, 1959-60-61, BY COUNTY OF RESIDENCE

Such adjusted maps are very useful in permitting the visual study of epidemiologic patterns. The geographic areas can be redrawn propor-tionate to any appropriate population of interest. For example, in a study of case fatality from coronary disease one might plot the cases on a map drawn to reflect the number of coronary care units or hospital beds in each area. It should be emphasized, however, that the epi-demiologist or public health planner cannot employ mapping in lieu of the precise calculation of specific or adjusted rates. On the contrary, the maps may best serve as a useful adjunct or summary of the numerical data.

An example of this is afforded by our mapping of death rates from cardiovascular disease among white and nonwhite males forty-five to sixty-four years of age in the period from 1959 to 1961 (Figures 5–6 and 5–7). A rather consistent pattern is seen: among whites the death rates tend to be higher in the eastern counties than in the western counties, and the area of consistently highest rates is the Upper Coastal Plain. The magnitude of the geographic gradient is such that the western part of North Carolina has rates in the lowest octile of all state economic areas, and the Upper Coastal Plain has rates in the highest octile of the United States (Sauer and Brand 1968). There is also a gradient according to size of population within the mountain and Piedmont area, although this is not readily evident from the map (Tyroler and Cassel 1964). However, the highest rates in the state were not found in the

Figure 5–6. Death rates from major cardiovascular diseases.* White males age forty-five to sixty-four. (1959–60–61).

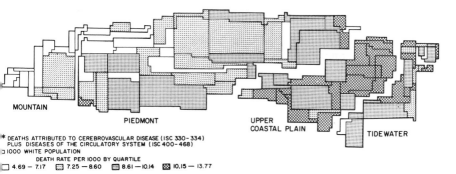

MOUNTAIN

PIEDMONT   UPPER
                       COASTAL PLAIN
                                        TIDEWATER

* DEATHS ATTRIBUTED TO CEREBROVASCULAR DISEASE (ISC 330–334)
  PLUS DISEASES OF THE CIRCULATORY SYSTEM (ISC 400–468)
⊐ 1000 WHITE POPULATION
          DEATH RATE PER 1000 BY QUARTILE
☐ 4.69 – 7.17   ▨ 7.25 – 8.60   ⊞ 8.61 – 10.14   ▨ 10.15 – 13.77

Figure 5–7. Death rates from major cardiovascular diseases.* Nonwhite males age forty-five to sixty-four. (1959–60–61).

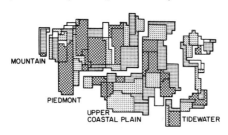

MOUNTAIN

PIEDMONT
        UPPER
        COASTAL PLAIN   TIDEWATER

* DEATHS ATTRIBUTED TO CEREBROVASCULAR DISEASE (ISC 330–334)
  PLUS DISEASES OF THE CIRCULATORY SYSTEM (ISC 400–468)
☐ 1000 NON-WHITE POPULATION
          DEATH RATE PER 1000 BY QUARTILE
☐ .00 – 9.35   ▨ 9.49 – 12.29   ⊞ 12.31 – 15.21   ▨ 15.24 – 28.57

populous counties, but in the less populous counties of the coastal plain. Among nonwhites the pattern differed: death rates were highest in the Piedmont and in the most populous counties.

There is some evidence that the west-east gradient observed in whites is not mere happenstance: similar findings were reported by Hamilton (1955) in his analysis of the 1950 mortality experience. There is also some evidence that variations in diagnostic practices cannot account for the differences in stroke mortality between the various counties of North Carolina. The relationship between death rates from cerebrovascular disease, arteriosclerotic heart disease, and other heart disease in this state was also studied and the findings compared with those of a national study (Kuller et al. 1969).

The high-rate counties of North Carolina are part of a large belt of southeastern coastal United States counties which have high cardiovascular and cerebrovascular death rates, compared with the rest of the United States (Sauer et al. 1966; Rose 1962; Acheson 1966; Sauer 1962). We are now developing procedures to determine whether the high death rates are due to higher incidence, higher case fatality rates, or a combination of both.

The observed differences in mortality rates among the various subpopulations in North Carolina have suggested a number of ecologic investigations into the possible roles of the physical and social environment. An example is our study of the relationship between cardiovascular disease mortality and hardness of drinking water. An inverse association between the two has been found in a number of studies in the United States (Schroeder 1960; 1966), England (Morris et al. 1961; Crawford, Gardner, and Morris 1968), Sweden (Biörck, Boström, and Widström 1965), and elsewhere. The association could not be confirmed in two other studies (Lindeman and Assenzo 1964; Mulcahy 1964). Because of the potentialities for coronary disease prevention which might be realized through control of water hardness, the validity of this association is an attractive subject for investigation.

In a recent study, data on coronary disease mortality and on average county water hardness from municipal and rural ground water sources in North Carolina were compared (Brittain 1968). No simple relationship of average water hardness to coronary heart disease mortality could be demonstrated. In fact, the findings contrasted somewhat with the usually reported inverse relationship: the Highlands area with the softest water had the lowest rate and the coastal plains area with highest death rate had an intermediate degree of water hardness (Table 5–4). Thus, differences in average water hardness cannot account for regional differences in coronary disease death rates, if water hardness were protective in North Carolina as it has been reported to be elsewhere.

TABLE 5–4. AVERAGE WATER HARDNESS AND DEATH RATES FROM CORONARY HEART DISEASE—REGIONS OF NORTH CAROLINA

Region	Average hardness (ppm in $CaCO_3$)	Average annual death rate (per 100,000) white males aged 55–64, 1956–64		
		Arteriosclerotic heart disease	Coronary heart disease	Cerebrovascular disease
		(I.S.C.[a] 420)	(I.S.C. 420.1)	(I.S.C. 330–334)
Highland	23	752	585	147
Piedmont	61	932	778	172
Coastal plain	51	1,062	877	247
Tidewater	163	919	713	218

[a] I.S.C. refers to nosological rubric in the Manual of the International Statistical Classification of Diseases, Injuries and Causes of Death, W.H.O., Geneva, 1957.

Data from the 44 North Carolina hospitals which subscribed to the PAS System* in 1967 were analyzed in a study of case fatality from myocardial infarction. During the first six months of 1967, 1,921 patients out of 113,324 were discharged with a diagnosis of acute coronary occlusion. Of these, 552 died in the hospital, giving an over-all case fatality rate of 29 per cent. This figure is consistent with national estimates made in the period prior to the development of coronary care units (Friedberg 1956). The rates of case fatality among the different hospitals ranged from a low of 14 per cent to a high of 80 per cent. At the time of this study only 7 per cent of patients received cardiac monitoring. This number has increased considerably and continues to increase with the opening of new coronary care units. Whether their use will substantially affect case fatality remains to be seen.

However, differences in survivorship of coronary patients in several hospitals at one point in time or in one hospital at different times may also reflect differences in admission policies, diagnostic practices, and the age-race-sex composition of the patient population, in addition to random statistical variation (Oliver et al. 1967). It is hoped that the development of epidemiologic surveillance by supervisory nurses (described earlier) will permit adjustment for most of these potentially confounding variables. It must also be remembered that hospitalized cases represent a relatively small fraction of all fatal episodes of myocardial infarction. In North Carolina from 1956 to 1964, only 38 per cent of all deaths certified to coronary disease occurred in a hospital. Thus, control of this disease cannot be realized through improvement in hospital care alone.

* Professional Activity Study of the Commission on Professional and Hospital Activities, Ann Arbor, Michigan.

POTENTIALS

We are entering a period of national concern and innovative interest in the organization and delivery of health care services. There is and there will continue to be an ever increasing flood of technical and scientific developments issuing from medical center clinics and research laboratories; and there is and there will continue to be a growing awareness of and demand for these developments by those practitioners and patients who do not now have access to them. Comprehensive health planning and regional medical programs are but two of many organizational responses to these trends.

The potentialities for epidemiologic service and research in these enterprises are limitless. The examples of cardiovascular disease epidemiology in southeastern communities were chosen to illustrate some of the currently available methods and also some of the problems in realizing these potentialities. The manifestations and distributions of disease in communities and the identification of populations at differing risk provide the raw materials of descriptive epidemiology which is mandatory for program planning, priority allocation of limited resources, and monitoring for evaluation of change over time. In addition to such well-recognized methodologic concerns as measurement reliability and validity and survey participation, there are formidable problems concerned with determining the appropriateness of different units of study for different purposes.

The Charleston study, for example, illustrates the fallacy of assuming genetic homogeneity in a community, despite its relatively circumscribed physical setting and the presence of putatively similar individuals of common origins. An epidemiologic study of genetic variables in a community must also consider social factors, since the determinants of genotype frequencies include marriage and mating patterns, physical and social isolation, and differential exposure to malnutrition and disease. In view of these factors, the definition of a study population in terms of its environment must differ for different purposes. The study of familial aggregation of blood pressure in Evans County, for example, estimated the distribution of elevated blood pressure and might be of value in planning for primary and secondary prevention in that community. However, the related individuals ascertained in the survey represent only those who have survived and remained in Evans County. In fact, unless all migrants and decedents are traced no one community at any point in time is suitable for a holistic approach to the epidemiologic study of disease etiology. A practical alternative is the study of various communities with differing characteristics, utilizing individually appropriate epidemiologic techniques. When the results of such diverse studies coincide, valid inferences on hypothesized relationships in disease may often be made.

In contrast to research on etiology, community studies on health services and administration are usually directed to strictly defined geopolitical entities. The reason for this is that such entities are the local or regional units for the organization and delivery of health services. Very recently, the establishment of regional medical programs has greatly accelerated the demands on the epidemiologist for community health planning and evaluation (Tyroler and Smith 1968).

Epidemiologic surveillance on a continuing basis will be an integral feature of the Regional Medical Program. As already indicated, there are formidable methodologic and theoretic problems in securing valid epidemiologic information about a region such as North Carolina. A diversity of sources is required, including cross-sectional and prospective community surveys and medical records from physicians, clinics, hospitals, nursing homes, industries, and schools. Some of these records will be the by-product of routine health service functions while others will be produced explicitly for, and under the direction of, the regional program. The sampling methods for obtaining these records, their optimal form and content, and the necessary data processing procedures, all require research. Research is also needed in methods for appraising and improving the quality and completeness of each data source. Record linkage techniques can yield information on the various routes taken by patients to and through the health services of a region. For persons who do not utilize these services, however, community sampling, rather than record surveys is required.

One approach to the problems discussed above might be to select several communities for study, estimate the desired morbidity rates, utilizing routinely available data, and then determine the actual rates by special survey. If there is good agreement between the estimated and observed rates of disease, and this is replicated in a heterogenous group of study samples, the model could be adapted for routine use. This would involve maintaining a few comprehensive survey centers in selected communities of each region, similar to that in Evans County.

References

Acheson, R. M. 1966. Mortality from cerebrovascular disease in the United States. In *Public Health Monograph No. 76, Cerebrovascular Disease Epidemiology. A Workshop*, pp. 23–40. P.H.S. Pub. No. 1441. Washington: U.S. Government Printing Office.

Acheson, R. M. and Fowler, G. B. 1967. On the inheritance of stature and blood pressure. *J. Chronic Dis.* 20:731–45.

Biörck, G., Boström, H., and Widström, A. 1965. On the relationship between water hardness and death rates in cardiovascular disease. *Acta Med. Scand.* 178:239–52.

Boyle, E., Griffey, W. P., Nichaman, M. Z., and Talbert, C. R. 1967. An epidemiologic study of hypertension among racial groups of Charleston County, South Carolina. The Charleston heart study, Phase II. In *The Epidemiology of Hypertension*. Edited by Stamler, J., Stamler, R., and Pullman, T., pp. 193–203. New York: Grune & Stratton.

Boyle, E., Thompson, C., and Tyroler, H. A. 1968. An epidemiologic study of the prevalance of the sickle cell trait in adults of Charleston County, South Carolina. *Arch. Environ. Health* 17:891–98.

Brittain, R. C. 1968. An ecological study of the relationship between water hardness and coronary heart disease mortality rates in the state of North Carolina. (Unpublished data.)

Cochran, R. R. 1963. Hyposthenuria in sickle cell states. *Arch. Intern. Med.* 112:222–25.

Crawford, M. D., Gardner, M. J., and Morris, J. N. 1968. Mortality and hardness of local water supplies. *Lancet* 1:827–31.

Femi-Pearse, D. and Odunjo, E. O. 1968. Renal cortical infarcts in sickle cell trait. *Brit. Med. J.* 3:34.

Friedberg, C. K. 1956. *Diseases of the Heart.* 2d ed. Philadelphia: W. B. Saunders.

Hamilton, C. H. 1955. Ecological and social factors in mortality variation. *Eugen. Quart.* 2:212–23.

Hayes, G., Tyroler, H. A., Cassel, J. C., McDonough, J. R., and Hames, C. G. 1967. Family aggregation of blood pressure in Evans County, Georgia. Paper presented at The American Heart Association Conference on the Epidemiology of Cardiovascular Diseases, Chicago.

Johnson, B. C., Epstein, F. H., and Kjelsberg, M. O. 1965. Distributions and familial studies of blood pressure and serum cholesterol levels in a total community—Tecumseh, Michigan, *J. Chronic Dis.* 18:147–60.

Kuller, L. H., Bolker, A., Saslaw, M., Paegel, B. L., Sisk, C., Borhani, N., Wray, J. A., Anderson, H., Peterson, D., Winkelstein, W., Jr., Cassel, J., Spiers, P., Robinson, A. G., Curry, H., Lilienfeld, A. M., and Seltser, R. 1969. Nationwide cerebrovascular disease mortality study. *Am. J. Epidem.* 90:536–85.

Levison, M. E. and Haddon, W. 1965. The area adjusted map. An epidemiologic device. *Public Health Rep.* 80:55–59.

Lindeman, R. D. and Assenzo, J. R. 1964. Correlations between water hardness and cardiovascular deaths in Oklahoma Counties. *Am. J. Public Health* 54:1071–77.

McDonough, J. R., Hames, C. G., Stulb, M. S., and Garrison, G. E. 1963. Cardiovascular disease field study in Evans County, Georgia. *Public Health Rep.* 78:1051–59.

———. 1965. Coronary heart disease among Negroes and Whites in Evans County, Georgia. *J. Chronic Dis.* 18:443–68.

Morris, J. N., Crawford, M. D., and Heady, J. A. 1961. Hardness of local water supplies and mortality from cardiovascular disease in the County Boroughs of England and Wales. *Lancet* 1:860–62.

Mulcahy, R. 1964. The influence of water hardness and rainfall on the incidence of cardiovascular and cerebrovascular mortality in Ireland. *J. Irish Med. Ass.* 55:17–18.

Oliver, M. F., Julian, D. G., and Donald, K. W. 1967. Problems in evaluating coronary care units. *Am. J. Cardiol.* 20:465–74.

Pollitzer, W. S. 1968. The Negroes of Charleston (S.C.); a study of hemoglobin types, serology, and morphology. *Am. J. Phys. Anthrop.* 16:241–63.

Pollitzer, W. S., Menegaz-Bock, R. M., Ceppellini, R., and Dunn, L. C. 1964. Blood factors and morphology of the Negroes of James Island, Charleston, South Carolina. *Am. J. Phys. Anthrop.* 22:393–98.

Rose, G. 1962. The distribution of mortality from hypertension within the United States. *J. Chronic Dis.* 15:1017–24.

Rucknagel, D. L. and Neel, J. V. 1966. The hemoglobinopathies. *Prog. Med. Genet.* 1:158–260.

Sauer, H. I. 1962. Epidemiology of cardiovascular mortality—geographic and ethnic. *Am. J. Public Health* 52:94–105.

Sauer, H. I. and Brand, F. R. 1968. Geographic differences in cause-specific death rates. Paper presented at the Meeting of the Society for Epidemiologic Research, Washington, D.C., 10 May 1968.

Sauer, H. I., Payne, G. H., Council, C. R., and Terrell, J. C. 1966. Cardiovascular disease mortality patterns in Georgia and North Carolina. *Public Health Rep.* 81:455–65.

Schroeder, H. A. 1960. Relation between mortality from cardiovascular disease and treated water supplies. *J.A.M.A.* 172:1902–08.

———. 1966. Municipal drinking water and cardiovascular death rates. *J.A.M.A.* 195:81–85.

Skinner, J. S., Benson, H., McDonough, J. R., and Hames, C. G. 1966. Social status, physical activity, and coronary proneness. *J. Chronic Dis.* 19:773–83.

Tyroler, H. A. and Cassel, J. 1964. Health consequences of culture change —II, the effect of urbanization on coronary heart mortality in rural residents. *J. Chronic Dis.* 17:167–77.

Tyroler, H. A. and Smith, H. L. 1968. Epidemiology and planning for the North Carolina Regional Medical Program. *Am. J. Public Health* 58:1058–67.

Winkelstein, W., Jr. 1966. Familial aggregation of blood pressure. Preliminary report. *J.A.M.A.* 195:848–50.

EDITORIAL COMMENTS

1. These three studies are distinguished by a single rationale for their initiation, viz., an apparently high cardiovascular disease incidence or mortality with suggestive racial differences. The execution of com-

munity studies in such presumed high-risk areas has the virtue of increasing the likelihood that predisposing environmental factors—if they exist—will be identified. Once such factors are found, studies to further test their relationship to disease will become necessary; in particular, longitudinal cohort investigations of morbidity in exposed and non-exposed persons. Evans County probably would be too small to permit such a study, but Charleston County or other larger defined areas in North Carolina would be appropriate.

2. The Evans County study illustrates how a small and remote community can be subjected to rigorous epidemiological investigation with expert guidance from afar (in this case, the School of Public Health at Chapel Hill). Of course, there was also a "convenience" factor in the choice of Evans County, viz., the enthusiastic co-operation of a local practitioner who also happened to be county health officer.

3. The evolution of the Charleston County study follows a not infrequent pattern in which epidemiological observations (based on mortality statistics for example) on unusual risks of disease are followed by specially designed studies to validate the observations. It would seem desirable and economical to incorporate into such studies tests for specific etiological hypotheses which might explain the unusual risks observed.

4. An interesting finding in the initial Charleston County survey was that too few Negroes in the higher social classes had been selected. The sample was then augmented with all the upper class Negroes in the county; a procedure which demonstrates a virtue of the sample survey method, i.e., the possibility of enlarging the sample. This option would not be available in a total population study of comparable size.

5. A weakness of the North Carolina studies at present is the absence of a denominator population, since not all of the state's hospitals are under surveillance. Consideration might be given to sampling the nonhospitalized population as well as admissions to the unmonitored hospitals.

6. The author suggests that comprehensive community studies, including clinical and preventive trials, might evolve from the Regional Medical Program. To the extent that this program increases the probability of identifying cases with a given disease and encourages area-wide record linkages between hospitals, this may well come to pass. The establishment of collaborative population laboratories in several communities with differing characteristics is another possible development in the Regional Medical Program. To be sure, community surveys will still be necessary to locate patients who do not make use of regular medical services.

CHAPTER 6

The rationale for undertaking this prospective study of cardiovascular disease, the initial methodologic design, the subsequent modifications, and the response rate over time are as relevant to investigators
today as they were twenty years ago when this pioneering study was
undertaken. The unique advantages of the cohort approach as well as
its shortcomings are well illustrated here.

THE FRAMINGHAM, MASSACHUSETTS, STUDY
TWENTY YEARS LATER

Tavia Gordon and William B. Kannel

INTRODUCTION

Since the end of 1948 the town of Framingham, Massachusetts, has
been the site of a long-term epidemiological study of cardiovascular
disease. The study has attempted to follow a cohort of 5,209 persons
by repeated re-examination at two-year intervals. The general philosophy
of the study was phrased in the original protocol in these terms:

If it is accepted:
That pathological change in or disordered function of the intimate
structures of the cardiovascular system resulting from stresses and insults of various types is reversible up to a degree or point which is inherent in the individual, and
That pathological or physiological change beyond that degree probably results in minute residual changes which are immeasurable by
methods now available, and
That continuous accretion of such residual changes results finally
in a clinically recognizable abnormality, and
That there is a wide variability in the individual response to many
stresses and insults,
It is hypothesized that the age of onset of degenerative cardiovascular disease is a function of three variables:

123

(1) Constitutional factors (including hereditary factors)
(2) Conditioning factors (including external environmental factors), and
(3) The time factor or length of time the conditioning factors must act on the constitutionally determined characteristics or interact with them to result in clinical cardiovascular disease.

The Framingham Heart Disease Epidemiology Study is designed to measure certain selected constitutional factors and certain of the conditioning factors in a large number of "normal" persons selected at random and to record the time during which these selected factors act and interact before clinical cardiovascular disease results.

Early History

The Framingham study plan has been formally described and evaluated a number of times. Pioneering studies, however, seldom arise through the rigid imposition of a perfectly designed plan, and it might be illuminating, at a time when the Framingham study is approaching maturity, to look back at its earliest beginnings.

The Heart Disease Epidemiology Study had its beginnings in October 1947 in a co-operative project of the Massachusetts State Department of Health (Dr. Vlado Getting, health commissioner), the Department of Preventive Medicine at the Harvard Medical School (Dr. David D. Rutstein, chairman), and the Heart Disease Demonstration Section of the U.S. Public Health Service (Dr. Bert R. Boone, chief). At the initiative of Dr. Joseph W. Mountin, assistant surgeon general, Drs. Lewis C. Robbins and Gilcin Meadors were detailed to organize a heart disease study in the Boston area. Working out of quarters at the Harvard Medical School and with the advice and assistance of the various co-operating organizations they canvassed opportunities for study populations. By December 1947 it was decided to initiate two programs, one to be known as the Cardiovascular Hygiene Demonstration under the direction of Dr. Robbins, the other to be known as the Heart Disease Epidemiology Study under the direction of Dr. Meadors. The first study was to be located in Newton, the second in Framingham, Massachusetts.

The purpose of the Newton program was to determine what existing knowledge of prevention, diagnosis, treatment, and rehabilitation of cardiovascular disease could be applied within community health programs. The purpose of the Framingham program, as it was originally conceived, was the development of case-finding procedures in heart disease. The potential of the Framingham program for epidemiological studies soon became apparent, however, and the program turned increasingly in that direction.

Because of the research orientation of the program, the question of including it among the activities of the National Heart Institute was raised. After a review by Dr. C. J. Van Slyke, director of the National Heart Institute, Dr. James A. Shannon, director for research, and Felix E. Moore, chief of biometrics, the National Heart Institute arranged to accept the transfer of the Framingham Heart Disease Epidemiology Study (as it was then called) on 1 July 1949.

In the meantime, operations had already begun at Framingham in a clinic located at the Framingham Union Hospital. The clinic was formally opened on 11 October 1948, but examinations had already begun by 29 September. By the time the study was transferred to the National Heart Institute more than 1,500 volunteers had been examined. A large amount of the groundwork for the later study had already been laid. A community had been selected for study and community participation had been obtained. Quarters had been prepared and the staff recruited. The first series of examinations had been designed and put in motion. The purposes and direction of the study had slowly taken shape.

It was already understood that the general epidemiological purpose of the study was the "determination of factors influencing the development of heart disease," and that the program would require repeated examinations of the study cohort. Important assistance in this early design came from a Technical Advisory Committee which included a number of outstanding physicians in cardiology, public health, and preventive medicine.* Other distinguished physicians, such as Howard Sprague and Conger Williams, joined this group later. The Technical Advisory Committee not only supplied technical advice but was also of help in recruiting expert assistance for the study operation.

When the Framingham Study became the responsibility of the National Heart Institute, a new study protocol and a sampling scheme was introduced. This was the work jointly of Mr. Moore and Dr. Meadors. Both the sampling scheme, which was finally spelled out in December 1949, and the study protocol, which was completed a month earlier, were really structural overlays on an ongoing study.

These were the beginnings. In April 1950 Dr. Thomas R. Dawber assumed direction of the study. Under his stewardship the study began a long period of growth and productivity. The formative period was by no means over but the study was well on its way.

* Edward F. Bland, M.D. (Massachusetts General Hospital); Laurence B. Ellis, M.D. (Boston City Hospital); James M. Faulkner, M.D. (Boston University Medical School); Burton E. Hamilton, M.D. (Boston Lying-In Hospital); Hugh R. Leavell, M.D. (Harvard School of Public Health); Samuel A. Levine, M.D. (Peter Bent Brigham Hospital); Benedict F. Massell, M.D. (New England Heart Association and Good Samaritan Hospital); Loren D. Moore, M.D. (Massachusetts Department of Public Health); Samuel H. Proger, M.D. (Pratt Hospital-Tufts Medical School); David D. Rutstein, M.D. (Harvard Medical School).

THE COMMUNITY

Framingham lies 21 miles west of Boston. When the study began in 1948 it was an industrial and trading center of 28,000 persons, including both built-up business and residential areas and outlying rural areas. There was a town meeting form of government.

It was in Framingham that the first community study of tuberculosis was undertaken; a program sponsored by the National Tuberculosis Association and the Metropolitan Life Insurance Company which began in 1917 and continued successfully for six years. This latter fact, together with an indication of community interest in the study, influenced the selection of the town to some extent.

The 20 years since 1948 have been a period of rapid change. The population of Framingham has doubled and there are now 10 precincts rather than 8. Like all other towns in the area, the sense of separateness from Boston has tended to diminish as economic ties have grown and open space has disappeared. Still, Framingham retains a large variety of local enterprise and a persistent identity.

METHODS

The choice of a sampling plan for this study was dictated by a number of considerations. The number of cases which could feasibly be studied— 6,000—was much smaller than the total adult population of Framingham. Therefore, some method had to be introduced to select persons and avoid the unknown biases of self-selection. The total sample had to be allocated in such a way as to yield the maximum information over the period that the study was to be carried out, and the plan had to be such that it could be acceptable to the community and could be carried out through the community organization.

One important decision that had to be made concerned the age-range of the study population. Clearly, if a very young group was studied, only a very small number would develop arteriosclerotic or hypertensive cardiovascular disease even in 10 to 20 years' time, and since this is a mobile age group they would be difficult to re-examine regularly over an extended period. On the other hand, in a very old group there would be too large a population with pre-existing cardiovascular disease. To balance these two effects, the age group thirty through fifty-nine years was selected for study. The population in this age-range was approximately 10,000. If 6,000 of this group were taken into the study, with the age-sex distribution existing in the town, it could be predicted (on the basis of the criteria of the study and tentative data available from a small volunteer group) that roughly 5,000 would be free of cardiovascular disease at the time of initial examination. Of these 5,000 it was estimated that approximately 400 would be found to have cardiovascular disease at the time of the fifth year after the initial examination, 900 at the end of the tenth year, 1,500 at the end of the twentieth year. (These numbers include, of course, persons who would be dead of the disease at the end of the specified period.) These numbers appeared to be large enough to insure statistically reliable findings, though it was recognized that even this number of cases would not be sufficient to carry out all of the detailed analyses which would suggest themselves in the course of the study.

There remained the problem of securing an actual listing of persons who would form the sample. The town of Framingham publishes annually a listing of all residents twenty years of age and over, based on a local census, and it was possible to use this list as a basis for sampling.

The Executive Committee advised that it would be desirable not to break up families. That is, if one member of a family was to be brought into the sample, all other family members resident in the same household should also be brought in, provided they were within the eligible age limits. This was arranged, and the sample was drawn in systematic fashion from a list which was first stratified by family size and by precinct of residence (eight precincts), and then arranged in serial order by address.

The sampling ratio was two-thirds, which would yield approximately 6,600 names. This would be 10 per cent over the number required for the study. It was thought that this would be sufficient to cover losses through refusal or by movement out of the town before examination. The list of residents twenty years of age and over on 1 January 1949 served as the sampling frame for precinct three. The list for 1 January 1950 served as the frame for the remaining seven precincts. Each list came in two forms, an alphabetic roster and a roster by address. The declared age, name, address, and precinct number were given for each person. The precinct list also specified the place of residence on the previous 1 January.

As a check on the completeness of the town lists, the Bureau of the Census matched the 1 January 1950 list against a sample of persons aged thirty to fifty-nine years, who appeared on the Framingham census schedules for 1 April 1950. Some 89 per cent of those on the census schedules were found on the town list.

The first examination determined the study in two ways: (a) in defining the cohort and (b) in characterizing it.

Defining the Cohort

In principal it would have been possible to go back to the entire sample on each examination cycle and eventually to bring in some part of the initial nonrespondents for characterization. This was not done. Some few of these people did come in later, either on their own initiative or in response to a special request, but it seemed obvious that only a scattering of the initial nonrespondents could be converted to regular participants, even with great exertion.

Nonresponse was substantially larger than anticipated: only two-thirds of the sample came in for examination (Table 6–1). Some people had moved, some were too ill to come in or had died before the end of the first examination cycle; most were simply nonco-operators.

It is clear from participation rates for later examinations that the initial volunteers (as indicated by their early appearance for the initial examination) were more co-operative over the long run than those persons who were initially more difficult to persuade (as indicated by their late appearance for the initial examination, that is, by higher case numbers) (Table 6–2). A more vigorous long-term pursuit of the initial nonrespondents, while it would have added more information about the sample, would probably have been of little help in evaluating characteristics requiring clinic follow-up.

It was decided to supplement the initial sample examinees not with a supplementary probability sample but with a set of volunteers. Those nonsample volunteers in the age-range of those who had been examined early in the study and were on the 1951 town lists were asked to return. If they did not return no efforts were made to bring them in at a later examination. Clearly it would have been better to hedge against a high level of nonresponse by drawing a supplementary probability sample at the outset and holding it in reserve until the need for it became apparent. The procedure actually used is another mark of the conceptual and operational difficulties that beset a pioneer enterprise.

TABLE 6–1. RESPONSE OF DRAWN SAMPLE AND NONRESPONSE BY REASON

Response and reason	Number of persons	Per cent of	
		Drawn sample	Nonrespondents
Total	6,532	100.0	—
Examined	4,494	68.8	—
Not examined	2,038	31.2	100.0
Moved from Framingham	426	6.5	20.9
Died	74	1.1	3.6
Ill or incapacitated	74	1.1	3.6
Refused	1,464	22.4	71.8

It was at first planned to re-examine only those volunteers who were "normal" on their initial examination. This plan, however, was not rigorously followed. While 13 people were eliminated for hypertensive or coronary heart disease, these omissions modified the clinical characteristics of the group only trivially.

This is another indicator of the conceptual problems in setting up the study. While the primary focus was on the development of disease in persons initially free of disease, it is perfectly clear in retrospect that any disease can be viewed either as a precursor or an end point. Thus, while we are interested in investigating the precursors of hypertension, we are also interested in hypertension as a precursor of coronary heart disease or cerebrovascular disease or other forms of cardiovascular disease. To have omitted all hypertensives from the study cohort would have crippled the study. Fortunately, this became apparent before any efforts were made to screen out diseased persons from the sample.

Characterizing the Cohort

The plan of a prospective study calls for measuring precursors of disease; that is, it requires that a person be characterized prior to the occurrence of an event. Thus, the completeness and precision of the characterization at initial examination is vital.

In point of fact, many key measurements were not made at the beginning of the Framingham study or they were made with inadequate precision. It was not until a year after opening the clinic that the laboratory was in full operation. While some procedures were under good control from the outset, others were not. In particular, serum cholesterol measurement, which has become one of the key measurements in the study, was not really in adequate control until late in the

TABLE 6–2. LOSS TO CLINIC FOLLOW-UP AS OF EXAM 8 ACCORDING TO REASON FOR LOSS AND EXAMINATION ORDER

Sample and order	Total		Dead		Moved		Refused	
	No.	Rate[a]	No.	Rate[a]	No.	Rate[a]	No.	Rate[a]
Total sample and								
nonsample volunteers	1095	210	531	102	237	45	327	63
Total sample	998	223	461	103	226	51	311	70
First 1,000		140		85		37		18
Second 1,000		195		99		53		43
Third 1,000		227		98		62		67
Fourth 1,000		264		104		52		108
Last 469	172	367	75	160	22	47	75	160
Nonsample volunteers	97	131	70	95	11	15	16	22

[a] Per 1,000.

first cycle of examinations. In the usual presentation of the Framingham results the majority of the serum cholesterol determinations are taken from the second examination cycle.

This is not the only deficiency in the initial examination. A history of cigarette smoking was not taken at first. After questions on this subject were introduced, they were modified as the staff gained experience. Thus, the quality of this information is uneven. In a few cases the initial information was not obtained until after the development of cardiovascular disease. While serum cholesterol has been found to change little after the development of cardiovascular disease, the same could hardly be assumed for cigarette smoking habits.

One other key measurement was different at the first examination (Exam I) than on later examinations, viz., blood pressure. Here the problems are somewhat different from those in the initial laboratory work and history items. Every examined person had his blood pressure taken in a well-standardized fashion. However, the initial examination seemed to have a pressor effect on a large number of individuals and it was found that the average blood pressure for the study group dropped in subsequent examinations. This phenomenon is now well-recognized; it was not when the study began.

While it is always preferable to begin a study with highly precise and elegant measurements, it is not always possible. Even studies that begin after a long period of planning are often beset by procedural difficulties. The more attentive the investigators, the more explicit these difficulties are likely to become. The planning period for the Framingham study extended well through the initial cycle of examinations. The examination itself grew as new ideas and resources became available. In addition, many of the instruments were poorly standardized at that time. Serum cholesterol measurement, for example, was not a standardized laboratory procedure in 1949. Studies of cigarette smoking were not the epidemiological staple they are today.

The chief hazard of imprecise measurements (but not the only one) lies in the possibility that real relationships will appear weaker than they should. As more reliable measurements become available and additional follow-up accumulates, it is important to re-examine the data. In Framingham this has been done a number of times. Later serum cholesterol measurements, for example, have been found to exhibit substantially the same relationship to coronary heart disease as the earlier, less precise, measurements; and the same is true of later more systematic histories of cigarette smoking. The ability to re-examine findings on the basis of new measurements is one of the attractive features of longitudinal studies. Indeed, it might be reasonable to consider measurement problems as one of the justifications for longitudinal studies. Such studies allow for the introduction of new instruments as they become available and for a gradual, systematic increase in precision as this becomes possible.

What has in fact happened in the Framingham study is that with the passage of time new hypotheses have been tested as an interest in these arose or as usable techniques became available. It was not until Exam 4, for instance, that a diet history was introduced. Physical activity histories were first taken at Exam 4. Protein-bound iodine was measured in Exams 4 and 5. A formal psychological questionnaire was not developed until Exam 8 and was administered during Exams 8 and 9.

Re-examination

The study design required that persons in the cohort be called back for re-examination at two-year intervals. Originally, the possibility of annual examinations had been considered but, fortunately, never attempted: the initiation of biennial examinations proved difficult enough. The first examination series began on 29 September 1948. The second series got under way with scattered examinations early in 1951, but did not begin in earnest until May of that year, more than two and one-half years after the first series had begun.

Repeated Examination

While there are other sources of information in this study, the chief one is the clinic examination. It is only on this basis that repeated observations of personal characteristics can be made; a standard examination is also the only means for obtaining uniform information on clinical status. Thus, adequacy of follow-up must be judged primarily by the rate at which the cohort returns for examination.

Of the original cohort of 5,209 persons, 4,678 were still alive at the time they were scheduled for Exam 8 (Table 6–3). Of these, 4,030 or 86.1 per cent took Exam 8. (The comparable figure for Exam 7 was 87.2 per cent; the net loss on successive examinations is now very low).

Another 42 persons who had missed Exam 8 returned for a later examination by the end of 1966 (Table 6–4). By the end of March 1968 this number had risen to 91 persons.

A large number of people took every possible examination (Table 6–5). Some 3,597 persons took all of the first 7 examinations; 3,436 took all of the first 8. This is 74.9 per cent, respectively, of the surviving cohort. These figures, high as they are, actually represent an understatement of the measure of co-operation. Because of a delay in calling back the SX group (nonsample volunteers) for their second examination, 237 volunteers were rescheduled so late for Exam 2 that it was felt impolitic to ask them to come in shortly thereafter for a regularly scheduled third examination. When allowance is made for this group, there are 79 and 78 per cent with a complete examination series through Exams 7 and 8, respectively.

TABLE 6–3. NUMBER SURVIVING IN COHORT AND NUMBER RECEIVING EXAMINATION AT EACH OF THE FIRST EIGHT EXAMINATIONS

		Number examined		
Exam	Number surviving	Total	Sample	Volunteers
1	5,209	5,209	4,469	740
2	5,177	4,792	4,052	740
3	5,125	4,416[a]	3,935	481[a]
4	5,073	4,541	3,843	698
5	4,990	4,421	3,750	671
6	4,895	4,259	3,593	666
7	4,803	4,191	3,551	640
8	4,678	4,030	3,402	628

[a] The indicated drop is an artifact arising from the arbitrary decision that volunteers would not be followed if they did not take Exam 2. Some 237, however, were recalled so late for Exam 2 that they were not called in for Exam 3.

TABLE 6–4. NUMBER OF PERSONS ACCORDING TO EXAMINATION STATUS AT EXAM 7 AND AT EXAM 8

	Both	Sample	Volunteers
Total receiving Exam 1	5,209	4,469	740
Examined, Exam 7	4,191	3,551	640
Not examined, Exam 7	1,018	918	100
Alive, Exam 7	612	569	43
Took later exam[a]	132	107	25
Did not take later exam[a]	480	462	18
Reside in Framingham	276	265	11
Reside outside Framingham	204	197	7
Dead: Exam 7	406	349	57
Took last possible exam before death	317	274	43
Missed last possible exam before death	89	75	14
Examined, Exam 8	4,030	3,402	628
Not examined, Exam 8	1,179	1,067	112
Alive, Exam 8	648	606	42
Took later exam[a]	42	30	12
Did not take later exam[a]	606	576	30
Reside in Framingham	355	337	18
Reside outside Framingham	251	239	12
Dead, Exam 8	531	461	70
Took last possible exam before death	410	354	56
Missed last possible exam before death	121	107	14

[a] Covers experience through 1966.

TABLE 6–5. NUMBER OF PERSONS ACCORDING TO EXAMINATION STATUS AT EXAM 7 AND AT EXAM 8 AND THE NUMBER OF BIENNIAL EXAMINATIONS RECEIVED

EXAM 7

Number of exams received	Received Exam 7 Both	S[a]	SX[b]	Did not take Exam 7 Alive or dead Both	S	SX	Alive at Exam 7 Both	S	SX
1	—	—	—	198	198	—	140	140	—
2	16	16	—	172	155	17	104	99	5
3	27	27	—	167	145	22	99	98	11
4	52	48	4	162	142	20	90	82	8
5	93	87	6	177	148	29	92	76	16
6	406	189	217	142	130	12	87	84	3
7	3,597	3,184	413	—	—	—	—	—	—
Total	4,191	3,551	640	1,018	918	100	612	569	43

EXAM 8

Number of exams received	Received Exam 8 Both	S	SX	Did not take Exam 8 Alive or dead Both	S	SX	Alive at Exam 8 Both	S	SX
1	—	—	—	184	184	—	121	121	—
2	14	14	—	175	158	17	101	96	5
3	13	13	—	169	150	19	98	90	8
4	25	22	3	161	142	19	82	77	5
5	53	48	5	178	157	21	88	80	8
6	92	78	14	151	129	22	74	65	9
7	397	190	207	161	147	14	84	77	7
8	3,436	3,037	399	—	—	—	—	—	—
Total	4,030	3,402	628	1,179	1,067	112	648	606	42

[a] S = Sample.
SX = Nonsample volunteers.

As anticipated, there has been a difference between the sample and SX groups in the rates of re-examination. Of the former, 84.9 per cent of the survivors received Exam 8; of the latter, 93.7 per cent. The SX group were volunteers in the first place, and thus more likely to co-operate; in defining the SX group only those volunteers who returned for a second examination when requested were retained. By contrast, the greatest loss in the sample was suffered at Exam 2. Some 385 persons still alive at that time did not take this examination; 184 of them never returned for a later examination.

By Exam 8, 531 persons in the original cohort had died. As might be anticipated, the number of deaths has mounted with each successive examination. Nearly 2 per cent of those alive at Exam 6 died before they were scheduled for Exam 7. In the next two years mortality loss was 2.6 per cent. Losses between succeeding examinations can be expected to increase rapidly.

Deaths constitute both a loss and a gain to follow-up. When reckoning the number who will be available for future observations, they constitute a loss. On the other hand, death is one of the end points of the study. Moreover, knowing a person to be dead provides a firm assurance that the person is not and will not be lost to follow-up. With the living it is sometimes difficult (particularly for those missing some examinations) to be certain whether one of the clinical end points has been reached.

The 648 persons not taking Exam 8, even though they were alive at the time it was due, took a varying number of earlier examinations. Some 84 persons took the preceding 7 examinations but missed the eighth; 121 persons took Exam 1 and never returned. A number varying between 74 and 101 persons missed 2, 3, 4, or 5 examinations.

It is surprising to find that where the person remains alive the likelihood of re-examination is about the same in one age-sex group as another (Table 6–6). It is also a little surprising to note that essentially permanent loss to follow-up for reasons other than death has been relatively constant from one examination to another (Table 6–7). The clear exception to this is a greater than average loss just after the first examination. The other apparent exception, for those receiving Exam 7 but not Exam 8, includes some persons who are not permanently lost to follow-up but will return when additional time has elapsed, or have already returned.

TABLE 6–6. NUMBER AND PER CENT OF PERSONS RECEIVING EXAM 7 AND EXAM 8 BY SEX AND AGE AT EXAM 1

| | | | Per cent of specified age-sex group | | | |
| | | | Of all persons at entry | | Of survivors at exam | |
Age at Exam 1	Number receiving Exam 7	Number receiving Exam 8	Exam 7	Exam 8	Exam 7	Exam 8
Men	1,811	1,741	77.5	74.5	87.0	86.5
29–34	332	322	84.9	82.4	87.1	85.0
35–39	380	376	86.2	85.3	89.4	89.3
40–44	343	333	81.5	79.1	87.5	87.9
45–49	274	261	76.5	72.9	87.0	85.9
50–54	261	247	70.0	66.2	85.0	86.4
55–62	221	202	62.8	57.4	84.4	83.1
Women	2,380	2,289	82.8	79.7	87.5	85.9
29–34	397	396	87.4	87.2	89.6	89.4
35–39	493	479	84.4	82.0	86.6	85.8
40–44	438	413	85.5	80.7	88.7	85.2
45–49	379	363	84.2	80.7	89.2	86.4
50–54	338	333	78.8	77.6	86.0	87.2
55–62	335	305	75.5	68.7	84.4	80.7

TABLE 6–7. NUMBER OF PERSONS NOT RECEIVING EXAM 8 ACCORDING TO LAST BIENNIAL EXAMINATION RECEIVED

Last biennial exam	Persons receiving exam 1			Alive at exam 8			Dead at exam 8		
	Total	Sample	Volunteers[a]	Total	Sample	Volunteers[a]	Total	Sample	Volunteers[a]
Total not taking Exam 8	1,179	1,067	112	648	606	42	531	461	70
Exam 1	184	184	—	121	121	—	63	63	—
Exam 2	132	115	17	64	59	5	68	56	12
Exam 3	130	119	11	71	69	2	59	50	9
Exam 4	134	114	20	62	54	8	72	60	12
Exam 5	169	157	12	74	72	2	95	85	10
Exam 6	156	136	20	75	69	6	81	67	14
Exam 7	274	242	32	181	162	19	93	80	13

[a] Volunteers had to return for their second biennial examination in order to be included in the cohort. These examinations are all considered Exam 2, although in some instances the examination was more than three years after Exam 1.

Loss Due to Moving, Disability and Refusal

There were 606 persons in the cohort who, though still alive when scheduled for their eighth examination, did not appear for examination then or (up to the end of 1966) later. Perhaps 10 per cent of this group can be expected to return at some future time; the remainder will probably not return.

Of these 606 persons, 355 still lived in Framingham. This includes some people who could not come in for examination and some who would not. What the proportion was of each it is impossible to say. It is clear, however, that there were some persons with serious disability in this group. One evidence of this is the fact that nearly 23 per cent of those who have died missed their last scheduled examination while alive.

The fact that a person fails to appear for re-examination does not mean that he is completely lost to follow-up. Considerable effort is made to keep track of his clinical status by various forms of community surveillance. Still, nothing short of re-examination provides the same assurance. Uncertainty about the clinical status of those persons who have moved from the area may remain fairly high.

On the other hand there is no direct evidence that loss to examination has led to any substantial loss of information about the appearance of new coronary heart disease (CHD). In fact, Tables 6–8 and 6–9 indicate that the incidence reported after loss to examination is only slightly less than might be expected had these people continued to take repeated examinations. These tables compare CHD experience among

TABLE 6–8. NUMBER OF PERSONS LOST TO EXAMINATION AFTER MOVING FROM FRAMINGHAM WHO DEVELOPED NEW CHD WITHIN THE 14-YEAR FOLLOW-UP

Exam at which loss first recorded	Total	1–2	2–3	3–4	4–5	5–6	6–7	7–8	Number with pre-existing CHD	Total number lost
2	4	—	1	1	1	—	—	1	1	47
3	1	—	—	—	—	—	1	—	—	36
4	1	—	—	—	—	1	—	—	—	32
5	3	—	—	—	—	1	2	—	—	33
6	4	—	1	2	1	—	—	—	1	40
7	1	—	—	—	1	—	—	—	—	34
8	3	1	—	—	—	—	2	—	1	19

Losses between exams 2 and 8	Number of CHD events	
	Before loss	After loss
Actual	8	9
Expected[a]	10.5	14.9

Losses between exams 3 and 7		
Actual	5	5
Expected[a]	6.9	10.7

[a] Expected numbers obtained by applying age-sex-exam specific rates for total cohort to the population lost at each examination.

TABLE 6–9. NUMBER OF PERSONS LOST TO EXAMINATION WHILE STILL RESIDENT IN FRAMINGHAM WHO DEVELOPED NEW CHD WITHIN THE 14-YEAR FOLLOW-UP

Exam at which loss first recorded	Total	1–2	2–3	3–4	4–5	5–6	6–7	7–8	Number with pre-existing CHD	Total number lost
2	10	—	2	1	1	—	3	3	2	104
3	5	2	—	1	1	—	—	1	1	51
4	4	—	2	1	—	—	—	1	—	56
5	3	—	—	1	—	2	—	—	1	38
6	4	—	—	1	—	—	2	1	1	52
7	5	1	—	—	—	2	1	1	—	46
8	8	1	1	2	2	—	2	—	2	39

Losses between exams 2 and 8	Number of CHD events	
	Before loss	After loss
Actual	17	22
Expected[a]	20.5	29.8

Losses between exams 3 and 7		
Actual	9	12
Expected[a]	11.4	16.6

[a] Expected numbers obtained by applying age-sex-exam specific rates for total cohort to the population lost at each examination.

those persons whose examination series lapsed, with the CHD experience for the total population. Table 6–8 gives counts for people who moved from Framingham and, presumably for that reason, did not return for examination. Table 6–9 gives counts for people who stopped coming in for examination while still resident in Framingham and who never returned.

There was a slight deficit in CHD incidence in both these groups, even while they were taking examinations. In part, this was accounted for by the fact that a person who is already dead cannot "move" or "refuse," so that cases of CHD first manifest at death are not included in counts before loss.

On a priori grounds one would assume that persons who moved out of Framingham were likely to be healthier than average at the time that they moved, and that persons who stopped coming while still resident in Framingham would include some persons who were seriously, even terminally, ill. However, both those who moved and those who did not had fewer cases of CHD reported after they stopped taking examinations than would be expected on the basis of the total cohort's experience.

Taking the reckonings in Tables 6–8 and 6–9 at face value, loss to examination has resulted in a 3 per cent deficit in the reports of CHD incidence in the 14 years since the study began. Since a clinic examination was required for the diagnosis of angina pectoris, this fact would be sufficient to explain the entire deficit in CHD incidence after loss to examination. It is obvious that failure to return for examination has not as yet introduced any serious bias in the counts of new CHD.

FINDINGS

We will not attempt to summarize the findings that have emerged to date; instead, we will present some highlights. Detailed references to the Framingham studies are given in the bibliography.

Age

It is well established that cardiovascular mortality rises over the age-range (twenty-nine to seventy-six years) traversed by the Framingham cohort during the first 14 years of the study. Thus it is not surprising to find that the incidence of these diseases, in general, rises over the full age span. In particular, the incidence of cerebrovascular disease and intermittent claudication increases without apparent break, as does the blood pressure of the surviving cohorts. For systolic pressure this is not surprising; almost all cross-sectional data have shown this. It is noteworthy, however, that diastolic pressure also rises to age seventy-four years—since cross-sectional data (including cross-sectional data from Framingham) have generally shown a leveling out at about fifty-five years. The difference represents the selective effect of mortality on cross-sectional data, persons with higher blood pressures being less likely to survive to older ages. When blood pressure changes are viewed longitudinally, of course, changes can be measured only in persons who are remeasured—that is, only in survivors.

The one notable exception to the tendency of cardiovascular disease incidence to rise with age is coronary heart disease in men. CHD incidence in males rises to age fifty-five years and then rises no further. This phenomenon is evident for each specific form of CHD except CHD death. The possibility that this represents some study artifact cannot be ruled out, but so far none has been uncovered. It would be highly desirable, of course, to have this finding duplicated in another cohort study.

Sex

While sex is associated with strong cardiovascular disease differentials, cardiovascular disease incidence does not have a uniform sex ratio. Coronary heart disease is predominantly a male disease, although this preponderance diminishes with age. Men and women are equally likely to develop cerebrovascular disease, while intermittent claudication has an intermediate sex ratio. Thus, while sex is clearly a factor in cardiovascular disease incidence, it does not have the relatively clear and simple effect that age does.

Blood Pressure

Blood pressure has a dual role in the Framingham study. Hypertension (that is, elevated blood pressure) is one of the major end points of the study. It is also one of the major factors involved in the development of other cardiovascular diseases.

The incidence of hypertension secondary to other conditions is very low. The study of hypertension in this general population sample has proved to be almost exclusively a study of essential nonmalignant hypertension. Most hypertension that has appeared in the Framingham cohort has developed insidiously among persons whose initial blood pressures were just below the hypertensive range. Very few persons had an abrupt onset of this condition. Our analysis to date has uncovered nothing really effective in predicting the development of hypertension other than an initially above average blood pressure.

As a risk factor in the development of cardiovascular disease, however, blood pressure has more than lived up to expectations. The Framingham data indicate blood pressure elevation to be the most ubiquitous of the factors leading to major cardiovascular disease. What is more, the data indicate that the probability of a cardiovascular illness developing increases in proportion to the blood pressure level over the full range, from the very lowest pressures to the very highest, and without any obvious jump in risk at any level. When cardiac pathology finally intervenes, however, the graduation of responses is less clear.

Serum Cholesterol

The Framingham study indicates that serum cholesterol elevation is associated with an increased risk of coronary heart disease at younger ages but that this association decreases with age. For men, the association persists at least to age fifty-eight years, though in an attenuated form. Brain infarction appears to exhibit a similar association with serum cholesterol level, but since this is a disease with low incidence under age sixty years, the exact form of the relationship is less well defined than it is for coronary heart disease. Intermittent claudication, a disease with even lower incidence in young persons, has not been shown to be related to serum cholesterol level on the basis of the Framingham data.

Multiple Factors

In the analyses of the Framingham data, the possibility has first been considered that where several factors are related to the development of a disease these factors have a simple additive effect. Sometimes this seems to fit the data very well. For example, in men forty-five to sixty-two years of age the effects of blood pressure and serum cholesterol on the incidence of coronary heart disease appear to be additive in a simple linear sense. In other cases this model is clearly not appropriate. We have already indicated that in men, age and cholesterol are interacting factors in the development of coronary heart disease. So also is blood pressure and definite left ventricular hypertrophy by electrocardiograph, for in men with this ECG finding, blood pressure elevation does not appear to increase the incidence of CHD.

POTENTIALS

One of the aspects of the Framingham study that requires a much more systematic evaluation than it has yet received is the natural history of the cardiovascular diseases. It is clear, for example, that the presence of one cardiovascular disease generally leads to a heightened incidence of other cardiovascular diseases. This general impression requires, however, a more systematic exploration. It must be recognized, of course, that the Framingham study will never allow a clear delineation of any but the major sequences of cardiovascular diseases.

One likely contribution of the Framingham study may be a clearer segregation of the differing manifestations of coronary heart disease. One of the early puzzles of the Framingham study was the weakness of the evidence associating cigarette smoking with the incidence of CHD, in face of the strong evidence from death studies. When coronary heart disease manifest only by angina pectoris was excluded, a clear relationship to cigarette smoking was found. There is reason to believe that other similar differentials are likely to become evident as the data are subjected to closer scrutiny.

Still the dominant feature of the data is not the distinctions but the kinship of the major cardiovascular diseases. For example, a linear combination of measurements designed to be effective in discriminating cases of coronary heart disease is also effective in discriminating cases of intermittent claudication or cerebrovascular disease. This is not unexpected: the major etiological processes for these various diseases have long been presumed to be similar.

The success of such epidemiological studies in uncovering indicators and risk factors of cardiovascular disease has long been apparent. Still, there is more unexplained than explained and a good deal more work to be done.

Bibliography of Framingham Study Publications

Cornfield, J. 1962. Joint dependence of risk of coronary heart disease on serum cholesterol and systolic blood pressure: A discriminant function analysis. *Fed. Proc.* 21:58–61.

Cornfield, J., Gordon, T., and Smith, W. W. 1961. Quantal response curves for experimentally uncontrolled variables. *Bull. Int. Statist. Inst.* 38:97–115.

Dawber, T. R. 1960. Summary of recent literature regarding cigarette smoking and coronary heart disease. *Circulation* 22:164–66.

———. 1963. Coronary heart disease: Morbidity in the Framingham study and analysis of factors of risk. *Bibl. Cardiol.* 13:9–24.

———. 1965. Heart attack—what's the risk? *Today's Health* 46:62–64.

Dawber, T. R. and Kannel, W. B. 1958. An epidemiologic study of heart disease: the Framingham study. *Nutr. Rev.* 16:1–4.

———. 1961. Susceptibility to coronary heart disease. *Mod. Conc. Cardiovasc. Dis.* 30:671–76.

———. 1962a. Application of epidemiology of coronary heart disease to medical practice. *Mod. Med.* (3 Sept.): 85–101.

————. 1962*b*. Atherosclerosis and you: Pathogenetic implications from epidemiologic observations. *J. Am. Geriat. Soc.* 10:805–21.

————. 1962*c*. Computers in epidemiologic research. Uses in the Framingham study. *Circulation Res.* 11:587–89.

————. 1963. Coronary heart disease as an epidemiologic entity. *Am. J. Public Health* 53:433–37.

————. 1966. The Framingham study. An epidemiological approach to coronary heart disease. *Circulation* 34:553–55.

Dawber, T. R., Kannel, W. B., and Friedman, G. D. 1963. The use of computers in cardiovascular epidemiology. *Prog. Cardiovasc. Dis.* 5:406–17.

————. 1966. Vital capacity, physical activity and coronary heart disease. In *Prevention of Ischemic Heart Disease: Principles and Practice.* Edited by Rabb, W., pp. 254–65. Springfield: C. C Thomas.

Dawber, T. R., Kannel, W. B., Kagan, A., Donabedian, R. K., McNamara, P. M., and Pearson, G. 1967. Environmental factors in hypertension. In *The Epidemiology of Hypertension.* Edited by Stamler, J., Stamler, R., and Pullman, T. N., pp. 255–88. New York: Grune & Stratton.

Dawber, T. R., Kannell, W. B., Love, D. E., and Streeper, R. B. 1952. The electrocardiogram in heart disease detection. A comparison of the multiple and single lead procedures. *Circulation* 5:550–66.

Dawber, T. R., Kannel, W. B., and Lyell, L. 1963. An approach to longitudinal studies in a community: the Framingham study. *Ann. N.Y. Acad. Sci.* 107:539–56.

Dawber, T. R., Kannel, W. B., and McNamara, P. M. 1963. The prediction of coronary heart disease. Read at 72d Annual Meeting of Association of Life Insurance Medical Directors of America, October 1963.

Dawber, T. R., Kannel, W. B., Pearson, G., and Shurtleff, D. 1961. Assessment of diet in the Framingham study: Methodology and preliminary observations. *Health News* 38:4–6.

Dawber, T. R., Kannel, W. B., Revotskie, N., and Kagan, A. 1962. The epidemiology of coronary heart disease—the Framingham enquiry. *Proc. Roy. Soc. Med.* 55:265–77.

Dawber, T. R., Kannel, W. B., Revotskie, N., Stokes, J., III, Kagan, A., and Gordon T. 1959. Some factors associated with the development of coronary heart disease: Six years' follow-up experience in the Framingham study. *Am. J. Public Health* 49:1349–56.

Dawber, T. R. and McNamara, P. M. 1967. Coronary heart disease: Identification of susceptible individuals. In *Atherosclerotic Vascular Disease. A. Hahnemann Symposium.* Edited by Brest, A. N. and Moyer, J. H., pp. 130–46. New York: Appleton-Century-Crofts.

Dawber, T. R., Meadors, G. F., and Moore, F. E., Jr. 1951. Epidemiological approaches to heart disease: The Framingham Study. *Am. J. Public Health* 41:279–86.

Dawber, T. R. and Moore, F. E. 1952. Longitudinal study of heart disease in Framingham, Massachusetts: An interim report. In *Research in Public Health,* pp. 241–47. Papers presented at the 1951 Annual Conference of the Milbank Memorial Fund. New York: Milbank Memorial Fund.

Dawber, T. R., Moore, F. E., and Mann, G. V. 1957. Coronary heart disease in the Framingham study. *Am. J. Public Health* 47:4–24.

Dawber, T. R., Pearson, G., Anderson, P., Mann, G. V., Kannel, W. B., Shurtleff, D., and McNamara, P. 1962. Dietary assessment in the epidemiologic study of coronary heart disease: The Framingham study. *Am. J. Clin. Nutr.* 11:226–34.

Doyle, J. T., Dawber, T. R., Kannel, W. B., Heslin, A. S., and Kahn, H. A. 1962. Cigarette smoking and coronary heart disease: Combined experience of the Albany and Framingham Studies. *New Eng. J. Med.* 266:796–801.

Doyle, J. T., Dawber, T. R., Kannel, W. B., Kinch, S. H., and Kahn, H. A. 1964. The relationship of cigarette smoking to coronary heart disease. *J.A.M.A.* 190:886–90.

Friedman, G. D., Kannel, W. B., and Dawber, T. R. 1966. The epidemiology of gallbladder disease: Observations in the Framingham study. *J. Chronic Dis.* 19:273–92.

Friedman, G. D., Kannel, W. B., Dawber, T. R., and McNamara, P. M. 1966. Comparison of prevalence, case history and incidence data in assessing the potency of risk factors in coronary heart disease. *Am. J. Epidem.* 83:366–78.

————. 1967. An evaluation of follow-up methods in the Framingham Heart Study. *Am. J. Public Health* 57:1015–24.

Gordon, T., Moore, F. E., Shurtleff, D., and Dawber, T. R. 1959. Some methodologic problems in the long-term study of cardiovascular disease: Observations on the Framingham study. *J. Chronic Dis.* 10:186–206.

Hall, A. P. 1965. Correlations among hyperuricemia, hypercholesterolemia, coronary disease and hypertension. *Arthritis Rheum.* 8:846–52.

Hall, A. P., Barry, P. E., Dawber, T. R., and McNamara, P. M. 1967. Epidemiology of gout and hyperuricemia: A long-term population study. *Am. J. Med.* 42:27–37.

Higgins, I. T. T., Kannel, W. B., and Dawber, T. R. 1965. The electrocardiogram in epidemiological studies; reproducibility, validity, and international comparison. *Brit. J. Prev. Soc. Med.* 1953–68.

Kagan, A., Dawber, T. R., Kannel, W. B., and Revotskie, N. 1962. The Framingham study: A prospective study of coronary heart disease. *Fed. Proc.* 21:52–57.

Kagan, A., Gordon, T., Kannel, W. B., and Dawber, T. R. 1959. Blood pressure and its relation to coronary heart disease in the Framingham study. In *Hypertension: Drug Action, Epidemiology and Hemodynamics. Proceedings of the Council for High Blood Pressure Research.* Vol. 7, pp. 53–81. New York: American Heart Association.

Kagan, A., Kannel, W. B., Dawber, T. R., and Revotskie, N. 1963. The coronary profile. *Ann. N.Y. Acad. Sci.* 97:883–94.

Kahn, H. A. 1961. A method for analyzing longitudinal observations on individuals in the Framingham heart study. *American Statistical Association. Proceedings of the Social Statistics Section*, 1961, pp. 156–60. Washington: American Statistical Association.

———. 1962. Use of computers in analyzing Framingham data. *Circulation Res.* 11:585–86.

Kahn, H. A. and Dawber, T. R. 1966. The development of coronary heart disease in relation to sequential biennial measures of cholesterol in the Framingham study. *J. Chronic Dis.* 19:611–20.

Kannel, W. B. 1964. Cigarette smoking and coronary heart disease. *Ann. Intern. Med.* 60:1103–06.

———. 1966a. An epidemiologic study of cerebrovascular disease. In *Cerebral Vascular Diseases. Transactions of the Fifth Conference Held Under the Auspices of The American Neurological Association and The American Heart Association.* Edited by Millikan, C. H., Siekert, R. G., and Whisnant, J. P., pp. 53–66. New York: Grune & Stratton.

———. 1966b. *Habits and Coronary Heart Disease: The Framingham Study.* U.S. Dept. of Health, Education, and Welfare. P. H. S. Pub. No. 1515. Washington: U.S. Government Printing Office.

———. 1967. Habitual level of physical activity and risk of coronary heart disease: The Framingham Study. *Canad. Med. Ass. J.* 96:811–12.

Kannel, W. B., Barry, P., and Dawber, T. R. 1963. Immediate mortality in coronary heart disease: The Framingham study. *Proceedings of 4th World Congress of Cardiology.*

Kannel, W. B., Brand, N., Skinner, J. J., Jr., Dawber, T. R., and McNamara, P. M. 1967. The relation of adiposity to blood pressure and development of hypertension: The Framingham Study. *Ann. Intern. Med.* 67:48–59.

Kannel, W. B., Castelli, W. P., and McNamara, P. M. 1967. The coronary profile: 12-year follow-up in the Framingham Study. *J. Occup. Med.* 9:611–19.

Kannel, W. B., Castelli, W. P., and Cohen, M. E. 1958. The electrocardiogram in neurocirculatory asthenia (anxiety, neurosis or neurasthenia): A study of 203 neurocirculatory asthenia patients and 757 health controls in the Framingham study. *Ann. Intern. Med.* 49:1351–60.

Kannel, W. B., Castelli, W. P., Cohen, M. E., and McNamara, P. M. 1965. Vascular disease of the brain—epidemiologic aspects: The Framingham study. *Am. J. Public Health* 55:1355–66.

Kannel, W. B., Castelli, W. P., Friedman, G. D., Glennon, W. E., and McNamara, P. M. 1964. Risk factors in coronary heart disease: An evaluation of several serum lipids as predictors of coronary heart disease. *Ann. Intern. Med.* 61:888–99.

Kannel, W. B., Castelli, W. P., Glennon, W. E., and Thorne, M. C. 1962. Preliminary report: The determinants and clinical significance of serum cholesterol. *Mass. J. Med. Tech.* 4:11–29.

Kannel, W. B., Castelli, W. P., Kagan, A., Revotskie, N., and Stokes, J., III. 1961. Factors of risk in the development of coronary heart disease

—six year follow-up experience: The Framingham study. *Ann. Intern. Med.* 55:33–50.

Kannel, W. B., Castelli, W. P., and McNamara, P. M. 1966. Detection of the coronary-prone adult: The Framingham study. *J. Iowa Med. Soc.* 56:26–34.

Kannel, W. B., Castelli, W. P., Thomas, H. E., Jr., and McNamara, P. M. 1965. Comparison of serum lipids in the prediction of coronary heart disease. *Rhode Island Med. J.* 48:243–50.

Kannel, W. B., Kagan, A., Dawber, T. R., and Revotskie, N. 1962. Epidemiology of coronary heart disease: Implications for the practicing physician. *Geriatrics* 17:675–90.

Kannel, W. B., LeBauer, E. J., Dawber, T. R., and McNamara, P. M. 1967. Relation of body weight to development of coronary heart disease: The Framingham Study. *Circulation* 35:734–44.

Kannel, W. B., Widmer, L. K., and Dawber, T. R. 1965. Gefahrdung durch coronare herzkrankheit; folgerungen für die praxis aus 10 jahren Framingham-studie. [Susceptibility to coronary heart disease; preventive implications of 10 years of observation in the Framingham study.] *Schweiz. Med. Wschr.* 95:18–24.

Mann, G. V., Pearson, G., Gordon, T., Dawber, T. R., Lyell, L., and Shurtleff, D. 1962. Diet and cardiovascular disease in the Framingham study. *Am. J. Clin. Nutr.* 11:200–25.

Revotskie, N., Kannel, W., Goldsmith, J. R., and Dawber, T. R. 1962. Pulmonary function in a community sample. *Am. Rev. Resp. Dis.* 86:907–11.

Stokes, J., III, and Dawber, T. R. 1956. Rheumatic heart disease in the Framingham study. *New Eng. J. Med.* 255:1228–33.

————. 1959. The "silent coronary": The frequency and clinical characteristics of unrecognized myocardial infarction in the Framingham study. *Ann. Intern. Med.* 50:1359–69.

Thomas, H. E., Jr., Kannel, W. B., Dawber, T. R., and McNamara, P. M. 1966. Cholesterol-phospholipid ratio in the prediction of coronary heart disease. The Framingham study. *New Eng. J. Med.* 274:701–05.

Thomas, H. E., Jr., Kannel, W. B., and McNamara, P. M. 1967. Obesity: A hazard to health. *Med. Times* 95:1099–1106.

Truett, J., Cornfield, J., and Kannel, W. 1967. A multivariate analysis of the risk of coronary heart disease in Framingham. *J. Chronic Dis.* 20:511–24.

U.S. Department of Health, Education, and Welfare. 1967. *Epidemiology of Stroke.* Edited by Kannel, W. B., Troy, B. L., and McNamara, P.M. P.H.S. Pub. No. 1607. Washington: U.S. Government Printing Office.

Vander, J. B., Gaston, E. A., and Dawber, T. R. 1954. Significance of solitary nontoxic thyroid nodules: Preliminary report. *New Eng. J. Med.* 251:970–72.

Walker, S. H. and Duncan, D. B. 1967. Estimation of the probability of an event as a function of several independent variables. *Biometrika* 54:167–79.

EDITORIAL COMMENTS

1. Unlike the three cardiovascular disease studies of the Southeast, the Framingham study was not undertaken because of an unusual frequency of heart disease. Historical and practical considerations were paramount here. These included an earlier study of tuberculosis, community acceptance, and the availability of an annually compiled town list of adult residents. It is of interest, however, that only 89 per cent of the Framingham residents age thirty to fifty-nine who appeared in the 1950 federal census were also found in the town list of the same year. The degree to which this can be explained by mortality and emigration is not discussed.

2. Although it was at first intended to follow only presumably normal persons, the study was soon modified to include propositi with hypertension and other diseases. This illustrates two advantageous features of community studies: their amenability to modification and their utility in the simultaneous study of multiple-risk factors and multiple outcomes—in the words of the author, "any 'disease' can be viewed either as a precursor or an end point." The latter feature may be unique to the longitudinal community survey. It is even absent from the usual type of prospective investigation in which a specific hypothesis is tested by following cohorts of subjects with and without a given characteristic of interest.* The modifiability of prospective community studies is also demonstrated by the subsequent addition of smoking, dietary, and physical activity histories, as well as serum cholesterol and protein-bound iodine measurements to the Framingham study protocol.

3. The sample size was apparently arrived at by considering the total population, the estimated incidences of the major cardiovascular diseases, and the practical limitations to the number of persons who could be examined. Apparently because of the very sizable initial nonresponse rate (31.2 per cent), the sample was augmented with volunteers. The authors, who did not participate in the original study design, state that "it would have been better to hedge against a high level of nonresponse by drawing a supplementary probability sample at the onset and holding it in reserve." Despite its obvious limitations, the use of volunteer subjects is not a rare phenomenon. An example is the large prospective study of smoking and health sponsored by a national voluntary health organization (Hammond 1964).

---

* Of course, this feature might be approximated by prospectively following several cohorts of subjects with a variety of characteristics whose etiological relationship to a given disease is to be tested.

4. The sample size represented 60 per cent of the total number of eligible adults in Framingham. In retrospect, one might ask whether a follow-up of the total group would not have been advantageous. More detailed analyses would have become possible with the larger numbers and the volunteers could have been included without possible bias. However, the sample size was limited by the resources available to the investigators.

5. One advantage of longitudinal studies exemplified in Framingham is that a patient might miss one examination cycle but return for a subsequent one. This reduces the problem of nonresponse, although it does complicate the statistical analysis.

6. The Framingham study has been in progress for over twenty years. Much useful information has been acquired on the correlates of coronary heart disease, despite the inadequacy of sample sizes for detailed analyses. Unfortunately, there does not appear to be a practical way to augment the study population. This raises the question, alluded to elsewhere, of when a community study has outlived its usefulness. Specific answers to such a question are not easily found. In the case of such a pioneering and productive enterprise as the Framingham project, one might suggest the addition of new studies. For example, as the original cohort has aged its risks of stroke and other diseases of aging have increased. Perhaps these conditions could be added to the variables for study.

Reference

Hammond, E. C. 1964. Smoking in relation to mortality and morbidity. Findings in first thirty-four months of follow-up in a prospective study started in 1959. *J. Nat. Cancer Inst.* 32:1161–88.

PART III

SOCIAL SURVEYS

As a populous area with nonwhites concentrated in a large central city, and the relatively more affluent whites in the suburbs, Alameda County, California, is representative of urban America today. In this setting, the relationships between stress, social factors, and health are being investigated in a community laboratory. The principal instrument is a mailed questionnaire followed up, as necessary, with other modes of contact. Such problems as the relative value of physical examinations and response validity in self-evaluations of health are directly posed here.

HEALTH AND WAYS OF LIVING

The Alameda County, California, Population Laboratory

Joseph R. Hochstim

INTRODUCTION

The Human Population Laboratory, a research facility within the California Department of Public Health, was established in 1959 under a planning grant from the National Institutes of Health to conduct cross-sectional and longitudinal health studies in Alameda County. Since that time a number of methodological and pilot studies on the health and ways of living of a cross-section of the Alameda County population have been carried out.

For the purposes of these studies, health is regarded as a function not only of physical condition but also of mental, emotional, and social well-being. The latter are reflected in an individual's relations with spouse, children, and co-workers, and in his over-all performance as a citizen. The general hypothesis being tested is that physical, mental, and social health are correlated with the wide range of demographic, familial, economic, cultural, and environmental factors and personal habits which may be called "ways of living."

Experience in preventive medicine suggests that for the promotion of positive health, attention must be paid to an individual's total way of life rather than to his medical needs alone. For this reason, interest in the relations between disease and mental and social stress has grown. While the physical conditions of life have been greatly improved in recent years, there have been concomitant changes in the psychological and social environment which may foster new diseases and diminish the importance of old ones.

The long-term research objectives of the Human Population Laboratory are:

1. To assess the general level of physical, mental, and social health of a broad sample of individuals.

2. To ascertain whether particular levels of physical health tend to be associated with comparable levels of mental and social health.

3. To determine which of various personal habits and demographic, familial, cultural, and environmental variables are most strongly related to health.

These varied objectives require an interdisciplinary approach for their attainment. Accordingly, the research staff includes medical epidemiologists, sociologists, psychologists, survey research experts, and statisticians. The Laboratory constitutes an important resource for various planning, health and welfare agencies in the metropolitan area which utilize its published medical and social data. Within the State Department of Public Health other research groups call upon the Laboratory's technical assistance in designing studies, selecting samples, or carrying out field work.

THE COMMUNITY

Alameda County, a part of the San Francisco–Oakland Standard Metropolitan Area, is located on the east side of San Francisco Bay and has a population of a little over a million, almost entirely urban.

The principal city is Oakland, which is the county seat and a major center for commerce, transportation, communications, and related industries. Together with Berkeley and Albany immediately adjoining, it comprises about half the population of the county. The southern part of the county includes suburban cities which supply workers for Oakland as well as for the automobile assembly plants and other manufacturing concerns recently established in the South County area.

Alameda County nearly doubled its population between 1940 and 1965, with most of the increase taking place in South County. Twenty-one per cent of the population lived there in 1940, compared with 49 per cent at present (Figure 7–1).

Figure 7–1. Population trends for Alameda County and major subdivisions 1940–65.

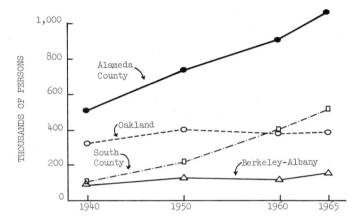

Oakland and Berkeley have remained relatively constant in total population, but the percentage of Negroes has increased. Between 1960 and 1965 the proportion of Negroes rose from 22 to 30 per cent in Oakland and from 17 to 21 per cent in Berkeley and Albany. The South County population continues to be almost entirely white (Figure 6–2).

As one might expect from this differential growth pattern, Oakland's population is much older than South County's. Sixteen per cent of Oakland whites are sixty-five years and older, compared with 5 per

Figure 7–2. Proportion of Negroes in major subdivisions of Alameda County, 1940–65.

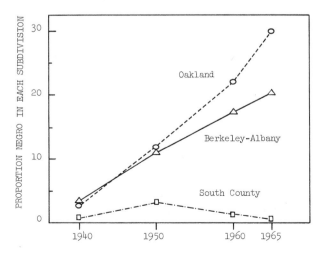

cent of the South County population. The proportions under twenty are, respectively, 28 per cent and 43 per cent. Oakland Negroes, however, are younger than the whites, 48 per cent being under twenty years of age. Oakland contrasts with South County in much the same fashion as other major urban centers differ from their suburban areas. Its proportion of divorced and separated people is double that of South County; its male unemployment rate is more than double; and nearly one-fourth of Oakland's children live in one-parent families, as compared with one-fourteenth in South County (Table 7–1). As these figures suggest, large numbers of poor people live in Oakland; and, in fact, part of the city has been designated as a target area for purposes of the federal antipoverty program. The Human Population Laboratory has collected descriptive data on people living in this depressed area and in the rest of the city. Representative findings on these groups will be presented below.

TABLE 7–1. SELECTED POPULATION CHARACTERISTICS—ALAMEDA COUNTY, SOUTH COUNTY AND OAKLAND, 1956

| | | | Oakland | | |
Characteristic	Alameda County	South County	All races	White	Negro
Age			Per cent		
Under twenty years	38	43	35	28	48
Sixty-five and older	9	5	12	16	4
Unemployed (male)[a]	3.9	2.5	5.6	4.5	8.3
Separated or divorced[b]	9	5	10	8	16
Children living with one parent[c]	14	7	23	13	37

[a] Based on men aged sixteen and older in the labor force.
[b] Based on people aged sixteen and over.
[c] Based on people under twenty who had never been married.

METHODS

For the purposes of this study, detailed information which is obtained most readily by questionnaire was needed, viz., data on socioeconomic status, family relations, personal habits, and other aspects of life style. It was decided to rely upon questionnaires for the data on health as well, rather than incur the expense of clinical examinations for the large number of persons involved. A baseline survey was conducted in 1965; the same sample will be resurveyed in 1971.

*The Sample**

An area probability sample of the adult population of Alameda County was drawn. This comprised 4,452 occupied housing units, 97 per cent of which were visited by an enumerator who had two responsibilities: (1) to secure demographic data on all household members (about 13,000 persons of all ages) and (2) to leave questionnaires for all persons twenty years of age and over and younger persons who had been married, with the request that they be filled in and returned in a week. A total of 8,083 adults were identified in this manner and questionnaires were eventually secured from 6,928 or 86 per cent of them.

Data Collection

Before embarking on the costly data-gathering process, the Laboratory carried out a series of preliminary studies. Of the three traditional methods of collecting information, viz., personal interview, telephone interview, and self-administered mail questionnaire, the personal interview is generally believed to have the highest response rate but also to be the most expensive. Telephone interviews are less expensive but suffer from sampling inadequacies while the least expensive mail questionnaires are said to be handicapped by relatively low response rates.

The possibility of combining the best features of the three techniques was investigated. The assumption was that the inexpensive mail technique could be employed to gather the bulk of the responses, while the hard-to-get part of the sample would be followed up with telephone or personal interviews. For this investigation three strategies of data collection were devised: In the "personal interview strategy" personal contacts were attempted first, with telephone and mail follow-up as needed; in the "telephone strategy" the initial telephone contact was supplemented with personal and mail inquiries; and in the "mail strategy" mail questionnaires were followed by telephone and personal interviews.

When tested with two independent samples, a highly comparable response rate was obtained from all three strategies. The proportion of questions left unanswered was only 2 per cent higher in the mail than in the other strategies, and, most important, the findings from the three strategies were virtually interchangeable. The major difference was in

---

* A detailed description of the sampling plan is given in Human Population Laboratory Series A, No. 7, 1966 (See References).

cost per completed questionnaire: the personal interview strategy was more than twice as expensive as the mail strategy (Hochstim 1967).

These results and the findings from other exploratory studies gave the Laboratory sufficient confidence in the mail strategy to adopt it as its basic method of data collection.

Questionnaire Content

Information was collected on general health, recent medical history, and style of life factors that might be correlated with sickness and health; marriage and parenthood; attitudes, feelings and worries; daily habits; spare time interests and activities; and employment status and other demographic characteristics. Since health was conceived as the general state of being sick or well—rather than in terms of specific diseases, discomforts, or disabilities—physical health was examined in terms of the individual's capacity to function in the various roles demanded of him in society.

Health has a subjective aspect as well as objective qualities. For this reason a number of subjective responses were included as indicators of physical health, viz.: whether the respondent is seriously bothered by an impairment, condition, or symptom; whether he feels his health is good, fair, or poor and how it compares with that of others his age; whether he feels he has more or less energy than others his age, and so on.

The relatively more objective indicators of physical health fell into four categories: (1) recurrent symptoms including headaches, coughing, pains in the stomach; (2) chronic conditions such as cancer, heart trouble, and arthritis; (3) impairments such as difficulty in seeing or hearing, or a missing limb; and (4) disability, defined as a reported restriction of movement, work capacity, or other activity.

The evaluation of mental health depended largely on several series of true-false items designed to measure ego resiliency, the presence of neurotic traits, and the sense of alienation or isolation known as "anomy." Respondents were also asked whether they had suffered from emotional or mental illness and whether they had visited a professional person for help with a mental or emotional problem. Other questions sought to elicit self-evaluations of general happiness, depression, restlessness, and other feeling states.

The indicators of social health included occupational adjustment as measured by satisfaction with present job, difficulties in relations with co-workers, and the number of changes of employer in the last ten years. Marital satisfaction was another index of social health, and still another was the individual's adjustment to the community—that is, whether he had voted or participated in other kinds of political activity, whether he belonged to any community service groups, and whether he depended on the community for financial support.

Physical, mental, and social health were expected to be related to life style, or "ways of living." Since health and life style were viewed as interdependent, either might affect the other, but in this research ways of living were treated as the independent variables. These included biological factors, family status, race, nativity, area of residence, socioeconomic status, social mobility, religion, personal habits, and use of medical care.

PROBLEMS

A number of methodological problems arose in the course of the Alameda County survey.

Will People Co-operate with a Long Mail Questionnaire Containing Many Personal Questions?

The experience of the Human Population Laboratory is that the great majority of persons will co-operate if they are properly motivated. In two preliminary surveys designed to test this method of data collection, response rates of 88 and 89 per cent were obtained in a mail strategy using questionnaires seven to eight pages long which took about 15 minutes to complete. The questionnaire planned for the baseline study, however, was 21 pages long and took about an hour to complete. Because of uncertainty that respondents would tolerate a self-administered questionnaire of such length, a pilot study was undertaken in which two versions of the questionnaire were tested: the 21-page version intended for use in the baseline survey, and a condensed one of 14 pages. Each version was administered to a randomly selected subsample of households.

The rates of return for the long and short forms were about equal, approximating 85 per cent. In the subsequent baseline study, the mail strategy achieved an 86 per cent response, even though the questionnaire was by then 23 pages long and took the respondent about an hour to complete.

Is the Personal Interview Follow-up Worth the Cost?

The high rate of return in the Human Population Laboratory surveys was due to persistent follow-up efforts, including personal interviews with individuals who did not respond to letters and telegrams. People who responded to the initial contact and mailed in their questionnaires immediately differed in a number of important respects from those who had to be interviewed. College-educated people and professional or technical workers were most likely to return questionnaires after the first contact, and white people were far more likely to do so than were persons of minority race.

Personal interviews were especially important in reaching people born in Mexico or of Mexican parentage: 42 per cent of these had to be interviewed as compared with 19 per cent of the entire sample (Table 7–2.) Language difficulties probably played a role here.

TABLE 7–2. FOLLOW-UP REQUIRED TO OBTAIN DATA, BY RACE—BASELINE STUDY, 1965

	Total	White	Negro	Oriental	Mexican	Other
All respondents	6,928	5,624	857	214	166	67
			Per cent			
Total	100	100	100	100	100	100
Returned questionnaire:						
Immediately	48	52	31	42	28	27
After letter	20	20	20	23	14	24
After telegram	13	11	20	14	16	19
Personal interview	19	17	29	21	42	30

These data indicate that persistent follow-up, including personal interview, is essential if disadvantaged groups in the population are to be proportionately represented. But the question remains: Is the reduction in nonresponse bias worth the cost? In a preliminary survey dealing with knowledge and use of the Papanicolaou test, the answer was an emphatic "yes": the addition of personal interviews definitely improved the estimates of the proportion of women knowing about and using the test (Hochstim 1967). The early respondents, those who returned their questionnaires promptly, were much more likely to know about the test and to have used it, than were the women who had to be interviewed.

To learn whether this observation held for other questionnaire items, estimates of various demographic characteristics were made at successive stages of data collection in the baseline study (Table 7–3). Without personal interviews the proportion of Negroes and the proportion of persons who had not gone beyond the eighth grade would have been seriously underestimated. The distribution of other characteristics, however, would not have been affected substantially.*

In regard to responses on disability, chronic conditions, and impairments there was hardly any difference between people who returned the

* The statements about findings in Tables 7–2, 7–3, and 7–4 are based on t-tests conducted at the level of .05.

TABLE 7–3. DEMOGRAPHIC CHARACTERISTICS ESTIMATED AT SUCCESSIVE STAGES OF FOLLOW-UP—BASELINE STUDY, 1965

Characteristics	Stages cumulatively			
	No follow-up	Letter only	Telegram also	Personal interview
All respondents	3,358	4,754	5,630	6,928
	Per cent			
Sex				
Male	44.8	45.4	45.8	45.6
Female	55.2	54.6	54.2	54.4
Age				
Under 30 years	23.6	23.3	23.3	23.7
30–44	30.3	31.1	32.1	32.2
45–64	31.3	31.8	32.2	31.3
65 and over	14.8	13.8	12.4	12.8
Race				
White	88.8	87.0	85.2	83.6
Negro	8.0	9.3	10.9	12.4
Other	3.2	3.7	3.9	4.1
Marital Status				
Married	73.4	74.4	75.1	74.5
Single	11.2	10.6	10.2	10.1
Separated or divorced	8.2	8.0	8.3	8.5
Widowed	7.2	7.0	6.5	7.0
Employment status				
Employed	55.1	56.4	58.4	58.2
Looking for work	2.0	2.4	2.4	2.6
Retired	9.1	8.3	7.4	7.7
Other (students, housewives, etc.)	33.8	33.0	31.8	31.5
Education				
Eighth grade or less	15.7	16.2	16.6	18.1
High school (9–12 years)	46.5	46.9	47.7	48.2
College (13 years or more)	37.8	37.0	35.8	33.8

mail questionnaires and those who had to be interviewed. The latter were more likely to consider themselves in fair or poor health, and a larger proportion of them had no health insurance or had never had a medical checkup but the over-all estimates were only slightly altered (Table 7–4).

The findings in Alameda County suggest that personal interviews are worth the additional cost when the research objectives include accurate estimates of such population characteristics as income level, race, ethnicity, and education, or when the variables of interest are associated with such factors, as in the question on the use of the Papanicolaou test. On the other hand, the prevalence of disability, chronic conditions, impairments or other complaints known to the respondent can apparently be estimated satisfactorily without personal interviews. Whether or not the reduction of bias achieved by interviewing is worth the cost must, therefore, be related to the specific objectives of the research (Hochstim and Athanasopoulos 1969). Personal interviews with a subsample of nonrespondents offer a quantitative solution to the problem.

TABLE 7–4. HEALTH CHARACTERISTICS ESTIMATED AT SUCCESSIVE STAGES OF FOLLOW-UP—BASELINE STUDY, 1965

| Characteristics | Stages cumulatively | | | |
	No follow-up	Letter only	Telegram also	Personal interview
All respondents	3,358	4,754	5,630	6,928
	Per cent			
Some disability	15.0	15.2	14.7	14.8
One or more chronic conditions	37.3	37.4	37.1	36.8
One or more impairments	10.1	9.7	9.3	9.2
One or more ailments	64.1	63.8	63.3	62.6
One or more health complaints	71.9	71.6	71.2	70.6
Never had a medical checkup	10.6	11.0	11.4	12.3
No health insurance	14.1	14.3	14.6	15.7
Rate own health "fair" or "poor"	16.4	17.7	17.9	18.5

How Much Bias Results from Nonresponse, Even after Intensive Follow-up?

As noted earlier, responses were not obtained from 14 per cent of the adults who had been enumerated. Because the study design required the enumerators to collect demographic information in the initial contact with each household, it was possible to estimate some effects of nonresponse. The nonrespondents were older and more likely to be male, single or widowed, and white than the respondents.* They formed so small a proportion of the total sample, however, that their effect on the population estimates was negligible (Table 7–5).

How Much of the Original Sample Can Be Traced Several Years Later and Induced to Participate in a Second Survey?

The 1964 pilot study utilized a sample of households that had been selected and enumerated in 1961. Some of the people in these households had moved in the interim: of the 749 we re-enumerated, 279 (37 per cent) had moved to a different address. A major effort was made to

---

* The appropriate Chi-square tests show the differences between respondents and nonrespondents on all four items to be significant at the level of .05.

locate these movers, and completed questionnaires were eventually received from two-thirds of them. The 470 persons still residing at their original addresses were all contacted, and 81 per cent completed the 1964 questionnaire. Thus, three years after the original enumeration, responses were obtained from 76 per cent of the people in the original sample, excluding those who were known to have died or who could not be classified as movers or nonmovers (Carrington 1969).

TABLE 7-5. SELECTED CHARACTERISTICS OF TOTAL ENUMERATED SAMPLE, RESPONDENTS, AND NONRESPONDENTS—BASELINE STUDY, 1965

Characteristics	Total enumerated sample	Question-naire respondents	Non-respondents
Total number of persons	8,083	6,928	1,155
	Per cent		
Sex			
Male	46.1	45.6	49.4
Female	53.9	54.4	50.6
Age			
Under 30 years	22.5	23.7	15.5
30–44	31.5	32.2	27.5
45–64	32.3	31.3	38.6
65 and over	13.6	12.8	18.5
Race			
White	84.4	83.6	89.1
Negro	12.0	12.4	9.2
Other	3.7	4.1	1.7
Marital status			
Married	74.2	74.5	72.1
Single	10.3	10.1	11.6
Separated or divorced	8.2	8.5	6.9
Widowed	7.3	7.0	9.0
Employment status			
Employed	57.8	58.2	55.2
Looking for work	2.5	2.6	1.9
Retired	8.1	7.7	10.4
Other (students, housewives, etc.)	31.6	31.5	32.3

Response Validity

To test the validity of responses to survey questions, one must have an independent source of confirmatory information. Survey research is expensive, however, and seldom justified if the information is already available elsewhere. Thus, response validity can rarely be tested. Nevertheless, circumstances permitted the Human Population Laboratory to assess the validity of several survey questions.

TABLE 7–6.   RESPONSE TO THREE-YEAR FOLLOW-UP PILOT STUDY SAMPLE, 1961–64

	TOTAL	Address in 1946	
		Same	Different
Number of respondents in 1961 survey	808		
Status in 1964:			
Not traced[a]	30		
Deceased	29		
Traced	749	470	279
		Per cent	
Traced in 1964	100	100	100
Completed questionnaire	76	81	67
Contacted, but did not complete			
questionnaire	19	19	19
Not contacted[a]	5	0	13

[a] May include some decedents.

In the baseline study, respondents were asked whether they had voted in the 1964 presidential election and, if they had, whether they had voted in Alameda County. The official voting records made it possible to validate the responses to these questions. In the subsample checked, the respondent's answer was verified in 94 per cent of the cases.

In a preliminary study (mentioned above) a sample of adult women were asked whether they had ever taken the Papanicolaou test for cervical cancer or, if not, whether they had ever had a pelvic examination. Those who reported either the test or the examination were asked to identify the physician or hospital involved. In 91 per cent of the cases the medical facility or physician had some record of the respondent, and in 84 per cent the questionnaire response was confirmed (Hochstim 1967).

Most recently, an attempt was made to validate the health questions asked in the baseline survey. The sample included nearly 1,000 subscribers to the Kaiser Foundation Health Plan in Oakland and Hayward, of whom 733 had taken either a multi-phasic screening examination or some other general physical examination not more than two years before the survey. With the co-operation of the Kaiser Foundation, physicians associated with the Human Population Laboratory reviewed the Kaiser records and attempted to rate each patient on certain variables used in the analysis of the survey data. They worked "blind," i.e., without knowledge of the patient's questionnaire responses.

Analysis of the consistency of ratings from the two sources is still in progress, and results are presently available for only one variable termed the "physical health spectrum." This is a classification of respondents into one of four groups: (1) those with some disability; (2) others who have no disability but report one or more chronic conditions; (3) respondents who disclaim any disability or chronic condition but who mention one or more symptoms; and (4) those who make no complaint about their health. These categories are conceived as segments of a continuum ranging from functional incapacity to excellent health.

The physical health spectrum was difficult to validate. For one thing, the questionnaire was designed to elicit information on minor disability, whereas the medical records, for understandable reasons, often failed to supply information of this type. Nevertheless, the physician evaluators were asked to estimate each patient's classification on the physical health spectrum from the medical records as best they could.

A total of 362 out of the 733 individuals (49 per cent) received the same rating on the basis of Kaiser records as they did from the questionnaire data (Table 7–7). An additional 38 per cent of the ratings agreed within one category. If the "some disability" and "chronic conditions" categories are combined to allow for the noncomparability of the data on restricted activity, 427 (58 per cent) of the respondents received the same rating from the two sources of information. This comparison, of course, is not an absolute measure of response validity. When ratings disagree, either record may be in error, or incomplete, or the two may simply contain different kinds of information, collected for different purposes at different times.

TABLE 7–7. PHYSICAL HEALTH SPECTRUM: RATINGS BASED ON QUESTIONNAIRES BY RATINGS BASED ON MEDICAL RECORDS—BASELINE STUDY, 1965

Rating based on questionnaire	Total	Rating based on medical record			
		Some disability	Chronic condition	Symptom only	No problem
Total	733	29	313	191	200
Some disability	93	*19*	55	14	5
Chronic condition	241	10	*167*	34	30
Symptom only	215	0	52	*87*	76
No problem	184	0	39	56	*89*

Reliability of Responses

A reliable indicator is one that consistently yields the same value as long as the condition being measured remains unchanged and changes its value only when the condition changes. Because some respondents in the 1964 pilot study had also participated in a study in 1961, the reliability of certain indicators could be evaluated. Answers to certain theoretically invariable questions asked of the same subjects in both surveys were compared. The consistency of responses to these seven questions was very high: only 30 out of a total of 2,381 answers changed—an average of one per cent (Table 7–8).

Marital status is not strictly invariant, but relatively few people would be expected to change their status during a three-year interval. Of 265 respondents, 241 (91 per cent) gave identical answers on marital status in the 2 surveys (Table 7–9). All but one of the 24 persons who gave different answers could have been reporting a true change. Only the one change from "divorced" in 1961 to "never married" in 1964 is obviously inconsistent.

A major study of response reliability is now under way. The consistency of responses to questions on physical, mental, and social health over a period of one to two weeks is being evaluated. This time interval is so brief as to preclude the likelihood of substantial changes in the respondents' health. The sample consists of the adults* living in approximately 1,000 Alameda County households. All procedures are as much like those used in the baseline study as is possible. An enumerator leaves

TABLE 7–8. CONSISTENCY OF RESPONSES TO SELECTED QUESTIONS—PILOT STUDY SAMPLE, 1961 AND 1964

Question	Number who answered both times	Per cent who answered consistently
Sex	265	100
Race	408	99
Born in the U.S.	400	99
Father born in U.S.	392	98
Mother born in U.S.	398	98
Father deceased by 1961	257	100
Mother deceased by 1961	261	99

TABLE 7–9. CONSISTENCY OF RESPONSES ON MARITAL STATUS—PILOT STUDY SAMPLE, 1961 AND 1964

Marital status in 1964	Marital status in 1961				
	Married	Widowed	Divorced	Separated	Never married
Total	217	17	9	4	18
Married	212	3	3	0	9
Widowed	3	14	0	1	0
Divorced	1	0	5	2	0
Separated	1	0	0	1	0
Never married	0	0	1	0	9

* For this survey, "adults" included all persons over nineteen years of age and all those sixteen to nineteen years old who had ever been married.

self-administered questionnaires for all adults in each household and returns on the following day to pick them up. On this visit he explains that the second part of the questionnaire will be sent by mail and that he will return one week later to pick it up. The second part is essentially a duplicate of the first part, namely a short (8-page) version of the (23-page) baseline questionnaire. It includes the items necessary for the calculation of the major summary measures. In a subsample of households the enumerator compares the two parts of the questionnaire and discusses the discrepancies with the respondent.

Analysis of these data will provide several kinds of useful information:

1. The proportion of respondents who answer inconsistently will be calculated for each of the major summary measures as a whole and for each original level of such measures. This will make it possible to compare the reliability of information on physical and social health, as well as to compare the reliability of respondents who reported good health originally with that of those who reported poor health.

2. Inconsistency rates will be computed for major subgroups within the sample. For example, Negroes will be compared with whites, older with younger people, well-educated with poorly educated, and so forth.

3. Attention will be paid to the distribution of the inconsistencies, to see whether they are randomly distributed among the available response categories or whether some directional bias is present.

FINDINGS

Health in a Depressed Area

Poverty and ghetto life are critical problems today, in Alameda County and elsewhere in the United States. A major objective of the Human Population Laboratory is to examine the high rates of physical and social impairment exhibited by poverty area residents. Of special interest is the comparative impact of three factors—income, race, and residence within or outside the poverty area—upon physical and social health. It was found, of course, that Negroes and others with inadequate income are at a disadvantage in many respects, but it was also observed that living in a poverty area is in itself a handicap (Hochstim et al. 1968).

The Oakland poverty area consists of a set of contiguous census tracts designated as a target for the federal antipoverty program because the male unemployment rate in 1960 was 9 per cent or higher. The area includes only 37 per cent of the total population of Oakland, but 77 per cent of its Negroes. The 908 people in the survey sample who lived in the poverty area were compared with the 1,672 who lived elsewhere in Oakland.

Thirty per cent of the poverty area residents were living on an inadequate family income, as compared with 12 per cent in the rest of Oakland (Table 7–10). The criterion of income adequacy was a combination of family size and family income. For instance, an income of $5,000–$6,000 was considered adequate for a family of one or two, marginal for a family of three to six persons, and inadequate for a family of more than six persons.

There were other indications of the economic deprivation of poverty area residents: they had higher rates of unemployment, a higher proportion on welfare, and a relatively low level of occupational and educational achievement (Table 7–11). Housing in the poverty area was less adequate than elsewhere in Oakland, and many more of its families lacked one parent (Table 7–12).

TABLE 7–10. FAMILY INCOME LEVEL BY AREA OF RESIDENCE—OAKLAND, 1965

Family income	Poverty area	Nonpoverty area
Total adults[a]	805	1,592
	Per cent	
Total	100	100
Inadequate	30	12
Marginal	23	16
Adequate	46	72

$$X^2 = 162.62, df = 2$$

[a] Excludes 103 adults in the poverty area and 80 in the nonpoverty area who gave insufficient information about income.

TABLE 7–11. ECONOMIC DEPRIVATION BY AREA OF RESIDENCE—OAKLAND, 1965

	Poverty area	Nonpoverty area
Total adults	908	1,672
	Per cent	
Unemployed[a]	11[b]	3
Receive unemployment, disability, or welfare payments	22[b]	7
Service workers or laborers[a]		
Men	36[b]	9
Women	42[b]	11
Eighth grade education or less	38[b]	17

[a] Based on the number of adults in the labor force.
[b] Difference significant at the level of $\leq .05$ (t-test).

TABLE 7–12. HOUSEHOLD CHARACTERISTICS BY AREA OF RESIDENCE—OAKLAND, 1965

Household characteristics	Poverty area	Nonpoverty area
Total households	600	1,106
	Per cent	
Do not own home	65[a]	44
Crowded (1.01 or more persons per room)	12[a]	4
Head and children but no spouse	14[a]	6

[a] Difference significant at the level of ≤.05 (t-test).

Alameda County Welfare Department records show that a dispropor-
tionate amount of the demand for community services comes from the
poverty area. The survey data also reflect its widespread physical and
social impairment. Poverty area residents were more likely than others
to report physical disabilities and chronic conditions. Thirty-four per
cent considered their health only fair or poor compared with 18 per
cent of those living elsewhere in Oakland (Table 7–13), despite the fact
that the over-all adult age distributions in the two areas were essentially
the same.

TABLE 7–13. HEALTH INDICES BY AREA OF RESIDENCE—OAKLAND, 1965

	Poverty area	Nonpoverty area
Total adults	908	1,672
	Per cent	
Some disability	16[a]	10
One or more chronic conditions	46[a]	38
Rate own health "fair" or "poor"	34[a]	18

[a] Difference significant at the level of ≤.05 (t-test).

Marital instability and general unhappiness were more common in
the poverty area than elsewhere in Oakland, and poverty area residents
were almost twice as likely as others to manifest a sense of rootlessness
or alienation, viz., anomy (Table 7–14).

Income and Residence

An important question is whether these higher rates of physical and
social impairment in the ghetto are associated solely with economic deprivation or whether they are also related to the more general conditions
of life in a depressed area. Physical health was strongly related to family
income in Alameda County. The lower the income the higher the propor-

tion reporting disability and chronic conditions and the higher the proportion who evaluated their health negatively (Table 7–15).

At the same time, the poverty area residents were more likely to
report health problems than were other Oakland residents at the same
income level. For disability and chronic conditions the differences between the areas were rather small. On self-evaluation of health, however, the differences between areas were at least as great as the differences between income levels.

The poorest people also reported more social problems: the less
adequate the income the higher the prevalence of marital and social

TABLE 7–14. MARITAL INSTABILITY AND GENERAL DISSATISFACTION BY AREA OF RESI-
DENCE—OAKLAND, 1965

	Poverty area	Nonpoverty area
Total adults	908	1,672
	Per cent	
Separated or divorced	18[b]	9
Marriage is "unhappy" or only "somewhat happy"[a]	30[b]	17
All in all, "not too happy"	16[b]	10
High anomy score	38[b]	20

[a] Based on married people only (550 in the poverty area and 1,156 in the nonpoverty area).

[b] Difference significant at the level of ≤.05 (t-test).

TABLE 7–15. HEALTH INDICES BY AREA OF RESIDENCE AND FAMILY INCOME LEVEL—
OAKLAND, 1965

	Poverty area			Nonpoverty area		
	Income level					
	Inade-quate	Mar-ginal	Ade-quate	Inade-quate	Mar-ginal	Ade-quate
Total adults[a]	242	189	374	197	256	1,139
	Per cent					
Some disability	27[b]	15	8	20[b]	10	7
One or more chronic conditions	54[b]	49[d]	39	52[c]	39	35
Rate own health "fair" or "poor"	46[b, d]	33[d]	25[d]	27[b]	21	15

[a] Excludes 103 adults in the poverty area and 80 in the nonpoverty area who gave
insufficient information about income.

[b] Within-area differences significant at the level of ≤.05 (F-test).

[c] Within-area difference nonsignificant after raw data were corrected by the indirect
method of age adjusting.

[d] Between-area difference for the indicated income group significant at the level of
≤.05 (t-test).

instability. Even within the same income level, however, poverty area residents were more likely than others to report separation, divorce, or an unhappy current marriage. Anomy, or alienation, was pervasive in the poverty area at all income levels; elsewhere it decreased with more adequate income (Table 7–16).

This suggests that poverty in the literal sense of inadequate income is not the distinguishing characteristic of the slum, but rather such factors as unemployment, employment in unskilled jobs, dependence on public support, and overcrowded living quarters. Low educational attainment and marital instability are also characteristic of the slum dweller. Morale is understandably low, as indicated by the relatively large proportion scoring high on anomy and rating their marriages unhappy or only somewhat happy. The subjective rating of health also may be, in part, an index of morale.

Race and Residence

Race is another aspect of poverty area life that bears on health, for minority racial status can be as much a handicap in our society as is lack of education or occupational skill. The survey findings were examined for evidence that racial composition might explain the differences between the two sections of Oakland in rates of sickness and social instability.

TABLE 7–16. MARITAL INSTABILITY AND GENERAL DISSATISFACTION BY AREA OF RESIDENCE AND FAMILY INCOME LEVEL—OAKLAND, 1965

	Poverty area			Nonpoverty area		
	Income level					
	Inade- quate	Mar- ginal	Ade- quate	Inade- quate	Mar- ginal	Ade- quate
Total adults[a]	242	189	374	197	256	1,139
	Per cent					
Separated or divorced	26[c, d]	17	10	16[c]	12	7
Marriage is "unhappy" or only "somewhat happy"[b]	39[c]	31	25[d]	25[c]	25	16
All in all, "not too happy"	21[c, d]	13	12	12	11	9
High anomy score	40	36[d]	37[d]	30[c]	25	18

[a] Excludes 103 adults in the poverty area and 80 in the nonpoverty area who gave insufficient information about income.

[b] Based on married people only.

[c] Within-area differences significant at the level of $\leq.05$ (F-test).

[d] Between-area difference for the indicated income group significant at the level of $\leq.05$ (t-test).

Negroes comprise a majority in the poverty area of Oakland: 58 per cent of total residents as compared with 8 per cent outside the area. But Negroes and whites in the poverty area were practically indistinguishable in income, education, unemployment rate, and dependence on community support; and both groups were quite different from their counterparts outside (Tables 7–17 and 7–18).

In only one respect did Oakland Negroes seem to be economically more deprived than whites living in the same area: they were much more likely to be in service occupations or unskilled jobs (Table 7–18).

TABLE 7–17. FAMILY INCOME LEVEL BY AREA OF RESIDENCE AND RACE—OAKLAND, 1965

Family income	Poverty area		Nonpoverty area	
	White	Negro	White	Negro
Total adults[a]	302	454	1,395	130
	Per cent			
Total	100	100	100	100
Inadequate	31	28	12	12
Marginal	24	23	16	19
Adequate	45	49	72	69

Within poverty area $X^2 = 1.8$, $df = 2$; not significant at level of .05.
Within nonpoverty area $X^2 = 10.6$, $df = 2$; significant at level of .05.
[a] Excludes 119 "orientals and others" as well as the 103 whites and 77 Negroes who gave insufficient information about income.

TABLE 7–18. ECONOMIC DEPRIVATION BY AREA OF RESIDENCE AND RACE—OAKLAND, 1965

	Poverty area		Nonpoverty area	
	White	Negro	White	Negro
Total adults	332	526	1,468	135
	Per cent			
Unemployed[a]	12[c]	10[c]	3	3
Receive unemployment, disability or welfare payments	21[c]	24[c]	6	8
Service workers or laborers[a]				
Men	20[b, c]	43	6[b]	32
Women	13[b]	52	7[b]	46
Eighth grade education or less	40[c]	38[c]	16	21

[a] Based on adults in the labor force.
[b] Within-area difference significant at the level of ≤.05 (t-test).
[c] Between-area difference for the indicated race significant at the level of ≤.05 (t-test).

In physical health, Negroes were at least as well off as whites (Table 7–19). The few Negroes who lived outside the poverty area appeared to be less susceptible to health problems not only because they were younger (68 per cent were under forty-five, compared with 46 per cent of the whites), but, perhaps, also because the most fit were the most likely to have escaped from the ghetto. The largest differences in health indices were between areas rather than between races. Compared with other members of the same race living elsewhere in Oakland, both Negroes and whites in the poverty area were much more likely to report health problems and to evaluate their health negatively.

TABLE 7–19. HEALTH INDICES BY AREA OF RESIDENCE AND RACE—OAKLAND, 1965

	Poverty area		Nonpoverty area	
	White	Negro	White	Negro
Total adults	332	526	1,468	135
	Per cent			
Some disability	18[a]	16	10[b]	5
One or more chronic conditions	48[a]	45[a]	39[b]	32
Rate own health "fair" or "poor"	32[a, c]	36[a]	18	22

[a] Between-area difference for the indicated race significant at the level of $\leq.05$ (t-test).

[b] Within-area difference nonsignificant after raw data were corrected by the indirect method of age adjusting.

[c] Within-area difference significant after raw data were corrected by the indirect method of age adjusting.

Negroes in both areas were more likely than whites to be unhappily married. In the poverty area they were also more likely to be separated or divorced and to suffer from alienation. But, again, poverty area residence has an independent effect on these variables: for each race, unhappiness and anomy were much more common in the poverty area than elsewhere (Table 7–20).

Thus, Negroes and whites living in the Oakland ghetto share economic, social, and psychological burdens in far greater measure than their counterparts elsewhere in the city. Negroes in both areas have lower-status jobs than whites and report more marital unhappiness, but in other aspects of economic deprivation and in the prevalence of poor health, they resemble their white neighbors more than they do other Negroes.

TABLE 7–20.   MARITAL INSTABILITY AND GENERAL DISSATISFACTION BY AREA OF RESIDENCE AND RACE—OAKLAND, 1965

	Poverty area		Nonpoverty area	
	White	Negro	White	Negro
Total adults	332	526	1,468	135
	Per cent			
Separated or divorced	13[b]	23[c]	9	10
Marriage is "unhappy" or only "somewhat happy"[a]	22[b]	35	16[b]	31
All in all, "not too happy"	14[c]	17[c]	10	8
High anomy score	32[b, c]	42[c]	20	23

[a] Based on married people only.
[b] Within-area difference significant at the level of ≤.05 (t-test).
[c] Between-area difference for the indicated race significant at the level of ≤.05 (t-test).

Income, Race and Residence

Within each area—poverty and nonpoverty—high-income whites resembled high-income Negroes more than they did low-income whites. Similarly, low-income Negroes resembled low-income whites more than they did high-income Negroes. Members of each race at a given income level, living outside the poverty area, were consistently better off than their counterparts inside the area. Regardless of income or residence, however, the Negroes were more likely than the whites to be in low-status occupations and to have unstable marriages.

These findings confirm that being poor or black is a handicap. They also show that residence in a poverty area is itself a major disadvantage, independent of income or race.

The Health of Married and Spouseless Mothers

A number of studies* have found that mortality and morbidity rates are higher among the divorced and widowed than among the married, but it is not known whether changes in marital status precede changes in health or vice versa. In seeking to understand the relation between health and marital status one may proceed from the assumption that marriage is not only the "normal" state, but also the least stressful state. As such, it would have a cushioning effect against illness. The separated, divorced, and widowed thus undergo greater life stress, which may either cause illness directly or reduce normal resistance to illness.

* See references at end of chapter.

Applying this line of reasoning to women, one would expect the impact of separation, divorce, or widowhood to be most severe for women who are raising children. Such women experience the parental stress of raising children without a father, the emotional stress of no longer having a mate, and often the economic stress of having to provide for a family without the help of a male breadwinner.

To test these assumptions, women in the Alameda County sample were divided into seven groups according to marital and parental status (Table 7–21). Single women with children, women married to someone other than the head of household, and spouseless women who were not heads of their own households were excluded because of their small numbers or because their parental status could not be determined.

After the data were adjusted for age by the indirect method, the seven groups were compared on a number of indicators of general health (Berkman 1969). Only two of the seven life-style groups showed health patterns consistently and distinctly different from the average: spouseless mothers now raising children had significantly higher rates of illness; married mothers now raising children had significantly lower rates (Table 7–22). The other five types—including separated, divorced, and widowed women who had never had children and those whose children had left home—had average or approximately average health patterns.

The observed differences between married and spouseless mothers were consistent with socioeconomic differences between the two groups: the spouseless mothers were definitely more underprivileged and many more of them were Negroes (Table 7–23).

However, even when socioeconomic factors were held constant, morbidity was greater among spouseless mothers than married mothers— among those living outside the poverty area as well as those living inside, among those with adequate incomes as well as those without, and among those keeping house as well as those working full time (Table 7–24).

TABLE 7-21. TYPOLOGIES OF FEMALE LIFE STYLES—ALAMEDA COUNTY SAMPLE, 1965

Parental status	Marital status
Never had children	and never married and now married to head of household and now head of household, without a husband
Has had children, but none at home now	and now married to head of household and now head of household, without a husband
Mothers now raising children	and now married to head of household and now head of household, without a husband

TABLE 7–22. HEALTH INDICES FOR MARRIED AND SPOUSELESS MOTHERS—ALAMEDA COUNTY, 1965

Age[a] and marital-parental status	Number	Per cent reporting each health problem		
		Some disability	One or more chronic conditions	"Fair" or "poor" health
Under 35 years				
Married mothers	690	4	19	13
Spouseless mothers	57	12[b]	28	26[b]
35–44 years				
Married mothers	569	8	26	13
Spouseless mothers	81	22[b]	37[b]	26[b]
45–54 years				
Married mothers	272	15	42	16
Spouseless mothers	48	25	58[b]	38[b]

[a] Women over 54 are not shown because few women of that age have children at home.

[b] Difference between married mothers and spouseless mothers significant at the level of $\leq.05$ (t-test).

TABLE 7–23. RACE AND SELECTED SOCIOECONOMIC CHARACTERISTICS OF MARRIED AND SPOUSELESS MOTHERS—ALAMEDA COUNTY, 1965

	Married mothers	Spouseless mothers
All mothers raising children	1,552	204
	Per cent	
Negro	10	37[b]
Living in the Oakland poverty area[a]	9	33[b]
With inadequate family income	7	39[b]
Receiving welfare payments	1	30[b]
Working full time	24	54[b]

[a] Based on Oakland residents only (132 married mothers and 63 spouseless mothers).

[b] Difference significant at the level of $\leq.05$ (t-test).

Negro women departed from this pattern and differed from white women in one respect. Although married Negro mothers were less likely than spouseless Negro mothers to report disabilities and fair or poor health, they reported almost as high a rate of chronic conditions.

Because it is only an assumption that certain life styles are more stressful than others, these findings do not necessarily confirm the association between stress and health. They are consistent with such an association, however, and they illustrate one approach to the understanding of health in terms of the variously stressful ways of living. A more immediate benefit of this study has been the identification of one group of women—the spouseless mothers—who report themselves to be distinctly sicker than others and who may constitute a group in special need of preventive and ameliorative health programs.

TABLE 7–24. HEALTH INDICES FOR MARRIED AND SPOUSELESS MOTHERS BY SELECTED SOCIOECONOMIC CHARACTERISTICS

	Number	Per cent reporting each health problem		
		Some disability	One or more chronic conditions	"Fair" or "poor" health
Negro				
Married	161	11	36	26
Spouseless	69	23[a]	39	38[a]
White				
Married	1,317	8	25	12
Spouseless	131	20[a]	44[a]	24[a]
Poverty area[b]				
Married	132	11	30	25
Spouseless	63	27[a]	48[a]	46[a]
Nonpoverty area[b]				
Married	291	6	24	13
Spouseless	48	17[a]	44[a]	23
Inadequate income				
Married	104	10	27	22
Spouseless	79	20	42[a]	34
Adequate income[c]				
Married	1,412	8	24	13
Spouseless	101	21[a]	42[a]	23[a]
Receiving welfare				
Married[d]	12	—	—	—
Spouseless	58	33	45	45
Not receiving welfare				
Married	1,456	7	26	13
Spouseless	143	16[a]	41[a]	23[a]
Working full time				
Married	366	7	29	13
Spouseless	110	13[a]	37	20
Keeping house				
Married	994	8	24	14
Spouseless	73	36[a]	48[a]	41[a]

[a] Difference between married mothers and spouseless mothers significant at the level of ≤.05 (t-test).
[b] Based on Oakland residents only.
[c] Includes "marginal" income.
[d] Too few cases to tabulate.

POTENTIALS

The Human Population Laboratory is collecting useful information about the living habits and health status of a large number of people. The mailed questionnaire has proved to be a relatively inexpensive method of gathering data, and the sample is large enough to permit adequate analysis by subgroups.

With these data one can begin to define the various styles of life that characterize our highly complex society and to investigate the relation between life style and health. Some aspects of this relationship have already been evaluated for poverty area residents and spouseless mothers. Negro men, career women, Orientals, school dropouts, and aging persons are other groups whose styles of life deserve study.

Because the mail questionnaire strategy of obtaining information has been tested and refined, a larger proportion of the original sample can be followed successfully than would otherwise be possible. Thus, longitudinal changes in health over time can be examined and perhaps related to concomitant variations in ways of living.

Data from the baseline study will be used eventually to construct a summary index of health. Such an index, based on a generic concept of disease, will facilitate scientific understanding of the relation between modern ways of life and corresponding patterns of disease.

The Human Population Laboratory's unified approach to the study of health and illness is in line with current thinking in medicine, psychology, and sociology. Its research seeks to relate health to the social, psychological, and cultural factors which must not be ignored in programs aimed at improving the total health of communities.

Acknowledgments

This study was supported by research grant CH 00076 from the Division of Community Health Services, U.S. Public Health Service. Dr. Lester Breslow is responsible for the concept and establishment of the Human Population Laboratory. The author wishes to express deep appreciation to Dr. Josephine W. Meltzer and to Miss Karen S. Renne for their helpful comments and suggestions during the preparation of this paper as well as for their very creative editing of the manuscript.

References

Berkson, J. 1962. Mortality and marital status—reflections on the derivation of etiology from statistics. *Am. J. Public Health* 52:1318–29.

California State Department of Public Health, Human Population Laboratory

Series A:

No. 1. Comparison of Three Information-Gathering Strategies in a Population Study of Socio-Medical Variables (September 1962).

No. 2. Cervical Cytology in Alameda County (January 1963).

No. 3. Evaluation of Three Approaches to Information Collection in an Epidemiologic Study of Cervical Cytology (May 1963).

No. 4. Alternatives to Personal Interviewing (May 1963).

No. 5. Sociocultural Aspects of Cervical Cytology in Alameda County (February 1964).

No. 6. The California Human Population Laboratory for Epidemiologic Studies (June 1964).

No. 7. Alameda County Population 1965 (April 1966).

No. 8. Demographic Fact Book of Alameda and Contra Costa Counties (June 1966).

Carrington, R. A. Mobility and change in a longitudinal sample (unpublished data).

Hochstim, J. R. Reliability of response in a sociomedical population study. (unpublished data).

———. 1967. A critical comparison of three strategies of collecting data from households. *J. Am. Statist. Ass.* 62:976–89.

Hochstim, J. R., Athanasopoulos, D. A., and Larkins, J. H. 1968. Poverty area under the microscope. *Am. J. Public Health* 58:1815–27.

LaHorgue, Z. 1960. Morbidity and marital status. *J. Chronic Dis.* 12:476–98.

McClosky, H. and Schaar, J. H. 1965. Psychological dimensions of anomy. *Am. Soc. Rev.* 21:14–40.

Meltzer, J. W. Reliability and validity of survey data on health (unpublished data).

National Office of Vital Statistics. 1955. *Vital Statistics, Special Reports. Mortality from Selected Causes by Marital Status: United States, 1949–51*, vol. 39, no. 7. Washington: U.S. Government Printing Office.

Renne, K. S. 1970 Correlates of dissatisfaction in marriage. *J. Marriage and the Family*, in press.

———. Health and marital experience in an urban population (unpublished data).

Sheps, M. C. 1961. Marriage and mortality. *Am. J. Public Health* 51:547–55.

Shurtleff, D. 1955. Mortality and marital status. *Public Health Rep.* 70:248–52.

———. 1956. Mortality among the married. *J. Am. Geriat. Soc.* 4:654–66.

Zalokar, J. B. 1960. Marital status and major causes of death in women. *J. Chronic Dis.* 11:50–60.

EDITORIAL COMMENTS

1. This is the first example encountered in the Casebook of studies in which the characteristics of the community are of primary rather than incidental interest. The social, economic, demographic, and physical attributes of Alameda County are independent variables which, together, constitute the ways of life to be investigated. The fact that several distinctly different ways of life are represented in Alameda County was appreciated by the investigators when the population laboratory was established. The selection of this community was, therefore, more than a simple matter of convenience.

2. While many questions on health were asked, no ascertainment was made of the prevalence of disease from sources other than the respondents themselves. Thus, perceptions of illness, rather than diagnosed diseases, were actually studied. We would hope that it might become possible to link the meticulously collected social data of Alameda County to objectively ascertained medical data. This would be of great value in validating the health responses, in distinguishing between perceptions and diagnoses of illness, and in detailing the relationships between health and ways of living. Checking the consistency of the "physical health spectrum" variable, as was done with data from the Kaiser Foundation Health Plan, represents a step in this direction.

3. The author's analysis of responses by ethnic group suggests that personal interviews were especially important in obtaining information from Negroes and Mexican-Americans. This may help to explain the difficulties encountered in Puerto Rico and Colombia with the use of survey instruments originally designed for studies in the United States.

CHAPTER 8

At a time when the social and behavioral aspects of illness have become subjects of growing concern, new methods for their investigation are being developed. The population of one ethnically heterogeneous district of Manhattan was sampled and interviewed on a large variety of health-related matters. An interesting feature of the Master Sample Survey is the provision for mutually beneficial collaboration between extramural research groups utilizing survey data and the permanent survey staff.

THE WASHINGTON HEIGHTS, NEW YORK CITY, COMMUNITY MASTER SAMPLE SURVEY

Paul W. Haberman

INTRODUCTION*

The Washington Heights Community Master Sample Survey was developed as a human population laboratory in response to the needs of a number of health research and service groups of the Columbia–Presbyterian Medical Center, the largest medical care facility in Washington Heights. The rationale for its development was largely practical. Many of the problem areas in sociomedical research can be approached only by large-scale community surveys which tend to be expensive and difficult to organize and administer. The availability of a permanent community survey core staff makes it possible for investigators to pursue their substantive research interests while being spared many burdens of organization and administration. Another advantage of this approach is that variables of interest to one researcher are often of interest to others working on related problems. For example, survey data relating to mental illness have proven useful in studies of alcoholism as well.

* Adapted in part from Gell and Elinson (1969).

177

The concentration of many studies in one geographically defined area and the existence of a permanent research staff also makes possible methodological investigation of the sample survey process itself. At a time when community studies are growing in number and significance this is a matter of considerable importance. Such problems as nonresponse bias, interviewer-respondent interaction, and response reliability and validity have already been examined by the Master Sample Survey staff.

Community surveys may also yield benefits in the planning and organization of community health services. Baselines can be established for the prevalence of various levels of disease-related disability, and the effectiveness of health services directed at these disabilities can be evaluated in the sampled population. No such assessments of the quality of community health services have yet been undertaken in Washington Heights.

More than 30 publications based upon the Master Sample Survey have already appeared in the literature. There have been two major foci of attention: (1) the role of socioeconomic status and ethnoreligious background in responses to illness and health services; and (2) the prevalence of untreated social pathology—mental illness, alcoholism, family disruption, etc.—in the community. In addition to these studies and to the methodological studies previously mentioned, the Master Sample Survey has also led to the development of various sociomedical indices and screening scores which are of general use in the field. Numerous civic and governmental bodies, such as city planning commissions, police and school departments, and religious and ethnic groups, have expressed interest in the community data generated by the sample survey. As a service to them, a handbook, now in its second edition, has been prepared (Elinson and Loewenstein 1963; Elinson, Haberman, and Gell 1968).

THE COMMUNITY

Location

New York City is divided into 30 Health Districts, each of which is subdivided into units known as health areas. While natural population groups and topographic boundaries were originally taken into consideration in these divisions, the health area boundaries now coincide with those of the census tracts. Comparable census and statistical data can thus be compiled by health areas and health districts.

The Washington Heights Health District is an administrative unit of the New York City Department of Health, located in the northwestern section of the borough of Manhattan (Figure 8–1). It extends nearly five miles from 134th Street northward to the end of Manhattan; and from the Hudson River, about one and one half miles at its widest point, to an eastern boundary along St. Nicholas and Bradhurst Avenues and the Harlem River. The Riverside Health District, which includes the main campus of Columbia University, is immediately to the south. The Central Harlem Health District is directly east of the southern part of Washington Heights. Numerous bridges on the north and east connect Washington Heights with the Bronx. On the west, the George Washington Bridge spans the Hudson River between Washington Heights and suburban Bergen County in northeastern New Jersey.

Figure 8–1. Washington Heights Health District, health areas—1960.

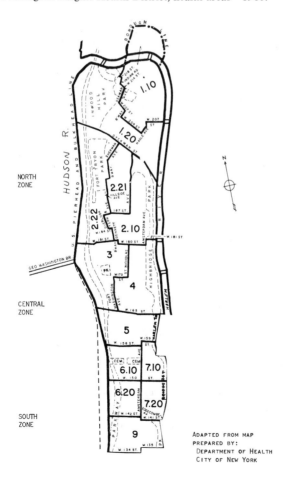

There are 13 health areas within the Washington Heights Health District. Because of the varying needs of investigators participating in the Master Sample Survey, the health district was divided into three zones which had boundaries coinciding with those of the health areas. The central zone, covering the area from 150th to 181st Streets, contains the Columbia–Presbyterian Medical Center and has been designated by the Columbia–Washington Heights Community Mental Health Project as a possible catchment area for future service programs. The south zone extends from 134th to 150th Streets, and the north zone from 181st Street to the borough line between Manhattan and the Bronx at 228th Street.

Demographic Characteristics

Washington Heights is essentially an urban residential area, with approximately 270,000 people and 100,000 dwelling units according to the 1960 U.S. Census. The social class range is, for the most part, from upper-lower to upper-middle class. As is the case with many other sections of New York City and other urban areas, Washington Heights is a community more or less in transition from middle to lower class. By 1960 the lower class area had become predominant.

The largest ethnoreligious groups are Jewish, Negro, Irish, and Puerto Rican. In 1960 Jews and Negroes each accounted for about one-quarter of the population in the health district. The Irish and Jewish are the older residents while the Negroes and Puerto Ricans are younger and newer arrivals. The proportion of Jews has declined, reflecting their exodus from Washington Heights and, in view of their relatively older ages, a higher mortality rate. At the same time there has been an increase in the proportion of Negroes and Puerto Ricans (Table 8–1) as well as persons from Cuba and the Dominican Republic. Compared with New York City as a whole, Washington Heights has more Negroes and Irish, fewer Italians, and similar proportions of Jews and Puerto Ricans.

Of the surveyed population, 18.4 per cent were less than 15 years old, 13.7 per cent were 65 years or older and the median age was 40.1 years. There were proportionally more persons (23.9 per cent) under 15 years and fewer (10.5 per cent) 65 years and over than in all of New York City, which had a median age of 35.1 years. The median size of a household in Washington Heights (2.6 persons) was slightly smaller than in the whole city (2.9 persons).

During the year preceding the Sample Survey the median family income in Washington Heights was $4,678, with a median per capita income of $1,799. More than one-quarter (28.2 per cent) of the families had an annual income of less than $3,000. The median education completed by persons twenty-five years or older was 11.2 years. Citywide, the median family income ($6,091) and the median per capita income ($2,100) were considerably higher, but the median years of education completed by persons twenty-five years or older (10.1 years) was lower.

Almost half (49.1 per cent) of the heads of families had lived at the same address for ten years or more prior to the Survey, while 9.7 per cent had moved within the past year. Eighty-five per cent of the heads of families had lived in New York City at least ten years, including 20.9 per cent who were born there. On the other hand, 39.1 per cent of all persons, and 47.3 per cent of the heads of families, were born outside of the United States. Residential mobility has been increasing in Washington Heights in recent years, in part reflecting the accelerated transition from middle to lower class character.

TABLE 8–1. POPULATION TRENDS 1930–60: WASHINGTON HEIGHTS HEALTH DISTRICT, BY ZONES

	Census year			
	1930	1940	1950	1960
Washington Heights Health District				
Total population	259,551	308,485	297,342	269,277
% Change	—	+18.9	−3.6[b]	−9.4
% Nonwhite[a]	11.2	13.5	20.9	24.1
% Puerto Rican[a]	—	—	4.3	8.4
North zone				
Total population	86,201	109,452	115,914	114,897
% Change	—	+27.0	+5.9	−0.9
% Nonwhite	0.9	0.6	0.5	3.5
% Puerto Rican	—	—	5.5	3.1
Central zone				
Total population	111,604	127,804	120,402	99,079
% Change	—	+14.5	−5.8[c]	−17.7
% Nonwhite	8.9	12.9	25.2	29.5
% Puerto Rican	—	—	4.3	10.0
South zone				
Total population	61,746	71,193	61,026	55,301
% Change	—	+15.3	−14.3[b]	−9.4
% Nonwhite	29.6	34.4	51.3	57.5
% Puerto Rican	—	—	2.0	16.5

[a] Nonwhite and Puerto Rican are not mutually exclusive. Approximately 1 per cent of Puerto Ricans herein are classified as nonwhites. Puerto Ricans are persons born in Puerto Rico and persons with at least one parent born in Puerto Rico.

[b] Decrease in population due entirely to revision of district boundaries in 1950. Reassigned population 99.4 per cent nonwhite.

[c] Half of decrease in central zone due to revision of boundary lines in 1950.

Source: U.S. Decennial Censuses, 1930–60.

Medical Facilities

The Columbia–Presbyterian Medical Center, New York City's largest voluntary hospital, is located in the central zone of the Washington Heights Health District. A district health center of the City Department of Health and the New York State Psychiatric Institute are among 12 hospitals and 10 other health facilities in the district.

METHODS

The primary aim of this project, as stated in the original proposal, is "to facilitate research on community health problems by developing and establishing a Master Sample Survey of a population living in a geographically defined area of New York City." With this in mind, operations have been set up in such a manner as to provide investigators with the opportunity to do community health research at minimal cost in time, money, and effort.

Sources of Data

The principal means of data collection employed in the Master Sample Survey was a household interview schedule or Family Form (See Appendix) containing questions about demographic, sociological, and health characteristics of all family members. Interviews conducted in selected dwelling units ("patterns cases") also included items on health services and patterns of referrals for medical care during the previous year. The units of analysis were families and family members. The informant was an adult who reported about all members of each sampled household.

Interviews were conducted in the home, usually with the wife as informant. Wives tend to be more accessible and, perhaps more knowledgeable about the health of family members. If the wife was not available, another responsible adult family member was interviewed but the informants were not randomized. It should be noted that about one-third of the households comprised a single adult who necessarily provided the information about himself.

Other primary means of data collection were questionnaires dealing with social factors in health behavior and attitudes and, for a subsample of adults in patterns cases households, interviews on psychophysiological symptoms and interpersonal relations. In addition, specific information was asked about all women who completed pregnancies in the preceding 24 months and about the health status of all children under age seven years. Survey reinterviews were conducted on subsamples of persons having selected characteristics, e.g., persons reporting an episode of serious illness in the preceding two months, problem drinkers, and persons with particular demographic characteristics.

Sampling Plan*

In designing the sampling plan for the Master Sample Survey, the following characteristics were considered desirable:

1. The design should permit the conduct of cross-sectional as well as longitudinal studies of both retrospective and prospective types.
2. The design should incorporate probability methods which permit the calculation of sampling errors.
3. The sample should be chosen on the basis of dwelling units. This is advantageous, first, because a sample of dwelling units is likely to remain valid for a number of years, especially if it is kept up-to-date, e.g., by sampling new construction. It has the additional advantage of permitting the study of meaningful subunits, such as heads of household, adult members, pregnant women, etc.
4. A minimum number of dwelling units should be drawn from any given residential structure in any subsample. This has the effect of increasing the statistical efficiency of the sample and minimizing interaction among respondents.
5. The sample should be self-weighting. That is, sample means and proportions should, without further weighting, provide estimates of the corresponding parameters for the universe, defined here as all persons residing in dwelling units in the Washington Heights Health District.

With these characteristics in mind, a stratified, two-stage cluster design was developed to yield a sample of 6,000 dwelling units out of the 100,000 or so in Washington Heights. The choice of design was complicated by the varying research needs of the participating investigators: some required a representative sample of the entire district, while others desired a sample of the central zone alone. The total of 6,000 sampled dwelling units included 4,000 from the central zone and 2,000 from the north and south zones combined. Although this did not comprise a self-weighting sample of any area, it could (after appropriate weighting) be used to represent the entire Washington Heights Health District.

* Adapted in part from Gell and Elinson (1969).

Ten sample strata were defined by geographical location (zone), average rent, and racial composition according to the 1950 U.S. Census. Clusters within these strata had an average of 50 dwelling units in the central zone and 100 in the north and south zones. First-stage sampling fractions for clusters within strata and second-stage sampling fractions for dwelling units within clusters were fixed so that the over-all sampling fraction for each stratum was 12 per cent in the central zone and 3 per cent in the north and south zones.

Limitations of time and money forced a reduction in the number of sampled dwelling units from 6,000 to 4,500. Sampling losses due to vacancies and demolition further reduced the number of units to 4,362, of which 3,329 (76 per cent) yielded interviews during 6 months of field work in 1960–61.

In order to reduce the nonresponse rate, one-third of the dwelling units not successfully interviewed were randomly selected for an intensive second effort: interviews in 210 additional units were obtained. These were assumed to be representative of all initial nonrespondents and were assigned a triple weight. The final weighted total of 3,959 dwelling units represented 91 per cent of the total eligible. These dwelling units contained 4,393 families and a total of 10,763 persons.

Sample Size and Composition*

In order to obtain a self-weighting representative sample of the entire health district, all dwelling units in the north and south zones and a 28 per cent random sample of those in the central zone were classified as patterns cases and designated for interviews on patterns of medical care. Interviews were obtained from 1,762 dwelling units representing 2,216 families and 5,344 persons. The patterns cases comprise self-weighting samples of each of the three zones, but the sample design precludes inferences specific to health area or smaller geographic subdivisions.

A comparison of the demographic information obtained from the Master Sample Survey and from the 1960 U.S. Census suggests that the sample is representative of Washington Heights in regard to the variables examined (Table 8–2). There were virtually no differences between the sample and the census populations with respect to sex, race, or age distribution. However, the sample had somewhat smaller proportions of persons reporting less than a high school education and of families with two or more persons reporting incomes of $6,000 and over. There was also a slightly larger proportion of blue collar workers among the sampled women.

* Adapted in part from Gell and Elinson (1969).

TABLE 8–2. DEMOGRAPHIC DATA FOR WASHINGTON HEIGHTS HEALTH DISTRICT, 1960–61, OBTAINED FROM MASTER SAMPLE SURVEY AND U.S. CENSUS

Demographic data, 1960–61	Master Sample Survey (patterns cases)	1960 U.S. Census (entire district)
Sex and race	(N = 5,344)	(N = 269,277)
All persons	*100%*	*100%*
White males	34.4	35.2
Nonwhite males	10.9	10.8
White females	41.0	40.7
Nonwhite females	13.8	13.3
Age at last birthday	(N = 5,344)	(N = 269,277)
All persons	*100%*	*100%*
Under 15 years	18.4	18.2
15 to 44 years	38.1	38.2
45 to 64 years	29.8	30.7
65 years and over	13.7	12.9
Median years of age	40.1 yrs.	40.4 yrs.
Education of persons 25 years and over	(N = 3,567)	(N = 189,644)
All persons 25 years and over	*100%*	*100%*
Grade school or none	35.7	39.8
Some high school	20.1	18.8
High school graduate	25.8	25.4
Some college or more	18.4	16.0
Median years of education	11.2 yrs.	10.6 yrs.
Family income for families of 2 or more persons[a]	(N = 1,370)	(N = 74,879)
All families with 2 or more persons	*100%*	*100%*
Under $4,000	26.6	26.1
$4,000 to $5,999	30.3	26.1
$6,000 to $9,999	32.1	33.5
$10,000 or more	11.1	14.3
Median family income	$5,547	$5,842

Occupation by sex	Males (N = 1,515)	Females (N = 1,176)	Males (N = 71,106)	Females (N = 52,252)
All persons reporting occupation[b]	*100%*	*100%*	*100%*	*100%*
Professional & technical workers; managers, officials, & proprietors	23.1	13.2	23.0	16.2
Clerical & sales workers	23.6	35.4	23.2	39.6
Craftsmen, foremen, & operatives	33.7	27.7	32.3	23.6
Service workers & laborers	19.7	23.6	21.5	20.5

[a] Family income for preceding year from all sources and before taxes.
[b] Persons sixteen years and over in Master Sample Survey, persons fourteen years and over in census.
Source: Elinson and Loewenstein (1963).

A self-weighting sample of persons twenty-one years of age and older in the Washington Heights Health District was developed by selecting a 60 per cent random sample of adults in patterns cases households. The 1,713 persons (1,883 after the addition of weighted cases from the one-third sample of second-effort interviews) who were interviewed are designated as "patterns respondents."

Those dwelling units in the central zone which had not been identified as patterns cases were designated as "non-patterns cases" and were interviewed in order to obtain a larger sample in the area adjacent to the Columbia–Presbyterian Medical Center. (Table 8–3). Interviews were obtained from 1,777 dwelling units in the nonpatterns sample, representing 2,177 families and 5,419 persons. It should be noted that the patterns and nonpatterns cases together do not comprise a self-weighting sample of the health district. Weights of 0.36 for the central zone and 0.64 for the north and south zones must be applied for this purpose. The various population samples which were interviewed in the Master Sample Survey of 1960–61 are shown in Table 8–4.

TABLE 8–3. RESPONSES TO INTERVIEW ATTEMPTS IN THE MASTER SAMPLE SURVEY, 1960–61

Housing units	Total cases	Patterns cases	Nonpatterns cases
Number selected	4,500	2,310	2,190
Sampling losses	−138	−68	−70
A) Eligible	4,362	2,242	2,120
B) Interviewed, 1st effort	3,329	1,636	1,693
C) Interviewed, 2nd effort	210	126	84
(from one-third sample of A–B)			
D) Not interviewed	823	480	343
Weighted response rate = $\dfrac{B + 3C}{A} \times 100$	90.8%	89.8%	91.7%

Interviews	Total cases		Patterns cases		Nonpatterns cases	
	Families	Persons	Families	Persons	Families	Persons
Interviewed, 1st effort						
A) Primary families	3,329	8,737	1,636	4,229	1,693	4,508
B) Additional roomers	377	463	169	215	208	248
Interviewed, 2nd effort						
C) Primary families	210	494	126	288	84	206
D) Additional roomers	19	27	11	12	8	15
Weighted total = $(A + B) + 3(C + D)$	4,393	10,763	2,216	5,344	2,177	5,419

TABLE 8–4. COMPOSITION OF SAMPLES INTERVIEWED IN THE MASTER SAMPLE SURVEY, 1960–61

Sample	No. of persons[a]	No. of families	Description
Total	10,763	4,393	Not a self-weighting sample; to compute rates for the entire district weight central zone cases by 0.356, and north and south zone cases by 0.644; includes triple-weighted cases
Patterns cases	5,344	2,216	Self-weighting sample of the district and each of its three zones.
Patterns respondents	1,883	—	Random sample of 60% of adults in patterns cases families
Central zone sample	5,419	2,177	Self-weighting sample of central zone only.

[a] Weighted as described in text.

A second household survey conducted in 1965–66 made it possible to study a number of demographic trends over time in the Washington Heights Health District (Elinson, Haberman, and Gell 1968).

PROBLEMS

The Master Sample Survey, like urban surveys in general, has experienced difficulties in the field because of the increasing reluctance of people to participate in surveys. This stems, perhaps, from a heightened desire for privacy or from the simple fear of opening doors to strangers. Another problem is exemplified by the regular underenumeration in the U.S. Census of adult Negro males in low income urban areas despite the legal constraints on nonrespondents.

Nonresponse and Response Bias

Nonresponse is a potentially serious problem which is sometimes dealt with by making additional efforts to interview nonrespondents. An assessment of the value of such additional efforts was made by comparing the frequency distributions of some 200 variables of interest in 2 subsamples of the Master Sample Survey: one which showed a 30 per cent nonresponse rate after a single interview effort and another in which the nonresponse had been reduced to 10 per cent by intensive additional effort (Loewenstein, Colombotas, and Elinson 1962). Differences between the subsamples in the distribution of the study variables were very few: for only 15 variables were there category differences as great as 3 per cent. These findings suggest that little bias has been introduced into the survey by virtue of nonresponse.

The relative roles of interviewers and subjects in nonresponse were investigated by reinterviewing a subsample of respondents having certain demographic characteristics (Dohrenwend and Dohrenwend 1968). That interview refusal is, at least in part, a function of the respondent was evident, since respondents who were unco-operative for some time before granting an interview were twice as likely as others to refuse reinterview. Refusal rates were significantly higher among older respondents and differed markedly among ethnic groups, being highest among the Irish. The role of the interviewer is shown by the successful completion of reinterviews after initial refusals when alternate interviewers were employed, and by the disproportion of randomly assigned respondents who were rated hostile or who refused to co-operate with particular interviewers. The respondent is responsible for some refusals, the interviewer for others.

The evidence suggests that nonresponse occurs when there is disparity in social status between interviewer and respondent. White, middle-class interviewers holding negative attitudes toward lower class persons tend to bias the answers of Negroes and of white lower class respondents more than do interviewers without negative attitudes (Dohrenwend, Colombotas, and Dohrenwend 1968). Interviewers may also bias the responses of respondents who have social status and personal characteristics similar to their own by conducting the interview on a personal, rather than a strictly professional basis and becoming embarrassed about asking certain questions. This hypothesis was tested by asking interviewers whether any questions had embarrassed them and whether they preferred to interview rich people or poor, whites or Negroes, and young or old persons. Their replies suggested that interview responses may be biased by the interviewer if there is too little or too much social distance between the interviewer and the respondent.

Women usually predominate in the field staffs of survey research organizations, in part because of their greater availability for part-time work such as interviewing. The possible effect of the interviewer's sex on one aspect of the survey data, viz., reporting of psychiatric symptoms (Langner 1962) was investigated. No significant differences were found in the reporting of psychiatric symptoms to male or female interviewers by respondents. This suggests that rationales commonly employed in hiring male or female interviewers need re-examination (Colombotos, Elinson, and Loewenstein 1968).

Response Reliability and Validity

Reliability and validity of interview responses are of crucial importance in community surveys. A number of variables in the Master Sample Survey were subjected to analysis in these terms. Information about level of education was obtained from all adults in the Master Sample Survey and from a subsample reinterviewed about three years later. Educational level, classified into eight categories, was inconsistently reported by 37.9 per cent of the subsample. The degree of inconsistency was the same whether respondents reported for themselves both times or only in the reinterview situation (where each respondent was interviewed separately). Since the inconsistencies were rather evenly divided in both directions (upgrading and downgrading), the over-all frequency distributions of reported educational level showed little variation between the two surveys. Inconsistent responses occurred more often among older respondents, perhaps reflecting their diminishing accuracy of recall over time. Mis-statements were also more frequent among males, and most of the inconsistencies concerned only one educational level. By collapsing the number of educational categories from eight to three, the response variance between the two surveys was reduced from 37.9 to 21.1 per cent (Haberman and Sheinberg 1966). In contrast, the reporting of age was consistent to within one year among 87.7 per cent of the respondents.

From an epidemiologic point of view, a major problem in household morbidity studies has been the low degree of correspondence between interview response and the results of clinical evaluation or physical examination. This error is compounded in the case of socially unacceptable conditions, such as alcoholism, drug addiction, or venereal disease, which are often denied or concealed, resulting in serious underestimations. Evidence of such underreporting of alcoholism or problem drinking was obtained from an independent check on Master Sample Survey responses (Bailey, Haberman, and Alksne 1965), from reinterviews with Master Sample Survey respondents who were supposedly nonalcoholics (Bailey, Haberman, and Sheinberg 1966), and from a study of respondents denying a drinking problem who showed gross drinking or who admitted it outside the context of the survey (Haberman 1963).

Illustrative findings from the alcoholism studies are as follows:

1. Of the 13 Master Sample Survey cases with a primary or secondary diagnosis of alcoholism, or a history of intemperate drinking from the records of various mental hospitals in New York and

Bellevue Hospital, only 6 were acknowledged by the family informant to have a drinking problem (Bailey, Haberman, and Alksne 1965).

2. Of 343 presumed nonalcoholics matched with the alcoholics on sociocultural variables, 29 (8.5 per cent) admitted drinking difficulties on reinterview three years later. In all except one of these cases the time of onset of the alcoholism preceded the first interview (Bailey, Haberman, and Sheinberg 1966).

3. Interviewer observation rather than questionnaire responses accounted for one-quarter of the 132 respondents initially identified as probable alcoholics in the 1960–61 survey (Haberman 1963).

Considerable variation in the consistency or accuracy of survey responses was also noted with regard to retest scores on psychophysiological symptomatology (Haberman 1965a), marital happiness (Mayer 1966c) and reported body weight (Perry, Learnard and Schweitzer 1963).

The distribution of scores on 22 psychophysiological symptoms (Langner 1962) for a subsample of survey respondents reinterviewed after 3 years was quite consistent over the 2 periods, with the later scores being slightly higher. Despite the over-all comparability of the two scores, however, there was considerable variation among respondents which appeared to be related to the presence or absence of stressful situations. To an appreciable extent these personal stresses encompass current and temporary conditions rather than chronic disturbances (Haberman 1965a).

In reinterviews of married women, comparisons were made between the wife's rating of her marriage and the interviewer's rating. The respondent and interviewer gave the same rating (on a six-point scale) in only one-third of 81 cases. The interviewer rated the respondent's marriage lower in 58.0 per cent of the cases and higher in only 8.6 per cent. Thus, interviewers were seven times more likely to downgrade a marriage than to upgrade it. This tendency was observed in each of the seven interviewers in the survey (Mayer 1966c).

Body build, a subject of considerable epidemiologic interest, was also investigated in the Master Sample Survey. A random subsample of 400 households with at least 2 eligible adults was selected, and each subject was asked about his own age, height, and weight and those of a second subject in the household. After questioning, both subjects were weighed and height and skinfold thickness were measured. The correlation between self-reported and scale weight was very high (R=0.90) in the total sample. Women and younger persons tended to report more accurately. There was also a very high correlation between reported weights and scale weights for second subjects in the household. It may be concluded that reported weight, including that obtained from a second household source, can be substituted for actual scale weight in populations such as that of the subsample studied (Perry, Learnard, and Schweitzer 1963).

FINDINGS

Studies on Illness and Medical Care

A collaborating research group from the New York City Health Department studied the patterns in which the sampled Washington Heights population sought and received medical care. Their study variables included symptoms of illness, behavioral patterns when ill, utilization of health services, patterns of referral for medical care, attitudes toward interpersonal relationships, and social group memberships.

Klem (1965) investigated data on Washington Heights health insurance coverage and physicians' services shopped for and received. She found that 65 per cent of all patients and 84 per cent of all attended conditions received medical attention from only one physician, usually the family physician. Among persons sixty-five years of age and older there was almost no difference in physician's care received between those with and without insurance coverage.

Suchman and Rothman (1965) studied the use of dental care services and found a positive association between socioeconomic status and utilization of dental facilities as well as substantial differences among ethnic groups. This led to their development of a sociological hypothesis to explain the relationship between dental care and sociocultural factors on the basis of membership in "parochial" or "cosmopolitan" social groups.

Different ethnic groups showed significant variability in knowledge about disease, attitudes toward medical care, and behavior during illness which was found to be related to the form of social organization within the ethnic group (Suchman 1964; 1965b). The form of social organization was found to be more important than either ethnicity or social class in relation to medical care orientation. Members of ethnocentric and socially cohesive ("parochial") groups tended to display less knowledge about disease, skepticism toward professional medical care, and dependency during illness. On the other hand, members of "cosmopolitan" groups were more apt to have a scientific health orientation.

The sociomedical sophistication of survey respondents was correlated with their social class and ethnic group membership. Each of these factors, in turn, was found to be related to symbols of the physician's social status, including the appearance of his office and its location (Rosenblatt and Suchman 1966).

In another study a subsample of survey respondents reporting a serious illness in the preceding two months was intensively reinterviewed as to initial symptoms, deliberations and decisions on seeking medical care, hospitalization, convalescence, and attitudes and behavior while ill (Suchman 1965c; 1966).

Studies on Alcoholism

A participating research group from the National Council on Alcoholism used the Master Sample Survey to estimate the prevalence and distribution of family problems related to alcoholism in an urban community. Their data included information on personal and family difficulties associated with excessive drinking as well as interviewer observation of problem drinkers as described above (see Problems). The over-all alcoholism rate in the Master Sample Survey was 19 per 1,000 with a ratio of 3.6 men to one woman and an increased prevalence in the lower socioeconomic groups (Bailey, Haberman, and Alksne 1965). The alcoholics revealed evidence of emotional strain and impairment by various psychological measures, especially as regards guilt and depression. The findings would seem to be applicable to urban, noninstitutionalized alcoholics who are still functioning in the community but who are socioeconomically and psychologically vulnerable.

A follow-up study of alcoholics, comparison group persons, and their respective spouses was also undertaken. The two comparison groups consisted of persons reported in the Master Sample Survey to have stomach ulcers or some other chronic stomach trouble and persons without either a drinking problem or chronic stomach trouble who were matched with the alcoholics on sex, age, marital and family status, education, and ethnic group. This study differed from previous ones in that the alcoholic subjects were selected from a community at large rather than from a specific clinic, social agency, or skid row. Unfortunately, reinterviews indicate that a number of control respondents had been misclassified as nonalcoholic (Bailey, Haberman, and Sheinberg 1966).

The alcoholics and their families were compared with the control groups on marital interaction (Sheinberg, Bailey, and Haberman 1969), psychological symptoms (Haberman 1965b), and childhood symptoms in respondents' children (Haberman 1966). Many more signs of disturbance were noted among the alcoholics and their families than in the comparison groups. A subsample of the alcoholics who had reported reduced and moderate drinking at the time of the first reinterview were followed up, together with their spouses, in a third round of interviews. Half of the 12 subjects were judged to have developed the ability to drink within normal limits (Bailey and Stewart 1967).

Other Studies

Requests are frequently received from investigators who wish to utilize Master Sample Survey subsamples in their research. For example, the Institute of Welfare Research of the Community Service Society of New York was interested in reinterviewing a subsample of women who were white, native-born, from fifteen to forty-four years of age, currently married for the first time, and classified as lower or middle class according to education and their husbands' occupation. The availability of the Master Sample Survey provided a list from which a subsample with these demographic specifications could be selected.

Among the questions explored were the differences between working and middle class wives in the extent to which they reveal their marital difficulties and in the persons to whom they confide. The data suggested that persons with whom a middle class wife talks gain a more complete picture of her difficulties than a comparable group of confidants in lower class circles. In the middle class, friends and relatives are apt to be equally knowledgeable about the wife's difficulties, whereas in the lower class, relatives are more likely to be knowledgeable about such difficulties than friends. Moreover, the middle class husband's relatives are more likely to be knowledgeable about the wife's difficulties than comparable relatives within the lower class (Mayer 1966a; 1967b).

Other studies based on the Master Sample Survey include investigations on congenital neurological disease and cardiovascular diseases. Both of these studies were conducted by research groups in the Columbia University School of Public Health and Administrative Medicine.

Second-Wave Household Survey

Two different methodologic approaches to the collection of data on utilization and costs of health care services were investigated in the second wave of the household survey (1965–66). In the first, interviewers inquired about services and charges by each medical facility used for each reported medical condition during the previous year. In the second, interviewers asked about services and charges by each reported facility irrespective of medical condition. The findings are currently undergoing analysis.

The other two participating research groups, from the Columbia University School of Public Health, are concerned with respondents' perceptions of selected mental health items and with the relations of the health of children to their environment. Subsamples of the 3,805 persons living in Master Sample Survey households have been reinterviewed to test the usefulness of community surveys for estimating the incidence of abortions and to explore the social, emotional, and physical problems of adolescents.

Core Staff Activities

In collaboration with the New York Community Mental Health Board, the survey core staff also developed and carried out a city-wide survey of the "Public Image of Mental Health Services" in New York City (Elinson, Padella, and Perkins 1967). In addition, a step-by-step account of the Master Sample Survey has served as the basis of a research training seminar for Ph.D. students at the School of Public Health. Selected aspects of the Master Sample Survey have also been considered in other doctoral-level seminars at the School.

POTENTIAL

The greatest potential of the Master Sample Survey which has yet to be realized lies in its use in the planning, organization, and evaluation of health care services. At present, medical and hospital services in Washington Heights are not well organized to meet the needs of the local population, except for the Columbia–Washington Heights community mental health program and the clinics in the district health center of the New York City Health Department.

As part of the recent affiliation between Columbia University and the Harlem Hospital Center, a patient care and program evaluation unit has been developed. In contrast to the Master Sample Survey, the main objective of this unit is to assess the impact of the Harlem Hospital Center on the health of the people of Harlem. Toward this end organizational and methodologic features of the Master Sample Survey are being examined and adapted.

The existing data of the Washington Heights Master Sample Survey, have not been fully utilized. The data are permanently stored in research archives at the Columbia University School of Public Health and Administrative Medicine and are available to qualified investigators with the permission of the original investigators. As a member of the Council of Social Science Data Archives, the Columbia University School of Public Health and Administrative Medicine Research Archives also exchanges information with other council members about other data sources and analytic methods.

Acknowledgments

The Master Sample Survey is supported by a grant from the Health Research Council of the City of New York, Contract Number U-1053, to Columbia University School of Public Health and Administrative Medicine, Jack Elinson, Ph.D., principal investigator. Several of the studies reported here were supported by U.S. Public Health Service Grant No. CH-00128 and Health Research Council Contract No. U-1318.

*References**

Bailey, M. B., Haberman, P. W., and Alksne, H. 1965. The epidemiology of alcoholism in an urban residential area. *Quart. J. Stud. Alcohol* 26:19–40.

Bailey, M. B., Haberman, P. W., and Sheinberg, J. 1966. Identifying alcoholics in population surveys: A report on reliability. *Quart. J. Stud. Alcohol* 27:300–15.

Bailey, M. B. and Stewart, J. 1967. Normal drinking by persons reporting previous problem drinking. *Quart. J. Stud. Alcohol* 28:305–15.

Colombotas, J., Elinson, J., and Loewenstein, R. 1968. Effect of interviewers' sex on interview responses. *Public Health Rep.* 83:685–90.

Crandell, DeW. L. and Dohrenwend, B. P. 1967. Some relations among psychiatric symptoms, organic illness, and social class. *Am. J. Psychiat.* 123:1527–38.

Dohrenwend, B. P. 1966. Social status and psychological disorder: An issue of substance and an issue of method. *Am. Soc. Rev.* 31:14–34.

Dohrenwend, B. S. 1967. Social status, stress, and psychological symptoms. *Am. J. Public Health* 57:625–32.

Dohrenwend, B. S. and Dohrenwend, B. P. 1966. Stress situations, birth order, and psychological symptoms. *J. Abnorm. Psychol.* 71:215–23.

———. 1968. Sources of refusals in surveys. *Public Opinion Quart.* 32:74–83.

Dohrenwend, B. S., Colombotas, J., and Dohrenwend, B. P. 1968. Social distance and interviewer effects. *Public Opinion Quart.* 32:410–22.

Dohrenwend, B. P. and Chin-Shong, E. 1967. Social status and attitudes toward psychological disorder: The problem of tolerance of deviance. *Am. Soc. Rev.* 32:417–33.

Elinson, J. and Loewenstein, R. 1963. *Community Fact Book for Washington Heights, New York City, 1960–61.* Columbia University School of Public Health and Administrative Medicine. (Processed.)

Elinson, J., Haberman, P. W. and Gell, C. 1968. *Community Fact Book for Washington Heights, New York City, 1965–66 and 1960–61.* Columbia University School of Public Health and Administrative Medicine. (Processed.)

---

* Includes publications based on Master Sample Survey which have not been referenced in this chapter.

Elinson, J., Padilla, E., and Perkins, M. E. 1967. *Public Image of Mental Health Services, New York City.* Mental Health Materials Center for New York City Community Mental Health Board. (Processed.)

Gell, C. and Elinson, J. eds. 1969. Washington Heights master sample survey. *Milbank Mem. Fund Quart.* 47:1–308.

Haberman, P. W. 1963. Differences between families admitting and denying an existing drinking problem. *J. Health Hum. Behav.* 4:141–45.

———. 1965*a*. An analysis of retest scores for an index of psycho-physiological disturbance. *J. Health Hum. Behav.* 6:257–60.

———. 1965*b*. Psychophysiological symptoms in alcoholics and matched comparison persons. *Community Ment. Health J.* 1:361–64.

———. 1966. Childhood symptoms in children of alcoholics and comparison group parents. *J. Marriage Family* 28:152–54.

Haberman, P. W. and Sheinberg, J. 1966. Education reported in interviews: An aspect of survey content error. *Public Opinion Quart.* 30:295–301.

———. 1967. Implicative drinking reported in a household survey: A corroborative note on subgroup differences. *Quart. J. Stud. Alcohol* 38:538–43.

Klem, M. C. 1965. Physician services received in an urban community in relation to health insurance coverage. *Am. J. Public Health* 55:1699–716.

Kolb, L. C., Bernard, V. W., and Dohrenwend, B. P. eds. 1969. *Urban Challenges to Psychiatry.* Boston: Little, Brown and Co.

Langner, T. S. 1962. A twenty-two item score of psychiatric symptoms indicating impairment. *J. Health Hum. Behav.* 3:269–76.

Lendt, L. A. 1960. *A Social History of Washington Heights, New York City, Columbia-Washington Heights Community Mental Health Project, Columbia University.* (Processed.)

Loewenstein, R., Colombotas, J. and Elinson, J. 1962. Interviews hardest-to-obtain in an urban health survey. *American Statistical Association. Proceedings of the Social Statistics Section, 1961,* pp. 160–66. Washington: American Statistical Association.

Loewenstein, R. and Elinson, J. 1964. Sampling variation of age-adjusted rates. *American Statistical Association. Proceedings of the Social Statistics Section, 1964,* pp. 9–15. Washington: American Statistical Association.

Mayer, J. E. 1966*a*. *The Disclosure of Marital Problems: An Exploratory Study of Lower and Middle Class Wives.* Institute of Welfare Research, Community Service Society of New York. (Processed.)

———. 1966*b*. *Other People's Marital Problems: The "Knowledgeability" of Lower and Middle Class Wives.* Institute of Welfare Research, Community Service Society of New York. (Processed.)

———. 1966*c*. Marital happiness appraised by self, friends, and interviewers. *Public Opinion Quart.* 30:454–55.

———. 1967*a*. The invisibility of married life. *New Society* (London) 9:272–73.

———. 1967*b*. Disclosing marital problems. *Soc. Casework* 48:342–51.

Perry, L. S., Learnard, B. A., and Schweitzer, M. D. 1963. Accuracy of reports of body weight. *Circulation*, 28:668–69.

Rosenblatt, D. and Suchman, E. A. 1964. Blue collar attitudes and information toward health and illness. In *Blue Collar World*. Edited by A. Shostak and W. Gomberg, pp. 324–33. Englewood Cliffs: Prentice-Hall.

————. 1966. Awareness of physician's social status within an urban community. *J. Health and Hum. Behav.* 7:146–53.

Sheinberg, J., Bailey, M. B., and Haberman, P. W. 1969. The alcoholic family: Marital interaction in the conjugal family. *Milbank Mem. Fund Quart.* 47:168–74.

Srole, L., Langner, T. S., Michael, S. T., Opler, M. K., and Rennie, T. A. C. 1962. *Mental Health in the Metropolis: The Midtown Manhattan Study*; *Thomas A. C. Rennie Series in Social Psychiatry*, vol. 1. New York: McGraw-Hill.

Suchman, E. A. 1964. Sociomedical variations among ethnic groups. *Am. J. Soc.* 70:319–31.

————. 1965a. Social factors in medical deprivation. *Am. J. Public Health* 55:1725–33.

————. 1965b. Social patterns of illness and medical care. *J. Health Hum. Behav.* 6:2–16.

————. 1965c. Stages of illness and medical care. *J. Health Hum. Behav.* 6:114–28.

————. 1966. Health orientation and medical care. *Am. J. Public Health* 56:97–105.

Suchman, E. A. and Rothman, A. A. 1965. Utilization of dental services. *N. Y. State Dent. J.* 31:151–58.

Washington Heights Health District Master Sample Survey, Family Form*

TIME INTERVIEW BEGAN: _____

1. a. What is the name of the head of this household? (Enter name in column 1)
   b. What are the names of all other persons who live here? (List all persons who usually live here, and all persons staying here who have no usual place of residence elsewhere. List these persons in the prescribed order.)
   c. Do any (other) lodgers or roomers live here?   __ No   __ Yes   (List)
   d. Is there anyone else who lives here who is now in a hospital, or in a nursing home, in a rest home, or in any other place of this sort?   __ No   __ Yes   (List)
   e. Away on business?   __ No   __ Yes   (List)
   f. On a visit?   __ No   __ Yes   (List)
   g. Is there anyone else staying here now?   __ No   __ Yes   (List)
   h. Do any of the people in this household have a home elsewhere?
      __ No   (Leave on questionnaire.)
      __ Yes   (Apply household membership rules; if not a member, delete.)

2. Sex

3. In what month and year were you born? How old does that make you on your last birthday?

   (If 16 years old or over, ask:)

4. Are you now married, widowed, divorced, separated, or never married?

   (If female and ever married, ask:)

   a. How many times have you been married?
   b. What (is) (are) the dates(s) of your (first) (second) (etc.) marriage?

---

* Source: Gill, C. and Elinson, J., eds., The Washington Heights Master Sample Survey, Appendix 3, in *Milbank Mem. Fund Quart.*, vol. 47, no. 1 (January 1969), part 2.

(If 16 years old or over, ask:)

5. What is the highest grade you attended in school?
   a. Did you finish the _____ grade (year)?

(If 16 years old or over, ask:)

6. What were you doing most of last week—
   (For males:) working, looking for work, going to school, or something else?

   (For females:) working, looking for work, keeping house, going to school, or something else?

(If 16 years old or over, ask:)

7. What were you doing most of the past 12 months—
   (For males:) working, looking for work, going to school, or something else?

   (For females:) working, looking for work, keeping house, going to school, or something else?

(If 'working" or "looking for work" in past week, ask:)

8. a. What kind of work do you usually do?
   b. In what kind of business or industry is this work done?
   c. Is this full-time or part-time?
   d. Do you work for yourself or someone else?

(If working for yourself:)

   1. How long have you been working for yourself?

(If working for someone else:)

   2. How long have you been working for your present employer?

(If "working," ask:)

   e. Is there a doctor or a nurse at work where you can get medical attention?

(If "looking for work" in past week, ask:)

9. How many weeks has it been since you last worked?

(If "retired" in past week, ask:)

10. What kind of work did you usually do when you were employed?
   a. How many years has it been since you last worked?

11. Where were you born?
   (If U.S., ask:)

   a. In what city and state were you born?

   (If not U.S. or Puerto Rico, ask:)

   b. Are you a U.S. citizen?

   (If 21 or over, ask:)

12. What is your religion?
   (If Jewish:) Is that Orthodox, Conservative, Reformed or none of these?
   (If Protestant:) What denomination is that?
   a. About how often do you go to (church) (synagogue) (services)?
   b. Did you happen to go to (church) (synagogue) (services) last week?

13. Now, about the father of Mr(s). _____ (HOH)— what kind of work did he do most of the time when Mr (s). —————(HOH) was under 21?

14. Where was Mr(s). _____'s father born?
   __ U.S. (In what state was he born?)
      State: _____
   __ Puerto Rico   __ Other (Specify country.)
      _____

15. What country or countries did Mr(s). _____'s (HOH's) family originally come from?

16. Does your family have a family doctor?
      1 Yes
      1. What is his name and address?
         Name: _____
         Address: _____
         _____

      2. How long have you used him? _____ years
                  Go to b
      0 No
   a. Do you or anyone in the family have a doctor whom you usually call when someone in the family gets sick?
         0 No   1 Yes
      1. What is his name and address?
         Name: _____
         Address: _____
         _____

2. How long have you used him? _____ years
Go to b
b. Does your family have any other doctor whom you usually call when someone in the family gets sick?
   0 No   1 Yes
   1. What is his name and address?
   Name: _____
   Address: _____

2. How long have you used him? _____ years

17. I have some questions about health insurance. We don't want to include insurance that pays ONLY for accidents, but we are interested in all other kinds. Do you or any member of this household belong to:

a. Blue Cross?
   0 No   1 Yes
   1. Who is covered by this plan? __ Entire family
   2. How long have you been a member of Blue Cross? _____ years

b. Blue Shield?
   0 No   1 Yes
   1. Who is covered by this plan? __ Entire family
   2. How long have you been a member of Blue Shield? _____ years

c. Health Insurance Plan of Greater New York (i.e., HIP)?
   0 No   1 Yes
   1. Who is covered by this plan? __ Entire family
   2. How long have you been a member of HIP? _____ years
   3. What is the name of the HIP group where you are a member?
   (If same for all covered, enter here; otherwise enter in each person's column:)
   Name:

d. Group Health Insurance (i.e., GHI)?
   0 No   1 Yes
   1. Who is covered by this plan?   __ Entire family
   2. How long have you been a member of GHI? _____ years

e. A Union health program?
   0 No   1 Yes (What is the name of the Union?)
   1. Who is covered by this plan?   __ Entire family
   2. How long have you been a member of this plan? _____ years
   3. What is the name of the union health program of which you are a member?
   (If same for all covered, enter here; otherwise enter in each person's column:)
   Name:

18. Do you have any (other) insurance that pays all or part of the bills when you go to the hospital?

      0 No   1 Yes

    1. Who is covered by this plan?   ___ Entire family
    2. How long have you been a member of this plan?   _____years
    3. What is the name of the plan?
       (*If same for all covered, enter here; otherwise enter in each person's column:*)
       Name:
    4. Does the plan pay any part of the surgeon's bill for an operation?

19. Do you have any (other) insurance that pays all or part of the bills for doctor's visits at your home or at his office?

      0 No   1 Yes

    1. Who is covered by this plan?   ___ Entire family
    2. How long have you been a member of this plan?   _____years
    3. What is the name of the plan?
       (*If same for all covered, enter here; otherwise enter in each person's column:*)
       Name:

20. Were you sick at any (other) time during the past month?
    (*Repeat question until respondent answers "No"*)

21. (Except for the past month, which we have already covered) were you sick at any (other) time in the past 12 months and talked to a doctor about it?
    (*Repeat question until respondent answers "No"*)

(*If between 45 and 64 years old, ask:*)

22. Have you had any of the following symptoms in the past 12 months?
    1. Acute indigestion or heartburn ....
    2. Shortness of breath ....
    3. Chest pain ....
    4. Palpitation___i.e., did you feel your heart beating hard? ....
    a. How many times did this bother you in the past 12 months?
    b. Is this something we have already covered?

23. Has anyone in the family—you, your, etc.—had any of these conditions during the past 12 months?
    (*Read each condition; for each condition ask:*)
    a. When was the first time this condition was ever noticed? (How many months or years ago?)

	No	Yes
1. Asthma	0	1
2. Hay fever	0	2
3. Tuberculosis	0	3
4. CHRONIC bronchitis	0	4
5. REPEATED attacks of sinus trouble	0	5
6. Rheumatic fever	0	6
7. Hardening of the arteries	0	7
8. High blood pressure	0	8
9. Heart trouble	0	9
10. Stroke	0	10
11. TROUBLE with varicose veins	0	11
12. Hemorrhoids or piles	0	12
13. Tumor, cyst or growth	0	13
14. CHRONIC gall bladder or liver trouble	0	14
15. Stomach ulcer	0	15
16. Any other CHRONIC stomach trouble	0	16
17. Kidney stones or CHRONIC kidney trouble	0	17
18. Arthritis or rheumatism	0	18
19. Mental illness	0	19
20. Diabetes	0	20
21. Thyroid trouble or goiter	0	21
22. Any allergy	0	22
23. Epilepsy	0	23
24. CHRONIC nervous trouble	0	24
25. Cancer	0	25
26. CHRONIC skin trouble	0	26
27. Hernia or rupture	0	27
28. Cirrhosis of the liver	0	28
29. (For men only) Prostate trouble	0	29

(After all conditions have been read, for each condition recorded, ask:)
b. Is this something we have already covered for the past 12 months?

24. Does anyone in the family have any of these conditions?

	No	Yes
1. Deafness or SERIOUS trouble with hearing	0	1
2. SERIOUS trouble with seeing, even when wearing glasses	0	2
3. Cleft palate	0	3
4. Any speech defect	0	4
5. Missing fingers, hand, or arm, toes, foot or leg	0	5
6. Cerebral palsy	0	6
7. Paralysis of any kind	0	7
8. REPEATED trouble with back or spine	0	8
9. Seriously confused or mixed up mentally	0	9
10. Club foot	0	10
11. Any PERMANENT stiffness or deformity of the foot, leg, fingers, arm or back	0	11

12. Mentally retarded 0   12
13. Any other condition present since birth 0   13

(After all conditions have been read, for each condition recorded, ask:)
a. Is this something we have already covered for the past 12 months?

25. Which member(s) of the family, including yourself, received dental care during the past 12 months?

    1 Entire family   0 No one in family

26. Which member(s) of the family, including yourself, received an eye examination for glasses during the past 12 months?

    1 Entire family   0 No one in family

27. Has anyone (else) in the family received any (other) medical attention in a child health station or a city health center in the past 12 months?

    0 No one in family

    (Repeat question until respondent answers "No")

28. Have you had any (other) medical attention—that is, have you visited a doctor, a clinic, or a health center, or been in a hospital for any (other) reason during the past 12 months (that we haven't already covered)?

    (Repeat question until respondent answers "No")

29. Are there any (other) health or medical services that you would have used for yourself or your family in the past 12 months if they were available?

    0 No   1 Yes

    a. For what purposes or conditions?
    b. What services would you have used if they were available?

30. Please look at this card and read each statement. Then tell me which statement fits you bet in terms of health.

    (Show Cards A-D, as appropriate)[1]
    (If "1," "2," or "3," ask:)
    a. Is this because of any of the conditions you have told me about?
    b. Which conditions?
    c. How long have you been this way?
    d. Please look at this card and read each statement. Then tell me which statement fits you best.
    (Show Card E)[2]

(Refer to Q. 1 and 3; if any child is under 2 years old, then ask the mother of that child:)

X No children in household under 2 years old.

31. I'd like to ask you some questions about your pregnancy with ——.

(If any female in the household is between 16–55 years old, ask 32 A and B:)

32. a. (Have you) (has anyone) (else) (in the household) been pregnant at any (other) time during the past 24 months?
       0 No   1 Yes (Who was pregnant?)
    b. Is anyone (else) in the household now pregnant?
       0 No   1 Yes (Who is pregnant?)

(Ask about each woman in the household 16 years old or over:)

33. How many times have you been pregnant all of your life?
    (If pregnant once or more, ask A, B, C:)
    a. How many of these pregnancies ended in miscarriages, abortions, or stillbirths?
    b. How many live births does that make?
    c. How many children are now living?
    (If the number of children listed under this mother as members of the household is not the same as the number of pregnancies, then ask:)
    d. What is the date of birth of your (first) (second) child or have you already given me this?

(Refer to Q. 1 and 3; if any child is 6 years old or under, then ask:)

X No children in household 6 years old or under

34. Now, I'd like to ask you some questions about the children in the house who are 6 years old or under—
       (Go to Children's Form)

35. Is anyone here taking care of children not in the family in this home during the day?
       __ Yes   __ No
    a. How many and how old are they?
    b. How often are they left here?

	Age	How many times a week left here?
1.	__	_____
2.	__	_____
3.	__	_____
4.	__	_____
5.	__	_____

    a. Is there anyone here who might be interested in taking care of children in this home during the day—children not in the family?

___ Yes   ___ No
1. Would anyone be interested in doing this for pay?
___ Yes   ___ No

(Ask 36 and 37 about all working mothers with any children 16 years old or under; mother is person No. _____)

___ No working mother with children 16 or under, skip to 38

36. Do you make any arrangements for having your children taken care of when you are working, or are they old enough to take care of themselves?
    0 Do not make arrangements   1 Yes—make arrangements

a. What arrangements do you make? *(If necessary, ask B, then circle code)*

(If children are taken care of by relative or baby sitter, ask:)
b. How old is he?
    1 Other relative—over 16 years old (e.g., brother or sister)
    2 Other relative—16 or under (e.g., brother or sister)
    3 Maid or housekeeper
    4 Neighbor or friend (circle only if child is taken care of at R's house, or at neighbor's or friend's house)
    5 Baby-sitter—over 16
    6 Baby-sitter—16 or under
    7 Day Care Home Operator (cares for fewer than 5 children in her home through the day or night)
    8 Nursery school or nursery school staff (cares for 5 or more children usually during the day only, but some also care for children at night)
    9 Playground or Club leader
    X Other arrangements (specify:)

_____

c. Do you pay for these arrangements?
    1 Yes   0 No

(Ask only if mother is respondent; person No. ——) —— Mother is not respondent

37. What is your biggest worry in providing care for your children when you have to be away?

38. Have you or any member of the household ever had difficulty because of too much drinking?
    0 No   1 Yes
a. Who is that? *(Enter persons' Nos. ___, ___, ___)*
b. (Have you) (has he) (has she) had any difficulty in the past 12 months?
    0 No   1 Yes
    1. When was the last time (you) (he) (she) had difficulty?

c. What kinds of difficulties (have you) (has he) (has she) had because of too much drinking? How about:

(Read statements and enter persons' Nos. to left of codes)
1 Your health
2 Your job
3 Money problems
4 Family arguments
5 Violence to members of family
6 Break-up of marriage
7 Trouble in the neighborhood
8 Trouble with the police
9 Other difficulties (Specify)

_____

d. (Have you) (has he) (has she) tried to get help? *(Enter persons' Nos.)*
    0 No   1 Yes
    1. Where (have you) (has he) (has she) tried to get help? *(Enter persons' Nos.)*

39. Is there anyone who has lived here in the past 12 months who spent any time in a nursing home, an old age, convalescent, or rest home, or special school, or in any other institution or place of this sort?
    0 No   1 Yes
a. Who is that? *Enter persons' Nos.* ___, ___, ___)
b. What is the name and address of the institution where he has spent any time?
Name: _____
Address: _____

40. Has anyone in the household spent any time in a hospital or institution because of mental illness during the past year?
    0 No   1 Yes
a. Who is that? *Enter persons' Nos.* ___, ___, ___)
b. What is the name and address of the institution?
Name: _____
Address: _____

41. Has anyone in the household spent any time in a hospital or institution because of mental illness during the past 10 years?
    0 No   1 Yes
a. Who is that? *Enter persons' Nos.* ___, ___, ___)
b. What is the name and address of the hospital or institution?
Name: _____
Address: _____

___ *(Check here if single-person household, and skip to 43)*

42. Now, I'd like to ask you some questions about your family life—most families divide up the work and responsibilities in some way. Who in your house generally: *(Enter persons' Nos. ___, ___, ___)*
    1. ___ Buys the groceries and household provisions
    2. ___ Prepares the meals
    3. ___ Washes the dishes
    4. ___ Makes the beds
    5. ___ Does the heavy housework
    6. ___ Empties the garbage
    7. ___ Decides how the family income will be spent
    8. ___ Takes care of paying the bills
    9. ___ Decides where the family will live
    10. ___ Decides what to watch on television

43. Who is the closest relative outside the household to whom you would turn in case of an emergency?
    Name: _____
    a. *(If necessary:)* How is he related to you?
    Relation: _____
    b. Where does he live? *(If in N. Y. C. ask for street address and borough; if outside N. Y. C., ask for city and state)*
    Address: _____

44. How many rooms do you have here altogether (including kitchen)?
    ___ rooms

45. How much rent do you pay each month? $_____

    (Ask about those who worked the past week or the past 12 months; see Q. 6 and 7:)

    X No one in family worked past week or past 12 months

46. How much did you earn before taxes in 19(59) (60)? *(Show Card F)*[s]
    In which of the groups on this card did your wages or salary fall during 19(59) (60)? Just give me the letter.
    Person No.:   ___ ___ ___ ___ ___
    Income Group: ___ ___ ___ ___ ___
    (Probe) Is this before taxes?   ___ Yes   ___ No

47. During 19(59) (60) in which group did the total income of your family fall, that is, yours, your ___'s, ___'s, etc? *(Show Card F)* Include income from all sources, such as wages, salaries, rents from property, pensions, help from relatives, etc. Just give me the letter. Income group: ___
    (Probe) Is this before taxes?   ___ Yes   ___ No

(If income A, B, C, or D, then ask:)
a. Does this include any public assistance or public welfare?
__ Yes __ No

48. a. How long has the head of the household been living at this address?
__ years
(If more than 5 years, skip to 49; if less than 5 years, ask:)
b. Where did he live before this? *(If N. Y. C. ask for street address and borough; if not N. Y. C. ask for city and state)*
Address: _____
How long did he live there? __ years
(If this period still covers less than 5 years, ask:)
c. And where did he live before that?
(If N. Y. C. get street address and borough; if not N. Y. C. get city and state)
Address: _____

49. How long has the head of the household lived in New York City?
__ years __ All his life

50. Do you think you may be moving within the next year or so?
0 No   1 Yes or Maybe
a. Why do you think you may be moving?

51. Thank you so much for giving us your time on this important research study. Just in case we need some additional information or in case I have made some mistake, when is the best time to reach you by phone?
Time _____ Telephone number _____
__ No telephone number

52. *(Check race of respondent:)*
1 White   2 Negro   3 Other *(Specify)* _____

53. How did the informant react to this interview? Was he cooperative __ or not? *(Continue on page 1, if necessary)*

54. Have you checked that the family number is correct on every form, and on every extra page? __ Yes

TIME INTERVIEW COMPLETED: _____

REFERENCES

[1] Card A
For: Workers and other persons except Housewives and Children
1. Not able to work at all.
2. Able to work but limited in amount of work or kind of work.
3. Able to work but limited in kind or amount of other activities.
4. Not limited in any of these ways.

Card B
For: Housewife
1. Not able to keep house at all.
2. Able to keep house but limited in amount or kind of housework.
3. Able to keep house but limited in kind or amount of other activities.
4. Not limited in any of these ways.

Card C
For: Children from 6 through 16 years old
1. Not able to go to school at all.
2. Able to go to school but limited to certain types of schools or in school attendance.
3. Able to go to school but limited in other activities.
4. Not limited in any of these ways.

Card D
For: Children under 6 years old
1. Not able to take part at all in ordinary play with other children.
2. Able to play with other children but limited in amount or kind of play.
3. Not limited in any of these ways.

[2] Card E
1. Confined to the house all the time, except in emergencies.
2. Able to go outside but need the help of another person in getting around outside.
3. Able to go outside alone but have trouble in getting around freely.
4. Not limited in any of these ways.

[3] Card F

A. Under $2,000	D. 4,000–4,999	G. 7,500– 9,999
B. 2,000–2,999	E. 5,000–5,999	H. 10,000–14,999
C. 3,000–3,999	F. 6,000–7,499	I. 15,000 and over

EDITORIAL COMMENTS

1. As in Alameda County, the social and behavioral aspects of illness are of primary importance in the Washington Heights studies. Another feature the two laboratories share is the absence of an independent procedure for ascertaining disease among the respondents.

2. Two valuable features of this laboratory are first, its permanent survey staff and data processing facilities and, second, its provision for collaborative studies between intramural and extramural research groups. The existence of a permanent core staff spares investigators many burdens of organization, administration, and staff recruitment, while collaborative study can result in considerable savings in overhead and other expenses for extramural investigators. Even with such facilities, however, investigators should participate in the design of the survey questionnaire in order for it to be maximally useful to them.

3. The Washington Heights survey is cross-sectional rather than prospective. This takes full advantage of the core facilities, while avoiding the high attrition from migration which would be expected in this metropolitan community.

4. As was true in Framingham, "limitations of time and money" forced a reduction in the sampled dwelling units from the number originally decided upon.

5. The studies on the effect of disparity in social status between interviewer and respondent are important. Among other things, they suggest the need for an independent determination of the frequency and typology of disease in the surveyed population.

6. Like most other large studies, the Master Sample Survey collected much data which have not been fully utilized. It is usually impossible to judge whether such unanalyzed information represents bonus material or whether the expense of its collection was negligible.

7. The interest expressed in the Master Sample Survey by city planning commissions, police and school departments and religious and ethnic groups suggests the impressive potential utility of this type of community laboratory. In this, the Rhode Island and Washington Heights surveys closely resemble one another.

CHAPTER 9

The smallest state in the Union is the community being studied by the Population Research Laboratory. Though staffed by members of a university sociology department, the laboratory collaborates closely with public officials and other interested parties in research on health and demography. Of special interest here is a sampling frame which contains a "surprise stratum" to adjust for unexpected changes in the size or location of the reference population.

THE BROWN UNIVERSITY, RHODE ISLAND, POPULATION LABORATORY: ITS PURPOSES AND INITIAL PROGRESS

Harold N. Organic and Sidney Goldstein

INTRODUCTION

A Population Research Laboratory has been established at Brown University for the execution of studies in community health, demography, and social structure. The laboratory is the outgrowth of a decade of extensive research in the university's department of sociology on various economic, social, and health characteristics of the state's population (Goldstein and Mayer 1958; 1961; 1964; 1965; Goldstein 1966; Pfautz 1962). These studies were essentially cross-sectional in orientation and their value for measuring changes over time was, therefore, limited. The desirability of a longitudinal approach and the advantages of Rhode Island as the setting for longitudinal studies were strong arguments in favor of creating a community laboratory in Providence. Another was the already established Center for Aging Research at Brown. This Center has followed a sample of 600 older couples (with the husband between the ages of sixty and sixty-four years) in the city of Providence through three rounds of interviews over a period of five years in order to assess changes in health status, medical expenses, social activities, and general adjustment to aging (Burnight 1965;

Burnight and Marden 1967). Experience with this sample argued strongly in favor of expansion to include the entire spectrum of adult ages as well as subjects residing outside the confines of the central city. The advantages of Rhode Island as a social science laboratory had already been recognized by the Department of Preventive Medicine at Harvard Medical School whose interest was in problems relating to the quality, effectiveness, and utilization of medical care facilities. Hospital records were a major source of data for this study and the need for follow-up studies in the field was readily acknowledged (Burgess et al. 1967).

In recent years there has been a convergence of the recognized needs for:

1. extending the cross-sectional statistical analyses of census and vital statistics data into longitudinal analyses;
2. broadening the population range encompassed in the sample of the Center for Aging Research;
3. obtaining more comprehensive and reliable data on health conditions, medical utilization, and the outcome of medical care.

To meet these needs the Population Laboratory was established and its major foci of interest were defined as:

1. current incidence and prevalence of illness and disability and their changes over time;
2. existing modes of providing, distributing, and utilizing health care services;
3. demographic, social, and environmental variables as they affect health and the utilization and outcome of health services.

THE COMMUNITY

Among community laboratories, this one is unusual in that it encompasses an entire state. Of course, Rhode Island's 1,214 square miles make it the smallest state in the Union, and it is, in fact, smaller than some of the other communities having population laboratories described in this Casebook.

At the time of the 1965 state census, Rhode Island had a population of 892,709 persons, representing a fifteen-fold increase since the first federal census in 1790 (Goldstein and Mayer 1962; U.S. Census 1966). This growth resulted from an interplay of births, deaths, and migration which affected not only the size of the population but its distribution by age, ethnicity, and other characteristics as well.

Rhode Island is, and has been for many decades, one of the nation's most urbanized states. By definition of the 1960 census, 86.4 per cent of its population live in urban places, a proportion equaled only by

California and exceeded slightly by New Jersey. Along with California, Rhode Island has the highest proportion (85.5 per cent) of the population living in metropolitan areas. Since the rural population is almost entirely nonfarm, the state is, in effect, a city-state in which the central cities and the smaller satellite cities have merged with their surrounding suburbs, and the suburbs in turn, have become increasingly indistinguishable from the villages and the more rural hinterland. This does not mean, however, that Rhode Island is uniformly settled: different parts of the state vary sharply in population density.

Central to the metropolitan area encompassed by most of Rhode Island and nearby parts of Massachusetts is the city of Providence, with a population of 187,000 persons. Early in the nineteenth century Providence emerged as one of the country's leading manufacturing centers, noted especially for textiles and metals. By 1900 its population had grown to 176,000, about 41 per cent of the total for the state. It continued to grow throughout the first four decades of the twentieth century and reached a peak of 253,000 persons in 1940. However, other parts of the state, including the city's suburbs, were growing more rapidly, and its proportion of the total population soon declined to 35.5 per cent. Providence began to lose population in the 1940's at an accelerating rate so that by 1960 it numbered 207,500 persons representing an intercensal decline of 16.6 per cent, the largest for a city of its size in the entire United States. This decline has continued into the 1960's, and in 1965 the 187,000 persons enumerated as residents of the city accounted for only 21 per cent of the state's population.

Several factors account for the stabilization and subsequent decline in the population of Providence. Like the state as a whole, the city was adversely affected by the decline of the textile industry. In addition, residential construction approached the far limits of the city by 1930 and was even further restricted by highway building and urban renewal programs in more recent years. Between 1950 and 1960 there was a net outmigration from the city of 61,000 people, mostly to the suburbs; an even greater loss was avoided because of a 20,000 excess of births over deaths. This pattern persisted from 1960 to 1965, during which time a net migration loss of 27,000 contributed to the city's decline to 187,000 persons.

In 1900 almost half of the metropolitan area's population lived in the central city; by 1965, a mere 15 per cent. The experience of Providence is not unique; it has, rather, presaged that of most other cities in the United States. Between 1950 and 1960 the population living in the central cities of the 212 metropolitan areas of the United States increased by only 11 per cent as compared with a growth rate of 49 per cent for those parts of the metropolitan areas outside the central city. In fact, more than one-quarter of the central cities have experienced actual population losses during the last decade, at the very time metropolitan populations were increasing rapidly. This phenomenon has also been observed in the other industrial cities of Rhode Island (U.S. Census 1961). The fact that Providence's demographic fluctuations have anticipated later developments in other American cities probably adds to its value, and that of the state, as a community laboratory.

Besides the redistribution of the population between city and suburbs, the composition of the population has undergone significant ethnic changes (Goldstein and Mayer 1963). The original Rhode Island colonists were English, and other population stocks were not welcomed at first. Nevertheless, there was a limited influx of Huguenots, Portuguese, Jews, Scots, and Negroes during the eighteenth century. Together with the remnants of the vanquished Indians, the presence of these ethnic groups marked the beginning of an increasing heterogeneity in the Rhode Island population, a trend which was soon to become evident in the United States as a whole. The arrival of the Irish in the early nineteenth century, followed by the French-Canadians after the Civil War, eventually resulted in a complete transformation in the originally homogeneous Anglo-Saxon Protestant population. This process continued with a massive influx from Italy and, to a lesser extent, from Eastern Europe and Portugal in the late 1800's and early 1900's. The 1905 state census showed for the first time that Catholicism had become the faith of the majority.

By 1910 the foreign-born constituted 33 per cent of Rhode Island's total population, and almost seven out of every ten inhabitants were either foreign-born or children of foreign-born. However, the interruption in immigration during World War I and the subsequent imposition of quotas resulted in a steady decline in both the number and the proportion of foreign-born. By 1960 only four out of every ten inhabitants were foreign-born or of foreign or mixed parentage. Among these, persons of Italian and of French-Canadian origin constituted the largest groups, followed by those from the United Kingdom and, to a lesser extent, from Ireland and Portugal.

Although Negroes represented as much as 10 per cent of colonial Rhode Island's population, the 25,444 nonwhites in 1965 constituted less than 3 per cent of the total, though nearly 60 per cent of them were concentrated in Providence. The state has not been as attractive to Southern Negro migrants as other Northern industrial centers because of the presence of a relatively large population of white working class immigrants. Among other ethnic groups present in sufficiently large numbers to permit specialized studies are the Armenians, Cape Verdeans, American Indians, East Europeans, Jews, and New England Yankees.

Being among the first cities in the United States to experience population decline—and a very high rate of decline—Providence has been the subject of a number of detailed investigations into the relation between population decline and the social and demographic structure of the city and suburbs. Underlying these studies was the hypothesis that outmigration would leave the city more homogeneous and thereby reduce its social class differentials. The analysis of many demographic and housing variables gave only partial support to this hypothesis (Goldstein and Mayer 1964). Although there was some evidence that the demographic changes were related to social class, the degree of change with migration was slight. Sociodemographic gradients persisted despite losses of population and residential movements within the city. The relatively modest effects of outmigration may be explained by the fact that as movement to the suburbs increased, the suburban areas themselves became more heterogeneous, while the participation of working class families in outmigration slowed the homogenization process within the city.

These earlier studies indicated that at the present stage of its metropolitan development the entire spectrum of social class may be found in both Providence and its suburbs (Goldstein and Mayer 1965). For persons of all social classes there are differences in the presumed merits of city and suburb as places in which to live, although these differences appear to be more significant to members of the higher social class. The great social and demographic heterogeneity of the city and the suburbs emphasizes the necessity for subjecting both to community study, rather than one or the other. In fact, one might also wish to include even the more peripheral areas beyond the suburbs in such analyses.

These considerations would appear to justify the use of the entire state as a community laboratory. A unique advantage of Rhode Island is that it has been entirely subdivided into census tracts, and detailed statistics on both the characteristics of the population and on vital events occurring therein are usually classified by census tract. In addition, the compact size of the state makes for a more economical survey operation. There are two other advantages in Rhode Island as a community laboratory. First, it is, for practical purpose, a closed system. The population secures almost all of its medical services within the state, and few medical services are rendered to residents of other areas. And, second, the existing medical facilities and practitioners, though not extremely numerous, are nevertheless sufficiently varied in specialty, organization, size, function, and location to permit valid comparisons in studies of medical outcome.

METHODS

The study methods include an analysis of public and institutional records and a series of 5 successive annual sample surveys of approximately 1,250 to 1,500 households comprising from 4,000 to 5,000 persons. Monthly or bimonthly contacts will be maintained with each sampled household during the year following the initial interview. Both cross-sectional and longitudinal data will, therefore, be available for the study of changes in medical behavior on the one hand and demographic and community structure on the other, as well as for analysis of their interrelations.

A special area of interest will be the relative values of alternative modes of follow-up contact including telephone, mail questionnaire, reinterview, and diary keeping. The reliability, appropriateness, and cost of each mode will be carefully assessed. In addition, an attempt will be made to maintain a simulated "continuous population register" beyond the first year after initial contact. Through a combination of periodic direct contacts, letters, and record checks, significant changes in the health or socioeconomic characteristics of the study population will be registered. In this fashion a cumulative population register of about 20,000 persons in 5,500 to 7,000 households will be generated and followed up.

The Sampling Design

The study design incorporates a clustered, multi-stage, stratified sample, with five successive annual surveys, thus permitting both cross-sectional and longitudinal investigations. The sample was made large enough to yield five independent samples of housing units—an efficient and economical feature. Taking 1,100 annual household interviews as an acceptable work load and estimating the identification, occupancy, and response rates as 98 per cent, 92 per cent and 85 per cent, respectively, a total list of 7,500 household addresses (1,500 for each of the 5 years) was required. Tabulations from the 1965 special census of Rhode Island indicated that there were about 300,000 housing units in the state. Therefore, an over-all sampling fraction of 1 in 40 for the 5 years, or 1 in 200 for each year, would yield the desired sample size.

Following the procedures outlined by Leslie Kish (1965) each of the state's 187 census tracts was assigned a stratification measure based upon its characteristics of ethnicity, nativity, and socioeconomic status. By arranging the tracts in rank order on these measures, and by assigning to each tract a probability of selection proportional to its size (number of housing units), tracts were systematically drawn at a fixed rate after a random start. Ninety-two tracts, constituting the Primary Sampling Units (PSU's) were drawn; these made up the first stage of the multi-stage frame.

In the second stage, each selected PSU was divided into chunks of approximately 30 housing units, as determined from published tract, block, and census enumeration district statistics, maps, and independent estimates made by the field staff. A sample of these chunks comprising a fixed sampling fraction constituted the second stage. From these chunks a third-stage sample of segments (blocks or smaller units) containing the aggregate 7,500 housing units was chosen. At the time of a household interview an adult respondent is randomly selected by means of a selection table which is equivalent to a table of random numbers. The interviews, which were begun in the fall of 1967, last about an hour and a quarter and, as already noted, provide baseline data on health and social characteristics. The periodic follow-up interviews will yield information on changes in health and medical behavior as well as on residence, occupation, and family composition.

The household interviews constitute the primary data source but they will be supplemented by others, including hospital record checks and vital events recorded by the State Department of Health. An experimental pilot project involving a validation by physicians of self-reported medical conditions has increased our confidence in the validity of the self-reporting procedure.

An additional virtue of the sampling design is its cumulability. An annual sample of approximately 1,000 households is not large enough, except in the case of relatively common complaints, to yield reliable incidence and prevalence rates. However, since the annual samples are self-representing and independent, they can be merged over a number of years to yield a greater number of cases suitable for analysis. Of course, it must be assumed in these circumstances that secular changes in rates are negligible.

Interview Schedules

Specially designed interview schedules are used in the initial household interview and in each of the follow-up contacts. The two major areas of inquiry on health concern general medical behavior and fertility behavior.

The general health questions relate to the respondent's present state of health, where and what types of medical resources he has utilized during the past year, and the identity of his physician and dentist. For those who have not consulted a physician or dentist in the past year, the time reference is changed from "the past year" to "ever in your lifetime." Two additional series of questions are then asked, both of which were first utilized in the 1955 nation-wide sample survey of the Health Information Foundation (Feldman 1966). In the first series a number of symptoms or conditions are mentioned and the respondent is asked whether he thinks these require the immediate attention of a health specialist of some kind; whether they should be attended to by ones' self or whether they are not serious enough to bother about. The purpose here is to probe the respondent's normative behavior relating to the specified conditions without regard to his actual experience. The latter is taken up in the second series of questions as well as in the monthly follow-up interviews. By combining the findings from the two series of questions and the follow-up contacts, normative, retrospective, and current behavior can be examined. The three behavioral modes need not be consistent, of course, and an analysis of the inconsistencies among various population subgroups may shed light on the utilization patterns of medical services.

In the initial interview schedule considerable attention is paid to the second major area of inquiry on health, i.e., fertility behavior. Of special interest is the experience of female respondents with the contraceptive pill, the reasons for its use, any observed side effects, and expectations for its future use. Directly related to these questions are others dealing with the respondent's menstrual history and the effects of the pill on the cycle. Current pregnancies are also reported and their progess is noted in subsequent follow-up contacts. New pregnancies that commence after the initial interview are followed in successive interviews, as are changes in birth control practices.

Areas of Research Interest

In its first year of operation, 1967–1968, the Population Laboratory focused upon three interrelated aspects of community health: (1) general medical behavior, past and present; (2) fertility behavior and neonatal death; and (3) mobility, including residential changes and travel to work.

Medical behavior was defined as the patterns of use or nonuse of medical care. It was assumed that such behavior will vary with the demographic and socioeconomic characteristics of the individual, his past experience with illness, and the specific nature of the health problem. The categories of medical care were considered to range from self-care and the advice of friends and family to the more organized forms of care, such as faith healers, irregular practitioners, osteopaths, and doctors of medicine. Among the questions asked were: What constitutes an adequate stimulus for individuals to seek medical care? What levels of care are typically sought, and in what sequence? What sources of information or patterns of referral are employed? These data on medical behavior will come largely from the monthly contacts following the initial household interviews. The frequency of these contacts will increase the probability that the respondents are reporting actual and recent behavior.

Fertility behavior and neonatal deaths are important indicators of life style and are also closely related to general health conditions. The specific questions asked on fertility include the following: How does family size and child spacing vary by socioeconomic status and residence? How are fertility and pregnancy wastage related to other medical problems in families? How are attitudes and practices relating to fertility control disseminated? What, if any, is the role of the medical profession in this communication process? How is the use or nonuse of such newly available birth control methods as the pill or the intrauterine device related to maternal health?

In recent years, infant mortality in the United States has declined at a slower rate than in a number of other Western countries. Intensive studies of possible ecological and sociodemographic factors underlying this pattern are planned and a three-stage study of infant mortality has already been initiated at the Population Laboratory.

In the first stage, all records of neonatal deaths in Rhode Island during 1965 and 1966 are being matched with their birth certificates, thus permitting a division of the certificates into two groups: those infants who survived the neonatal period and those who did not. These two groups will be compared in order to assess the impact of a variety of factors on survivorship. The second stage will consist of an analysis of hospital records, physicians' records, and interview with physicians caring for the mothers and infants. In the third stage, high-risk subgroups will be identified and prospective and retrospective studies of infant mortality conducted. Of special interest here will be the social and psychological factors which affect the type of medical care received by the mothers.

Studies of mobility have been included because of the direct and indirect impact of these processes on social behavior and health. Most changes of residence disrupt existing social ties and create problems of adjustment to the new physical and social environment (Kantor 1965; Wolpert 1966). Such problems may be particularly critical for children, especially when there are frequent residential changes. On the one hand, by permitting job changes without accompanying residential changes, commuting may reduce the mental, social, and health problems that stem from residential mobility. On the other hand, the greater separation of family members resulting from increased commuting distances may contribute to family disruption and may impede the social activities and the seeking of appropriate medical services by family members. The increased participation of women in the labor force may also have unanticipated consequences both for their personal well-being and for that of their families.

The mobility studies are still being developed. Among the data to be sought are the following items:

1. frequency, distance, and circumstances surrounding residential mobility;
2. labor force status and changes of employment;
3. distance, time, and mode of transportation employed by family members in their daily movements;
4. the effects of migration and daily movement upon the patterns of social participation of family members;
5. the effects of mobility and daily movement upon the patterns of referral and of securing and utilizing medical services;
6. relations among health, medical, and social problems and the extent of repeated residential and job changes.

Because of the longitudinal design of the study, it is anticipated that a considerable number of households will be identified at a time when moves are being contemplated or have recently been made, thus permitting detailed investigation of their rationales and effects.

PROBLEMS

It is essential that the sampling frame not be so rigid that shifts in population size, composition, or location render it obsolete. The Rhode Island frame was constructed in the spring of 1967 and is expected to last five years. It is continually being adjusted by field checks and communication with municipal planning boards on new construction, demolition, and vacancies. The possibility of future developments such as new housing subdivisions in suburban communities or high-rise apartments in central cities was taken into account in constructing the initial frame.

While a moderate degree of population shift can be adjusted for in these ways, larger or unpredictable changes can raise serious methodologic problems. To avoid this, a "surprise stratum" is employed. Any areal growth in excess of three times the expected number of housing units is transferred to the surprise stratum, which is then treated as a new chunk to be segmented, listed, and selected like other areal units.

Another problem is that of differential response rates by the various socioeconomic subgroups. High status subjects are often overrepresented among nonrespondents as, increasingly, are urban nonwhites. Every effort is made to ascertain the age, sex, occupation, and ethnicity of non-respondents and their households. Such information is gleaned from all available sources, including the initial household canvass, city directories, and inquiries from neighbors. Educated guesses may then be made as to the extent and direction of the nonresponse bias.

The Rhode Island community study shares another problem with most longitudinal investigations: on the one hand, there is a progressive attrition in response over time. People die, move away, or lose interest and refuse to grant further interviews. On the other hand, respondents who remain may, by virtue of their long association with the project, being to anticipate the lines of questioning and provide answers which, perhaps erroneously, they think are being sought. The dilemma is compounded by the paradox that special efforts to retain respondents may sensitize them to the study purposes; while the absence of such efforts may lead to high attrition rates.

Finally, there is the problem of conducting surveys of this type in subcommunities that are suspicious of or hostile to the larger society, its purposes, and its representatives. If difficulties in conducting survey operations in the Negro ghetto led to the exclusion of the small Negro community from the study universe, the loss would amount to about 3 per cent. Study findings could still be generalized to a community—the white community—with meaning and utility, but no knowledge would be gained about the subgroup most in need of improved health services. Although this problem may be a relatively minor one in Rhode Island, this is surely not the case in the larger urban centers and in many other cities of the nation.

Serious attention must be paid to its resolution by health workers and public administrators everywhere.

FINDINGS

At this writing the Population Research Laboratory at Brown University is in the first year of its program; the findings, therefore, are necessarily tentative.

The sample size, nonresponse categories, and final response rate for the initial interview are shown in Table 9–1. The over-all response of 82 per cent is consistent with rates from similar studies conducted among highly urbanized populations. The same is true for the distribution of non-responses by category.

Table 9–2 presents selected demographic characteristics of the respondents, their household members and comparable information on the general population taken from the latest available U.S. census publications. The household members represent a sample of the census popu-

TABLE 9–1. RESPONSES TO THE INITIAL INTERVIEW

Response		Number	Per cent
Completed interview		1,127	81.8
Respondent refused in person		156	11.3
Respondent not seen, household member denied access		35	2.6
Respondent not seen, landlord denied access		8	0.6
No contact after required number of calls		47	3.4
Language barrier, no interpreter available		4	0.3
Total eligible housing units		1,377	100.0
Original sample list of housing units		1,516	
Housing units discovered in field		6	
Total housing units		1,522	
Less ineligible housing units			
Respondent incompetent	25		
Housing unit vacant	120	145	
Total eligible housing units		1,377	100.0

lation; in fact, the degree of similarity between the two groups is striking. The differences between these groups and the respondents themselves reflect the fact that the latter had to be adults. The respondent group in general, therefore, was older; it had a higher proportion of females, reflecting their greater expectation of life; and it comprised more married and widowed, as well as fewer never married persons.

Tabulations on the demographic attributes of respondents to the follow-up interviews have not yet been made. However, it is likely that these will conform closely with the findings in the initial sample. This expectation is based upon the high completion rates in the first two follow-up rounds: 93 per cent and 94 per cent, respectively (Table 9–3).

In the follow-up rounds, the telephone was the primary mode of contact. All respondents who had telephones were called, while personal visits were made to persons without telephones and to those with whom telephone connection could not be made. The high completion rate of the first follow-up interview was not unexpected, since these respondents had been co-operative in granting the initial interview. The persons most resistant to interview had already removed themselves from the pool of potential follow-up respondents by being among the initial nonresponders. The success of contacts by telephone had previously been observed in the Alameda County Survey (Hochstim 1967).

Some preliminary data are now available on medical and fertility behavior. Table 9–4 relates to the normative prescriptions of the sample for a series of medical symptoms. For comparative purposes the national figures reported by Feldman (1966) are shown in parentheses. It appears that Rhode Islanders are somewhat less likely to suggest seeing

TABLE 9–2. AGE, SEX, RACE, AND MARITAL STATUS OF RESPONDENT—HOUSEHOLD
SAMPLE AND CENSUS POPULATION

Selected characteristic	Sample		Census population
	Respondent	Household	
Age in years			
Under 10	0.0%[a]	22.3%	19.5%
10–19	1.1	18.4	17.9
20–29	19.1	13.3	12.4
30–39	18.4	11.1	11.3
40–49	21.3	12.2	13.2
50–59	16.8	10.1	10.9
60–69	11.5	6.5	8.2
70–79	9.3	4.6	5.0
80 and over	2.5	1.3	1.8
Not ascertained	0.0	0.2	0.0
Total	100.0%	100.0%	100.0%
Number	(1,127)	(3,750)	(892,709)[b]
Sex			
Male	41.6%	48.3%	48.8%
Female	58.4	51.7	51.2
Total	100.0%	100.0%	100.0%
Number	(1,127)	(3,750)	(892,709)[b]
Race			
White	96.5%	96.1%	97.1%
Negro	3.0	3.5	2.6
Other	0.4	0.2	0.3
Not ascertained	0.1	0.2	0.0
Total	100.0%	100.0%	100.0%
Number	(1,127)	(3,750)	(892,709)[b]
Marital status			
Married	68.6%	63.0%	60.9%
Widowed	13.2	7.5	8.3
Separated	3.1	1.5	3.9
Divorced	4.2	2.0	2.0
Never married	10.9	26.0	24.9
Total	100.0%	100.0%	100.0%
Number	(1,127)	(2,611)[e]	(627,705)[d]

[a] Criteria for eligibility as respondent were adult status, defined either as twenty-one years of age or over, or being currently married. This accounts for the small per cent in the ten to nineteen year age group.

[b] Source: U.S. Census (1966), Table 3, pp. 97–103.

[e] Household sample, age fourteen and over.

[d] Census population, 1960, age fourteen and over. Source: U.S. Census (1961), Table 105.

TABLE 9–3. RESPONSE RATE: FIRST AND SECOND FOLLOW-UP INTERVIEWS

Response category	Per cent: first follow-up			Per cent: second follow-up		
	Nonre-sponse	Com-plete	Total	Nonre-sponse	Com-plete	Total
Telephone: Completed		80.1			82.5	
Refused	1.3			2.7		
Total	1.3	80.1	81.4	2.7	82.5	85.2
Household: Completed		13.1			11.2	
Refused	1.3			1.2		
Total	1.3	13.1	14.4	1.2	11.2	12.4
Other nonresponse[a]	4.2		4.2	2.4		2.4
Total	6.8	93.2	100.0	6.3	93.7	100.0
Number of cases	(76)	(1,051)[b]	(1,127)	(68)	(1,013)	(1,081)[b]
Per cent of original eligible housing units (1,377)	5.5	76.3[b]	81.8	4.9	73.6	78.5[b]

[a] Includes respondents who moved, could not be reached, or who were temporarily away from the state.

[b] Discrepancy between the number completed in the first follow-up and the total in the second follow-up is due to the fact that 30 nonresponses from the first follow-up were recouped in the second.

TABLE 9–4. OPINIONS OF INITIAL SAMPLE ON NEED FOR PROMPT MEDICAL ATTENTION FOR EACH OF TWELVE SELECTED SYMPTOMS

Now here are some conditions that people sometimes complain about. (SHOW CARD 6) READ LIST ALOUD WITH RESPONDENT. I'd like you to tell me which of those conditions you think a person should see someone about right away and whom would you see; which ones a person should take care of himself, unless they keep up or get worse; and which ones a person shouldn't bother much about because they are not usually important. For instance, a cough of several weeks. Do you think a person should see someone about that; or take care of it himself unless it keeps up or gets worse; or shouldn't bother about it?

Symptom	Per cent			
	See someone	Care for himself	Not bother	Don't know
Cough for several weeks	86 (87)[a]	11 (11)	3 (2)	*[b] (*)
Diarrhea or constipation	37 (71)	57 (26)	6 (2)	* (1)
Feeling of dizziness	63 (79)	24 (14)	12 (5)	* (2)
Frequent headache	68 (76)	27 (19)	4 (3)	1 (2)
Lump or discolored patches of skin	93 (93)	3 (3)	3 (2)	* (2)
Sore throat, running nose	25 (47)	69 (48)	6 (4)	* (1)
Backache fairly often	65 (69)	24 (21)	10 (8)	1 (2)
Rash or itch for a week or more	74 (79)	21 (17)	5 (3)	1 (1)
Severe shortness of breath	93 (92)	3 (4)	3 (3)	* (1)
Toothache	90 (89)	8 (8)	2 (2)	* (1)
Unexplained loss of 10 pounds or more	77 (81)	7 (8)	15 (9)	1 (2)
Feeling tired all the time	62 (83)	22 (11)	15 (5)	1 (1)

[a] Figures in parentheses taken from Feldman (1966), Table 4.3, p. 61.

[b] Asterisk (*) signifies less than 0.5 per cent. Rows do not always sum 100 due to rounding.

someone than was the national sample, especially as regards diarrhea or constipation and sore throat or runny nose. The reasons for these differences are unknown. Some may be forthcoming after the response categories have been cross-tabulated by age, sex, and various socio-cultural characteristics.

Retrospective reports on what the respondent did when afflicted by a number of conditions in the past year are summarized in Table 9–5, and comparisons are made with the national sample. The differences between the Rhode Island and national samples are not as marked as for

TABLE 9–5. EXPERIENCE OF INITIAL SAMPLE WITH TWENTY-SEVEN SELECTED SYMPTOMS AND CONDITIONS, AND MEDICAL CONSULTATION SOUGHT WITHIN PAST YEAR

(SHOW CARD 7) READ LIST ALOUD WITH RESPONDENT
28A. Which of these conditions have you yourself had at any time during the last year? (CHECK ALL THOSE MENTIONED UNDER COLUMN "HAS HAD." IF R "HAS NOT HAD" A CONDITION, BE SURE TO CHECK "HAS NOT HAD.")
Now, would you please tell me for each condition mentioned: Did you see a doctor (dentist) about condition in the past year?

Symptom/condition	Per cent			
	Had	Not had	Not ascertained[a]	Had and saw Dr.
Cough for several weeks	15	85	*	53 (49)[b]
Diarrhea or constipation	26	74	*	31 (44)
Feeling of dizziness	25	74	*	60 (56)
Frequent headaches	19	80	*	53 (50)
Lump or discolored patches of skin	8	92	*	75 (67)
Sore throat, running nose	36	64	*	28 (40)
Backache fairly often	23	77	*	52 (47)
Rash or itch for a week or more	13	87	*	58 (55)
Severe shortness of breath	11	89	*	74 (56)
Toothache	18	82	*	89 (77)
Unexplained loss of 10 pounds or more	5	95	*	60 (64)
Feeling tired all the time	31	69	*	47 (54)
Allergy	14	86	*	50
Arthritis, rheumatism	19	81	*	53
Asthma	4	95	*	60
Diabetes	4	96	*	100
Gall bladder, liver	4	96	*	86
Heart trouble	4	96	*	92
High blood pressure	13	87	*	90
Kidney trouble	4	96	*	90
Piles or hemorrhoids	15	85	*	39
Sinus trouble	20	80	*	41
Varicose veins	12	88	*	37
Indigestion	22	78	*	18
Cut finger	31	69	*	10
Have a temperature (over 101)	15	85	*	67
Inability to sleep	25	75	*	36

[a] Not ascertained. Asterisk signifies less than 0.5 per cent. Rows do not always sum 100 because of rounding.
[b] Figures in parentheses taken from Feldman (1966), Table 3.3, p. 46.

the normative prescriptions. However, in the cases of diarrhea or constipation and sore throat or running nose the local respondents again exhibited an independence of doctors that distinguished them from the national sample.

In regard to fertility control, a substantial majority of respondents and their spouses favored the practice. This was true for both male and female respondents and is particularly noteworthy in view of the Catholic majority in the state's population (Table 9–6).

Detailed questions about contraceptive methods ever or currently employed were asked only of female respondents. The methods used by 345 users among 581 ever-married females indicate a heavy reliance upon rhythm, abstinence, and withdrawal (Table 9–7). This is not surprising in view of the religious distribution of the population.

TABLE 9–6. ATTITUDE OF RESPONDENT AND SPOUSE TOWARD THE USE OF CONTRACEPTION IN 1,004 HOUSEHOLDS OF EVER-MARRIED RESPONDENTS (PER CENT)

Attitude toward use of contraception	Respondent[a]	Spouse[a]
Positive	67.9	61.9
Negative	22.9	20.4
Pro-Con	6.6	6.1
Refused to discuss	1.7	1.6
Don't know	0.4	8.7
Not ascertained	0.5	1.3
Total	100.0	100.0

[a] Respondent reported about his own attitude, whether or not presently married. In reporting spouse's attitude the subject was either the current spouse if married, or the last spouse if widowed, separated, or divorced.

TABLE 9–7. USE OF CONTRACEPTIVE METHODS BY EVER-MARRIED FEMALE RESPONDENT;

Method	Number of cases[a]	Per cent among 345 ever-married users	Per cent among 581 ever-married females
Rhythm	134	38.8	23.1
Abstinence	43	12.5	7.4
Rubber; condom	137	39.7	23.6
Withdrawal	95	27.5	16.4
The pill	85	24.6	14.6
I.U.D.; coil	8	2.3	1.4
Diaphragm	69	20.0	11.9
Douche	67	19.4	11.5
Jelly; creme	23	6.7	4.0
Suppositories	10	2.9	1.7
Foam; foam tablet	17	4.9	2.9
Sponge	0	0.0	0.0

[a] Sums to more than 345 due to use of multiple methods.

The contraceptive pill is of particular interest, as it was cited more frequently than the diaphragm as a preferred method. The characteristics and experience of pill users will be closely scrutinized, not only in the first year's sample but in successive years as well. In this manner, a sufficiently large group of pill users will be assembled for detailed study. Equally important, the follow-up interviews will provide a basis for detecting changes in contraceptive behavior, including adoption of new methods, abandonment of earlier practices, and the reasons for the changes.

Another subject of concern in this community study is fertility impairment. Self-reported fertility conditions of respondent and spouse are being classified (Table 9–8) and investigated. Special attention will be focused on those married couples who cannot conceive even though the wife is under fifty years of age. The follow-up interviews will permit the longitudinal evaluation of these couples as well as of other couples among whom fertility problems make their appearance—perhaps when they stop contraception in an effort to conceive.

POTENTIALS

It is too early to judge whether the Human Population Laboratory is fulfilling the hopes on which it was conceived. However, the high level of community co-operation elicited and the quality of the data already collected bode well for the project's ultimate success.

The incorporation of monthly follow-ups into the design will provide a unique opportunity to measure attitudinal or behavioral changes over time. For example, when public policies (such as the provisions of Medicare or Medicaid) are initiated or altered, the inclusion of appropriate questions in the next round of interviews will assure a rapid assessment of the public reaction. Such data should be of value to social and medical scientists as well as to government officials and others engaged in policy-making or execution.

TABLE 9–8. MARITAL AND CONCEPTION STATUS OF 1,004 HOUSEHOLDS OF EVER-MARRIED RESPONDENTS

Marital and conception status	Per cent
Respondent married, couple can conceive	48.1
Respondent widowed, separated, or divorced	22.4
Respondent married, wife under fifty years of age, but couple cannot conceive	6.3
Respondent married, wife over fifty years of age, classified "couple cannot conceive"	22.6
Respondent married, couple's conception status not ascertained	0.6
Total	100.0

A closely related potential is the opportunity for public agencies to utilize the Population Laboratory as a systematic data source. The laboratory's policy calls for co-operative research projects with other departments of the university and with public institutions outside the university. An example of such collaboration is the program undertaken with the State Health Department to code census tract identification on all of the state's birth and death records for the period 1960 to 1967. This information will benefit both the laboratory in its research and the health and social agencies of the state.

A unique opportunity was recently afforded the State Health Department to evaluate an aspect of its health education program with the co-operation of the Population Laboratory. An eight-page magazine supplement devoted to various aspects of diabetes was distributed as part of the Sunday newspaper. The two monthly follow-up interviews immediately preceding and immediately following the distribution of the supplement made possible a before and after experimental assessment of the effectiveness of newspapers in disseminating health information. In the absence of a community laboratory, no effort would have been made to include program evaluation as part of a public education campaign.

In a related development, the Governor's Commission on Vocational Rehabilitation is seeking to participate in a future monthly round. Although it is required by law to assess the prevalence and nature of disabling conditions in Rhode Island, the commission has no means at its own disposal to obtain such data. Inclusion of appropriate questions in a round of interviews will provide clues as to the extent of these conditions. It is anticipated that, as public awareness of the laboratory increases, the demands for its use by other state health and social agencies will also grow.

There should also be ample opportunity to utilize follow-up contacts for collecting specialized data on selected subsegments of the total sample. The 1,127 households in the first year's sample comprise 3,750 individuals of all ages and sociodemographic characteristics. Although only one individual in each household has been selected as respondent in the field survey and follow-up interviews, other household members might well serve as additional respondents or subjects of inquiry. For example, a survey of school dropouts could utilize the teenagers identified in the sample. Surveys of utilization of maternal health facilities could focus on women of childbearing age. Studies on adjustment to the problems of old age could be conducted on the approximately 400 older persons in the sampled households. In other instances it might be desired to survey selected households in greater detail. For example, special surveys of Jews, working class families, or recent migrants to the suburbs could be incorporated into the follow-up contacts once the subjects of interest were identified at the initial interview.

Another indirect but very important potential of the laboratory lies in the opportunities it can provide for training researchers in the social sciences and public health. After a year of academic preparation in research methods, doctoral candidates in sociology and demography at Brown University are now required to participate in a year's research practicum. A number of these students will satisfy this requirement by participating in the activities of the Population Laboratory. As research apprentices, they will take part in the decision-making and in the implementation of various phases of community study, including sample selection, schedule design, pretesting, field interviewing, follow-up contacts, code construction, data processing, and data analysis. Thus, whatever contributions the laboratory makes through its substantive findings and its methodological studies will be augmented by the training offered these students and the commitment they may make to careers in health-related research.

Acknowledgments

The Population Laboratory is supported by Grant CH 00212 from the U.S. Department of Health, Education, and Welfare, Public Health Service.

References

Burgess, A. M., Jr., Organic, H. N., Peterson, O. L., and Burnight, R. G. 1967. Medical care in Rhode Island: A report of studies planned and in progress. *Rhode Island Med. J.* 50:696–99.

Burnight, R. G. 1965. Chronic morbidity and the socio-economic characteristics of older urban males. *Milbank Mem. Fund Quart.* 43:311–22.

Burnight, R. G. and Marden, P. G. 1967. Social correlates of weight in an aging population. *Milbank Mem. Fund Quart.* 40:74–92.

Feldman, J. 1966. *The Dissemination of Health Information.* Chicago: Aldine.

Goldstein, S. 1966. Jewish mortality and survival patterns: Providence, Rhode Island, 1962–1964. *Eugen. Quart.* 13:48–61.

Goldstein, S. and Mayer, K. B. 1965. Demographic correlates of status differences in a metropolitan population. *Urban Stud.* 2:67–84.

———. 1958. *The Ecology of Providence: Basic Social and Demographic Data by Census Tract.* Providence: Brown University. (Processed.)

———. 1961. *The Ecology of Providence: II, Comparative Data on Social and Demographic Process, 1950–54 and 1955–59.* Providence: Brown University. (Processed.)

———. 1962. *Metropolitanization and Population Change in Rhode Island.* Providence: R. I. Development Council.

————. 1963. *The People of Rhode Island, 1960.* Providence: R. I. Development Council.

————. 1964a. Migration and the journey to work. *Soc. Forces* 42:472–81.

————. 1964b. Population decline and the social and demographic structure of an American city. *Am. Soc. Rev.* 29:48–54.

Hochstim, J. 1967. A critical comparison of three strategies of collecting data from households. *J. Am. Statist. Ass.* 62:976–89.

Kantor, M. B. ed. 1965. *Mobility and Mental Health.* Springfield: C. C Thomas.

Kish, L. 1965. *Survey Sampling.* New York: John Wiley & Sons.

Pfautz, H. W. and Wilder, G. 1962. The ecology of a mental hospital. *J. Health Hum. Behav.* 3:67–72.

U.S. Bureau of the Census. 1963. *U.S. Census of Population, 1960. Standard Metropolitan Statistical Areas.* Washington: U.S. Government Printing Office.

U.S. Bureau of the Census. 1961. *1960 Census of Population,* vol. 1, part 41. Washington: U.S. Government Printing Office.

U.S. Bureau of the Census. 1966. *Current Population Reports, Special Census of Rhode Island, 1 October 1965,* Series P-28, no. 1393. Washington: U.S. Government Printing Office.

Wolpert, J. 1966. Migration as an adjustment to environmental stress. *J. Soc. Issues* 22:92–102.

EDITORIAL COMMENTS

1. The Population Laboratory in Rhode Island represents an elaboration of ongoing research activities at Brown University, including those of the Department of Sociology, the Center for Aging Research, and the collaborative studies with the Department of Preventive Medicine at Harvard. Its study goals appear to be very similar to those of the U.S. National Health Survey, viz., morbidity from disease and disability; patterns of health care services; social and environmental factors in health; and health service utilization, etc.

2. The fact that Rhode Island is entirely subdivided into census tracts upon which federal and state statistics are based is a distinct advantage in community studies. This should facilitate record linkage between the vital statistics offices and the laboratory. Another advantage is the centripetal pattern of medical care in the state. This contrasts with the situation in Washington Heights which is much less of a closed system.

3. The sample size of 1,100 interviews per year represents what was thought to be an acceptable work load. No particular hypothesis-testing situation was considered in the determination, however.

4. A very important feature of the Rhode Island Population Laboratory are the plans to supplement the household interview data with

records from hospitals, physicians, and vital statistics registries. This will make it possible to estimate morbidity rates and trends, to validate questionnaire responses, and to undertake methodologic investigations of the sample survey process itself.

5. Two other useful features of the study are, first, the "surprise stratum" which will permit adjustments for rapid demographic changes and, second, the cumulative nature of the clustered samples which will permit the inclusion of additional households should this be required.

6. The extent of the laboratory's plans to trace nonrespondents is also impressive: city directories, inquiries from neighbors, and other sources are to be employed. Not all community studies have been able to devote this much attention to nonresponse.

7. The close relationship of the laboratory with the state's public health agencies is suggested by the following activities already undertaken: evaluation of a health education campaign on diabetes for the State Health Department; development of an interview round on disability for the State Commission on Vocational Rehabilitation; and the coding of census tract information on all state birth and death certificates.

PART IV

PSYCHIATRIC SURVEYS

Population samples from diversified rural and urban areas (Stirling County, Nova Scotia, and New York City) were utilized for studies of the relationship between the sociocultural environment and psychiatric disease. Psychiatrists, employing modified clinical criteria, estimated the likelihood that each respondent had a psychiatric disorder. Information was also assembled on a variety of symptom patterns reported by the respondents on personal interview. Correlations between the various symptoms and relationships between symptoms and clinically determined "caseness" were investigated by techniques of multi-factorial analysis.

COMPARISON OF FACTOR STRUCTURES IN URBAN NEW YORK AND RURAL NOVA SCOTIA POPULATION SAMPLES: A STUDY IN PSYCHIATRIC EPIDEMIOLOGY

Robert C. Benfari and Alexander H. Leighton

INTRODUCTION

The relationships between psychiatric disorders and the sociocultural environment have been under investigation in a rural area of Nova Scotia since 1948 (Leighton 1959). Stirling County was chosen because within its geographic boundaries there are communities with markedly contrasting characteristics—demographic, economic, sociocultural, and historical—which were thought to be of possible significance in the etiology or course of psychiatric disease. Several years later a similar investigation was undertaken in a highly urbanized population of New York City.

THE COMMUNITIES

Stirling County*

Stirling County comprises approximately 970 square miles of Nova Scotia, one edge dipping into the sea, the other into the forest that borders most of the northeastern extremes of the North American

* Condensed from Leighton et al, 1963.

continent. Between the shore and the forest there are strips and fingers of cleared land where subsistence farming is carried on. The principal occupations of the area are fishing, lumbering, and farming. An additional occupation is taking care of the tourists who come to admire the region's scenery, to enjoy its moderate climate, and to take advantage of the possibilities for sport and recreation.

The population consists of approximately 20,000 persons, of whom a little more than half are English-speaking, principally the descendants of migrants from New England in the late eighteenth and early nineteenth centuries. The balance are French-speaking Acadians, whose ancestors came from rural France in the seventeenth and eighteenth centuries. They have tended to stay together in one-half of Stirling County, while the English-speaking population inhabit the other half.

In the French half of the county, St. Malo, shore line settlements are now practically continuous. One, Mattapan, with a shipbuilding industry, is considerably larger than the rest. The English settlements show more tendency to clump into villages and even towns. The largest, Bristol, is a port and shopping center for the whole county. In addition to the French and English groups, there are also several settlements of Negro families, some of whom are descendants of escaped slaves while others arrived with English immigrants or, more recently, migrated from the West Indies.

While the entire county was included in the study, certain areas within it were selected for closer attention. The rationale was to identify English and French groups living in integrated and disintegrated social settings in order to test the hypothesis, that where the environment is disintegrated there will be more evidence of psychological difficulties. The town of Bristol, though sociologically heterogeneous, was also chosen for special study.

New York City

Several communities of New York City were sampled in such a manner as to assure the inclusion of socially integrated and disintegrated white neighborhoods. These included census tract areas from the Eastside of Manhattan, Canarsie and Park Slope in Brooklyn, as well as Queens.

METHODS

The rural sample from Nova Scotia was obtained by selecting respondents from each community of Stirling County in proportion to its population. No attempt was made to analyze the results according to the characteristics of the individual communities, although such cross-comparisons might be useful in future studies.

The 290 respondents for the New York survey were selected by a stratified sampling procedure from 8 of the 2,056 census tracts in New York City. These tracts were chosen after a winnowing process directed at obtaining those at the extremes of the integration-disintegration continuum (Hughes et al. 1960), predominantly white in their population composition. The intention was to maximize comparability with the Nova Scotia sample.

The criteria employed for the initial sampling were largely indices derived from New York City census tract data on socioeconomic deprivation, family disorganization, juvenile delinquency, cultural contrast, and racial composition. Since the environment of the respondents was of interest, in addition to their mental health, the selection procedure specified that two socially contrasting blocks be chosen within each census tract, rather than being scattered throughout the tracts. In this fashion 16 social blocks or neighborhoods were selected, each representative of the 2 extreme degrees of social integration which account for, perhaps, 5 to 7 per cent of the total population of New York City.

An important feature of this study were the criteria for "caseness," i.e., the bases for labeling the respondent a psychiatric case. Existing diagnostic classification schemes in psychiatry usually contain references to presumed causal factors. This has obvious disadvantages when the research aim is to explore etiology. In order to avoid this difficulty, a phenomenological diagnostic procedure was devised in which the criteria for assessment were the symptom patterns reported by the surveyed respondents and evaluated by specially trained psychiatrists. The 1952 Diagnostic and Statistical Manual of the American Psychiatric Association was used to classify the symptoms, but only after the removal therefrom of all causal assumptions.

Information on respondents was obtained from a number of sources, including:

1. A questionnaire interview.
2. Observations by the interviewer.
3. Impressions from local physicians (if available).
4. Hospital and other institutional records (if available).

Utilizing these data sources, the respondents were assigned as many symptom patterns as their records suggested. These were classified into nine major rubrics, some of which have been modified as the study has progressed (Table 10-1).

Each symptom pattern was recorded as to whether it was current at the time of the interview or whether it had occurred only in the past. Its duration was also noted. A judgment was then made as to the extent of

TABLE 10–1. DETAILED SYMPTOM PATTERNS UTILIZED IN STIRLING COUNTY AND NEW YORK CITY SURVEYS

Major symptom rubric	Detailed symptom pattern
I. Psychophysiologic disorders	1. Allergies 2. Cardiovascular reactions 3. Endocrine reactions 4. Gastrointestinal reactions 5. Genitourinary reactions 6. Headaches 7. Hemic and lymphatic reactions 8. Musculoskeletal reactions 9. Reactions of organs of special sense 10. Respiratory reactions 11. Skin reactions 12. Subjective body sensations 13. Weight disturbances
II. Psychoneurotic disorders	14. Anxiety reaction 15. Conversion reaction 16. Depressive reaction 17. Dissociative reaction 18. Fatigue state 19. Hypochondriacal reaction 20. Obsessive-compulsive reaction 21. Paranoid reaction 22. Phobic reaction 23. Tension state
III. Personality disorders	24. Compulsive personality 25. Emotionally unstable personality 26. Dependent or passive-aggressive personality 27. Inadequate personality 28. Paranoid personality 29. Schizoid personality 30. Other personality disorder
IV. Sociopathic disorders	31. Alcoholism 32. Antisocial reaction 33. Drug addiction 34. Dyssocial reaction 35. Sex deviation
V. Psychotic disorders	36. Affective psychosis 37. Paranoia 38. Schizophrenia 39. Other psychosis
VI. Mental deficiency	40. Mental deficiency
VII. Brain syndrome	41. Acute brain syndrome 42. Chronic brain syndrome
VIII. General motor disturbance	43. General motor disturbance
IX. Special symptom reactions	44. Special symptom reactions

impairment associated with each individual symptom pattern, with each major rubric, as well as for all symptoms combined. Finally, the psychiatrist's degree of confidence in the validity of the respondent's caseness was judged on a four-point scale ranging from high (A) to medium (B) to low (C) to absent (D). The latter, in effect, was the estimated probability that the respondent is, or was at some time in his life, a psychiatric case.

The data were examined utilizing techniques of multivariate analysis which have been made possible by the advent of high speed electronic computers. These techniques are particularly applicable to problems of classification such as, for example, determining the minimum number of detailed symptom patterns necessary for categorizing an individual as a psychiatric case (Benfari and Leighton 1968).

As discussed above, each respondent or group of respondents can be defined by 9 major symptom rubrics or 44 detailed symptom patterns (Table 10–1). The clustering of symptoms within given individuals or groups was of special interest.

Correlations between various symptoms and symptom clusters were examined by means of factor analysis. By this technique the number of variables (in this case, symptom patterns) in terms of which each individual can be described is reduced from 44 to a relatively small number of factors or symptom complexes. For each factor, coefficients of correlation between that factor and its constituent symptom patterns are calculated. These coefficients, which vary in value between +1.00 and −1.00, are termed "loadings." They measure the extent to which an increase in the score of a particular symptom pattern brings about an increase in the factor score.

It is customary to represent factors geometrically as reference axes in terms of which individual symptom patterns can be plotted. If a symptom pattern has a loading of 0.74 on one factor and 0.20 on another, for example, these factor loadings can be plotted on Cartesian co-ordinates. Points corresponding to the other component symptom patterns may be plotted in the same way, using the weights derived by the factor analysis. The reference axes are usually rotated in order to obtain the most satisfactory and easily interpretable pattern. In the present study, rotation was designed so that each symptom pattern had loadings on a minimum number of factors. It was hoped that this procedure would lead to what Cattell (1965) terms "unitary source traits" or symptoms. The observed number of factors actually exceeded two very often: this complicated the geometrical representation and the statistical analysis somewhat.

After computing the matrices of rotated factor loadings, the factors themselves were named and interpreted. This called for psychological insight rather than statistical inference. To discern the nature of a particular factor, for example, the symptom patterns having high loadings on that factor would be identified and attempts made to learn what attributes they have in common.

These methods, usually called "*R*-analysis," were applied to the various symptom pattern ratings in order to evaluate the relationships between symptom frequencies and to determine which symptoms occur in clusters. In the *R* technique one is dealing with correlations between symptoms in many individuals, i.e., common factors or shared characteristics. Another approach was also utilized, viz., the "*Q*-analysis," in which persons rather than symptoms are factor-analyzed (Mowrer 1953). This technique is designed to identify subgroups of persons with similar scores on a roster of symptoms. Thus, one can measure the extent of agreement between the clinical model of caseness (as judged by the psychiatrists) and the empirical model (based upon the factor analysis of symptom clusters).

PROBLEMS

Reliability

The extent of agreement between the evaluations of 283 Bristol respondents by 4 psychiatrists was rather high. On the *A, B, C,* and *D* rating of caseness the mean interpsychiatrist agreement was 67 per cent and the range was 65 to 72 per cent (Leighton et al. 1963). On the rating of degree of impairment the mean percentage was 78 and the range, 74 to 84 per cent. On the 7 main rubrics of symptom patterns, the mean interpsychiatrist agreement was 89 per cent, with a range of 79 to 98 per cent. When disagreements did occur, these most often involved only one grading step, such as between *A* and *B* or *B* and *C*.

The interpsychiatrist reliability in the urban survey of New York City was similar to that observed in Nova Scotia. As measured by product moment correlations, the correlation coefficients between raters ranged from 0.70 to 0.90 for the more common symptom patterns, both psychophysiological and psychoneurotic. Lower correlations (0.40 to 0.70) were found for the less easily diagnosed symptoms, such as psychotic reactions and personality disorders. For the most part, however, interpsychiatrist reliability was high enough to demonstrate a significant relationship between each possible pair of raters.

Validity

A serious problem in the use of instruments such as community surveys is their validity, i.e., whether they truly measure the phenomena under investigation. It was not possible to fully validate the survey questionnaire, if only because of the difficulties inherent in diagnosing psychiatric disorders. A number of validity checks were made, however, utilizing the method of triangulation, viz., gathering and comparing data from different sources, including resident physicians, existing clinic records as well as the questionnaires themselves, and direct psychiatric examination. Considerable agreement between the survey and clinical data was apparent (Leighton, Leighton, and Danley 1966).

Representativeness

In comparing the factor structures of the two samples it is necessary that the groups be comparable in such attributes as age, sex, and socio-economic status. These conditions were satisfied by the sampling procedures employed.

Nonresponse

Relatively low nonresponse rates were obtained. For the urban sample this was 15 per cent; for the rural sample, 7 per cent. Of course, it is possible that the two nonrespondent groups differed in the prevalence of psychiatric conditions, but this could not be ascertained.

FINDINGS

R–*Analysis*

The standard principal components factor analysis was computed for 290 respondents in the New York sample and for 100 cases drawn from the 1963 survey of Stirling County. A few of the 44 symptom patterns did not occur and were ignored. After the principal components solution, a biquartimax rotation was applied to the remaining factors in order to simplify the rows and columns of the factor matrix.

In the urban sample, 7 rotated factors accounted for 44.3 per cent of the total variance within the sample, the remaining 55.7 per cent being accounted for by a unique factor or factors, perhaps comprised of the lack of symptoms (Table 10–2). Factor I accounts for 29.5 per cent of the common factor variance. It appears to reflect an assortment of neuroses, as it comprises psychoneurotic as well as psychophysiologic symptoms.

Next in order of importance there are 2 distinct personality disorder factors (II and III) accounting, respectively, for 15.5 per cent and 12.9 per cent of the common factor variance. We have labeled factor II "personality disorder of the stormy type" in that it is constituted of the paranoid and emotionally unstable personality disorder symptom patterns. In addition to these a psychotic reaction symptom (schizophrenic reaction, undifferentiated) also loads on this factor, probably as a result of our inability to adequately distinguish psychotic symptoms of the paranoid and emotionally unstable types from schizophrenic symptoms. Factor III is a withdrawn personality disorder in that both schizoid and inadequate personality disorders have very high loadings on this factor.

TABLE 10–2. ROTATED FACTOR LOADINGS FOR VARIOUS SYMPTOM PATTERNS—URBAN SAMPLE, NEW YORK CITY

Factor	Symptom pattern	Loading	% variance accounted for by factor	
			Fractional[a]	Total[b]
I. Mixed neurosis			29.5	13.1
	Anxiety	.690		
	Subjective body sensations	.658		
	Depression	.637		
	Hypochondriasis	.621		
	Tension	.616		
	Fatigue	.598		
	Respiratory	.572		
	Cardiovascular	.556		
	Gastrointestinal	.540		
II. Personality disorder 1			15.5	6.9
	Paranoid personality	.795		
	Emotionally unstable	.623		
	Schizophrenic reaction	.598		
III. Personality disorder 2			12.9	5.7
	Schizoid	.828		
	Inadequate	.829		
IV. Psychosomatic 1			11.7	5.2
	Allergy	.663		
	Respiratory	.336		
	Brain syndrome	−.370		
	Cardiovascular	−.422		
	Musculoskeletal	−.475		
V. Psychosomatic 2			10.2	4.5
	Headache	.527		
	Genitourinary	.467		
VI. Undefined factors			10.2	4.5
	Psychoneurotic, other	.831		
	Drug and alcohol abuse	.708		
	Psychotic reaction, other	.424		
VII. Mental deficiency			9.9	4.4
	Mental deficiency	.680		
	Body weight	.426		
I–VII. All seven factors			100.0	44.3

[a] Proportion of common factor variance accounted for by given factor.
[b] Proportion of total variance accounted for by the common factors.

Two separate psychosomatic factors emerged from the analysis. Factor IV is a bipolar factor with symptom clusters of allergy plus respiratory symptoms or musculoskeletal plus gastrointestinal symptoms. Factor V is an interesting combination of genitourinary symptoms plus headaches. Eighty per cent of the respondents with high scores on this factor were women. Factor VI appears to be a cluster of undifferentiated symptoms, both neurotic and psychotic, that are also related to drug and alcohol abuse. The symptoms may be the underlying cause of the drug and alcohol abuse or, conversely, they may be their byproduct. Factor VII, accounting for 9.9 per cent of the common factor variance, is a syndrome made up of high loadings on mental deficiency and a more moderate loading on body weight disturbance. This unusual combination of symptom patterns may reflect the tendency of persons with symptoms of mental deficiency to be overweight, or vice versa.

In comparing the factor structure of the rural and urban samples it becomes evident that some symptom factors are common to both (Table 10–3). Factor I (mixed neurosis) appears in both and accounts for most of the common factor variance. The two psychosomatic factors appear to be similar in both samples. Allergy and respiratory symptoms comprise a psychosomatic factor in both the rural and urban areas. The second psychosomatic cluster has genitourinary symptoms as a common variable in both samples, although it is combined with different symptoms in the two groups: headache among females of the urban sample and gastrointestinal symptoms with body weight disturbances in the rural sample. The mental deficiency factor is more clearly defined in the urban population, while it is complexed with sociopathic symptoms in the Nova Scotia respondents. This may be a methodologic artifact in that sociopathy was not clearly assessed in the urban sample because of a relative lack of collateral information from physicians about the respondents. The types of personality disorders observed in the two samples are clearly distinct: a withdrawn and a stormy type in New York, and mixed types combined with sociopathic disorders in Nova Scotia.

An observation of possible theoretical importance is the emergence of Factor VIII in the rural sample. The interrelatedness of psychoneurotic depression and passive-aggressive personality disorder has been noted in the literature. It may be that the combination of these two symptom patterns indicates depression of the endogenous rather than of the reactive type. In the urban sample depression does not emerge as a single factor but, rather, is submerged in the mixed neurosis factor. Thus, it is not as easily interpreted as in the rural sample. Another factor which is noted in the rural population is one comprising brain

TABLE 10–3. ROTATED FACTOR LOADINGS FOR VARIOUS SYMPTOM PATTERNS—RURAL SAMPLE, NOVA SCOTIA

Factor	Symptom pattern	Loading	% variance accounted for by factor	
			Fractional[a]	Total[b]
I. Mixed neurosis			21.3	11.2
	Anxiety	.784		
	Tension	.735		
	Subjective body sensations	.671		
	Cardiovascular	.593		
	Headache	.539		
	Musculoskeletal	.493		
	Gastrointestinal	.490		
II. Psychosomatic 1			14.5	7.6
	Allergy	.647		
	Respiratory	.588		
III. Psychosomatic 2			10.4	5.5
	Genitourinary	.645		
	Body weight	.609		
	Gastrointestinal	.561		
IV. Sociopathy			12.3	6.5
	Sexual	.765		
	Mental deficiency	.660		
	Dyssocial	.654		
V. Sociopathy/personality disorder[a]			10.5	5.5
	Antisocial	.764		
	Personality disorder, other	.726		
VI. Sociopathy/personality disorder[b]			10.6	5.6
	Drug and alcohol abuse	.770		
	Inadequate personality	.720		
	Psychoneurotic, other	.500		
VII. Brain syndrome with concomitants			10.3	5.4
	Affective psychosis	.817		
	Brain syndrome	.780		
VIII. Psychoneurotic/personality disorder			10.1	5.3
	Depression	.644		
	Passive-aggressive	.616		
I–VIII. All eight factors			100.0	52.5

[a] Proportion of common factor variance accounted for by given factor.
[b] Proportion of total variance accounted for by the common factors.

syndrome and affective psychosis symptoms. The mood fluctuations which occur with brain syndrome may explain the clustering of these two symptom patterns in the rural sample. In the urban sample brain syndrome emerges as a bipolar factor, coupled with the psychosomatic syndrome of allergy and respiratory disorder. High scores on brain syndrome and musculoskeletal symptoms are associated with low scores on allergy or respiratory and vice versa. This is not readily interpretable. However, since brain syndrome increases with age it may imply that allergies and respiratory ailments related to allergies diminish with age.

The absence of a strong psychotic factor may be due in part to their relative infrequency in the populations studied or, perhaps, to the reluctance of the psychiatric raters to use these diagnostic categories in evaluations of questionnaire data.

Q-Analysis

To prepare for Q-analysis, the symptom pattern ratings of each respondent were converted to standardized scores, utilizing the mean and variance of the total sample as standards. The scores were then transposed so that the respondents became variables and the symptom patterns became units of analysis. Since the loadings of the factors in a Q-analysis represent the contribution of individuals to the factor cluster it would be impractical to list all the respondents and their separate loadings on each factor. Instead, the results of the Q-analysis are presented by including only persons having a loading of 0.50 or greater on any one factor.

In Table 10–4 are given the Q-analysis results on 116 respondents in the New York urban survey who were chosen so as to comprise a representative sampling of approximately equal numbers of each *A, B, C,* and *D* caseness rating. The distribution of respondents whose symptoms clustered in each of six factors as well as a zero loading group are cross-tabulated with ratings of caseness.

Factor I accounts for 30 per cent of the total common factor variance and distinguishes *A* and *B* cases from *C* and *D*'s. Factor V is a *B* factor (accounting for 10 per cent of common factor variance) and is related to psychosomatic disorder. Factors II and III distinguish *C* from the other cases and account for 40 per cent of the common factor variance. Factors VI, IV, and the zero loading are *D* factors accounting for 20 per cent of the variance. When one defines I as an *A* factor, V as a *B* factor, II and III as *C* factors, VI, IV, and zero as *D* factors there is 78 per cent agreement between these designated factors and the *A, B, C,* and *D* psychiatric rating of caseness. On the other hand, it is clear from the marginal totals that most of the *B* cases are submerged in Factor I with the *A* cases.

Since most of the factors accounted for differences between case and noncase, an additional Q-analysis of *A* and *B* cases alone was done to see whether there was a meaningful difference between the two groups based upon symptom patterns. Factors I and III were considered *A* factors; they consisted of the following symptom patterns:

TABLE 10-4. DISTRIBUTION OF RESPONDENTS ACCORDING TO CASENESS AND ROTATED FACTORS—URBAN SAMPLE, NEW YORK CITY (Q-ANALYSIS, BIQUARTIMAX ROTATION)

| Caseness category | Rotated factors | | | | | | ZERO Loading | TOTAL |
	I	V	II	III	VI	IV		
A	27	1	1	1	0	0	0	30
B	15	4	2	5	0	0	0	26
C	0	0	12	12	0	5	1	30
D	0	0	2	4	11	4	9	30
TOTAL	42	5	17	22	11	9	10	116
% Common Factor variance	30	10	20	20	10	10		
	Depression Anxiety Fatigue state Hypochondriasis Respiratory Gastrointestinal Subjective body sensations[a]	Skin Respiration Allergy Musculoskeletal Gastrointestinal[a]	Anxiety Skin or subjective body sensations[a]	Depression Tension state[a]	Skin Body weight disturbance[a]	Depression Psychoneurosis Other[a]	Zero loadings[a]	

THE ABOVE ARE SYMPTOMS THAT PREDICT PERSON CLUSTER BASED ON FACTOR SCORES.
[a] List of symptom patterns that predict person clusters based on factor scores.

Factor I: Depression
Gastrointestinal
Musculoskeletal
Subjective body
 sensations
Tensions

Factor III: Fatigue state
Genitourinary
Headache
Hypochondriasis
Subjective body
 sensations

Factors II and IV, constituting B factors were comprised as follows:

Factor II: Allergy
Respiratory

Factor IV: Anxiety
General motor
 disturbances
Hypochondriasis
Skin
Tension state

The distribution of these *A* and *B* factors among the 56 cases in the New York survey who received caseness ratings of *A* and *B* was then tabulated (Table 10–5). The agreement ratio was 75 per cent, indicating that good distinctions can be made between *A* and *B* cases in terms of symptom patterns.

TABLE 10–5. DISTRIBUTION OF RESPONDENTS CLASSIFIED AS *A* AND *B* CASES ACCORDING TO TWO SYMPTOM FACTOR SCORES (*Q*-ANALYSIS, BIQUARTIMAX ROTATION)

Caseness category	Rotated factors			
	I and III	II and IV	ZERO	TOTAL
A	25	5	0	30
B	7	17	2	26
Total	32	22	2	56

Symptom factors

Factor I: Anxiety
Depression
Gastrointestinal
Musculoskeletal
Subjective body sensations
Tension
% Common variance = 39

Factor II: Respiratory
Allergy
% Common variance = 23

Factor III: Fatigue state
Genitourinary
Headache
Hypochondriasis
Subjective body sensations
% Common variance = 23

Factor IV: Anxiety
General motor disturbance
Hypochondriasis
Skin
Tension
% Common variance = 15

From the Q-analysis, the following types were identified:

Two A factors,
Two B factors,
Two C factors, and
Three D factors.

Undoubtedly more types (as related to caseness) would emerge with larger sample sizes. We believe that the construct validity of the $ABCD$ model has been demonstrated by the congruence of the nine empirical factors and the four caseness categories.

POTENTIALS

The phenomena designated as symptoms in this report were not freely selected from nature but were, rather, limited by the questionnaire employed. Despite this, the factors that emerged were somewhat different from the usual clinical disorders and do not fit very well into any of the more traditional diagnostic categories. These findings are consistent with a position taken by one of us in considering the question of rethinking the nomenclature of psychiatric disorder (Leighton 1967). It seems significant that in both urban and rural samples the greatest amount of variance was accounted for by the combination of mixed neurosis and personality disorder symptoms (58 per cent and 41 per cent, respectively). It would seem that in adapting to ecological stresses both communities experienced similar symptom manifestations. These similarities are far greater than any of the observed differences. Of course additional studies would be required to confirm these general symptom factors, preferably in different age groups and cultures.

It is anticipated that the sociocultural environment, in addition to affecting frequencies, will also affect the expression of some symptom clusters. The observed differences in factors across the two cultural settings were, therefore, of interest; for example, the sociopathic/personality disorder factor in Nova Scotia and the schizothymia/cyclothymia personality disorder in New York City. Factor structures of the kind analyzed here could also be studied in private clinics, outpatient departments, and hospital wards of a given locality for whatever light might be shed on the problem.

Analysis of factor clusters also tells us something about the interrelationships between single symptom patterns that may be helpful in psychiatric classification. The distinctions between the two psychosomatic symptom clusters in the two samples, for example, may be related to malfunctions of the autonomic nervous system. The genitourinary, gastrointestinal and body weight cluster seems very similar to a psycho-somatic syndrome observed by Freeman (1946) and thought by him to reflect suppression of parasympathetic activity by excessive sympathetic activity. The other psychosomatic factor (allergy and respiratory) may thus be the result of increased parasympathetic activity. These are merely hypotheses which could be followed up by controlled physiological testing of respondents who are high in these factors. By the same reasoning, unitary symptom patterns might be related to maladaptations of normal systems. Suggestive leads such as these should be tested by the rigorous methods of epidemiology.

The intent of the present chapter has not been the presentation of substantive findings as such but, rather, the demonstration of an approach to community-based epidemiological surveys of psychiatric disorder. The ultimate aim would be to enlarge the data base both within a given cultural setting and across cultures to determine stable symptom clusters and to note unique symptom clusters due to variations in sociocultural determinants. Thus, one may ultimately hope to reach conclusions regarding the influence on health of the social environment in terms of qualitative and quantitative differences in symptom patterns.

References

American Psychiatric Association. 1952. *Diagnostic and Statistical Manual: for Mental Disorders*. Washington: U.S. Government Printing Office.

Benfari, R. C. and Leighton, A. H. 1968. *PROBE, A Multivariate Analysis of Stirling County Evaluation Procedure*. Harvard Report No. 91, Harvard School of Public Health. (Processed.)

Cattell, R. B. 1965. Factor analysis: An introduction to essentials II. The role of factor analysis in research. *Biometrics* 21:405–35.

Freeman, G. L. 1946. The physiological conquest of personality structure. In *Twentieth Century Psychology*. Edited by P. Harriman, pp. 405–28. New York: Philosophical Library.

Goldfarb, A., Moses, L., Downing, J., and Leighton, D. C. 1967. Reliability of psychiatrists' ratings in community case finding. *Am. J. Public Health* 57:2149–157.

Hollingshead, A. R. and Redlich, F. C. 1958. *Social Class and Mental Illness*. New York: John Wiley & Sons, Inc.

Hughes, C. C., Tremblay, M. A., Rapoport, R. M., and Leighton, A. H. 1960. *People of Cove and Woodlot: Communities from the Viewpoint of Social Psychiatry*, vol. II. *Stirling County Study of Psychiatric Disorder and Sociocultural Environment*. New York: Basic Books.

Langner, T. S. and Michael, S. T. 1963. *Life Stress and Mental Health: The Midtown Manhattan Study*, vol. II. *Thomas A. C. Rennie Series in Social Psychiatry*. New York: McGraw-Hill.

Leighton, A. H. 1959. *My Name is Legion: Foundations for a Theory of Man in Relation to Culture*, vol. I. *Stirling County Study of Psychiatric Disorder and Sociocultural Environment*. New York: Basic Books.

―――. 1967. Is social environment a cause of psychiatric disorder? In *Psychiatric Epidemiology and Mental Health Planning*. Edited by Monroe, R. F., Klee, G. D., and Brody, R. B., pp. 337–45. Psychiatric Research Report No. 22. Washington: American Psychiatric Association.

Leighton, D. C., Harding, J. S., Macklin, D. G., MacMillan, A. M., and Leighton, A. H. 1963. *The Character of Danger: Psychiatric Symptoms in Selected Communities*, vol. III. *The Stirling County Study of Psychiatric Disorder and Sociocultural Environment*. New York: Basic Books.

Leighton, A. H., Leighton, D. C., and Danley, R. A. 1966. Validity in mental health survey. *Canad. Psychiat. Ass. J.* 11:167–78.

McMahon, B., Pugh, T. F., and Ipsen, J. 1960. *Epidemiologic Methods*. Boston: Little, Brown and Company.

Mishler, E. G. and Scotch, N. A. 1963. Social-cultural factors in the epidemiology of schizophrenia: A review. *Psychiatry* 26:315–51.

Mowrer, O. H. 1953. *Psychotherapy Theory and Research*. New York: Ronald Press.

Srole, L., Langer, T. S., Michael, S. T., Opler, M. K., and Rennie, T. A. C. 1962. *Mental Health in the Metropolis: The Midtown Manhattan Study*, vol. I. *Thomas A. C. Rennie Series in Social Psychiatry*. New York: McGraw-Hill.

EDITORIAL COMMENTS

1. There have been a number of social surveys of mental illness in the United States during the past few decades (Jaco 1960). These have varied widely in their scope, methods, clinical definitions, and sources of data. In one type of study, questionnaire responses are utilized both for diagnostic classification of disease and for analysis of epidemiologic relationships. The Stirling County and the New York City surveys are of this type.

2. The reliability of caseness evaluations by the four participating psychiatrists was measured and found to be of a high order in both survey areas. A similar determination of response reliability in the sampled populations would also have been desirable, if circumstances permitted.

3. Two objectives appear to have been undertaken simultaneously in these studies: first, the development and validation of a system for classifying psychiatric symptoms and, second, the application of this system to study the relationships between psychiatric disorder and the sociocultural environment. Since no independent means were available for validating the symptom scores, it might have been preferable to

separate the epidemiological aspects of the survey from the methodological aspects.

4. Considering the criteria for the selection of the New York City sample, one wonders whether appropriate subsamples of the Washington Heights Master Sample Survey might not have served just as well as the specially drawn sample, if this were feasible.

5. A possible method for securing an objective verification of each respondent's mental health is given by the authors' suggestion for the "controlled physiological testing of respondents who are high in these (symptom) factors."

Reference

Jaco, E. G. 1960. *The Social Epidemiology of Mental Disorders: A Psychiatric Survey of Texas.* New York: Russell Sage Foundation.

CHAPTER 11

Not all epidemiologic studies require community-based samples for investigation. Patients hospitalized for a variety of reasons at one famous medical center (University-Community Hospital, New England) were selected for an intensive study of illness in its social setting. It was observed not only that illness affects social relationships but that the latter alter perceptions of illness. One may consider whether there are other methodologic approaches to such problems in addition to that described.

SOME REACTIONS TO THE IMPACT OF ILLNESS ON FAMILIES IN A NEW ENGLAND CITY

August B. Hollingshead

INTRODUCTION

An important and relatively unexplored area in medical research is the social setting in which diseases arise, are recognized, and are dealt with. This social setting is a function of the interactions of patients, families, physicians, and others at home and in the hospital. Whether a particular course of treatment is perceived as successful or not can be influenced by the interrelations between society and sickness. An in-depth study of such interrelations was conducted in a sample of patients hospitalized at an outstanding New England medical center.

THE COMMUNITY

The city in which the study was conducted is the center of a metropolitan area extending some 40 miles along the Atlantic Ocean on one side and some 10 to 20 miles inland on the other side. The area, integrated by manufacturing, financial, trade, and health institutions located in the city, is roughly rectangular in shape and encompasses some 500 square miles. The population is divided between the city with its 140,000 inhabitants and the suburban towns with a population of approximately 46,000.

Two major general hospitals care for the inpatient health needs of the metropolitan population. One is a large community hospital affiliated with a major school of medicine; the other is a middle-sized hospital operated by the Roman Catholic Church. The present study was centered in University-Community Hospital, which attracts some 93 per cent of its patients from the city and the surrounding towns. The remaining 7 per cent of the patients come from more distant places of residence.

METHODS

The propositus was a physically ill adult who had recently been admitted to the medical or surgical service of University-Community Hospital. An additional eligibility requirement was that he be a principal member of a family of procreation—defined as the husband or the wife of a spouse pair living in the same household. There were 225 families in the study, 113 represented by wives and 112 by husbands; each selected at random from among the aggregate of white married patients between forty and sixty-four years of age who were living with their spouses in the state and were conscious at hospital admission.

After the patients were selected, approval for their inclusion in the study was sought from the physicians of record as well as from the patients and their spouses. Once this was obtained, data were collected from patient, spouse, other family members, physicians, nurses, and ancillary medical personnel.

Questionnaire schedules were used in interviews with these persons and special attention was paid to the interactions between them and to the mood, intensity, and manifest feelings of each. The investigators were in direct face-to-face contact with patient, spouse, and family members for an average of 38 hours. In addition, about five or six hours were devoted to interviews with physicians, nurses, and hospital staff who were caring for the patient. After discharge from the hospital each patient was visited in his home periodically for two years in order to measure survivorship and degree of recovery from the illness or impairment.

The 225 patients sampled approximated 5 per cent of all study-eligible patients who were admitted to the hospital during the two-year period of case selection. They were divided randomly into 3 parts: 161 full-study families, 32 partial-study I families, and 32 partial-study II families. The full-study families were studied intensively in both the hospital and at home. The partial-study I families were studied less intensively in the hospital, but intensively after discharge. The partial-study II families were studied only in the home after the discharge of the principal member from the hospital. The 2 partial-study groups served as controls for the full-study families in order to determine if intensive study in the hospital influenced relations between the health professionals and the patient and, more indirectly, the relations of the health professionals to the family members of the patient. It may be noted that intensive study was not found to affect the relations of the health professionals to the patient or to the family members.

The assembled data were prepared for analysis by two different procedures. Specific items of information, both quantitative and qualitative, were coded and punched on Hollerith cards for machine processing. In addition, a 48-question assessment schedule was completed in order to summarize the respondent's experiences and the interviewer's observations. Each assessment item represented a consensus on a particular question arrived at by the two principal investigators.

PROBLEMS

Eleven physicians refused to grant permission for the inclusion in the study of 16 patients—8 men and 8 women. These patients had 4 characteristics in common:
1. They were all of high socioeconomic status.
2. They were all private patients (12 medical, 4 surgical).
3. They were all seriously ill (2 terminally).
4. Their physicians protected them from the study.

Five additional patients refused to participate in the study after their physician sponsors had given us permission to approach them. All were private patients, four women and one man. All faced major personal or social problems, and four of the five were afflicted with serious diseases: one who had advanced heart disease and a diseased gall bladder later died in the hospital; one had psoriasis and advanced arthritis; two were suffering from cancer, frightened, confused, and in pain. Four expressed the hope that they could co-operate later, but this did not come to pass as the enormity of their anxieties and debilitations engulfed them. A fifth patient refused to co-operate out of hand. He was a downwardly mobile, severely deteriorated, alcoholic with advanced cirrhosis of the liver. To be hospitalized was an insult to his dignity; to have his privacy invaded by the study was beyond his endurance.

The 21 nonrespondents represented 8.5 per cent of the 246 persons selected for study; 6.5 per cent were physician rejections and 2 per cent were patient rejections. Stated otherwise, 76 per cent of the rejections were by physicians in behalf of their patients and 24 per cent were patient rejections after the physician had given his consent for the study. It is significant that all of the rejections were among private patients. Moreover, even within the private accommodation category they were in the higher socioeconomic group.

Forty patients, one-quarter of the total, died before the field work was completed. This gives some indication of the number of very seriously ill persons who were included in the study.

FINDINGS

Sociobiographical Characteristics

The husbands of the study group had attained a mean age of fifty-four years and the wives fifty-one years. Eighty per cent of the husbands and wives were native Americans, two out of three having been born and reared in New England. The spouse pairs exhibited a high percentage of first marriages for both partners; only 18 per cent of either the husbands or the wives had been married before. There were children in 91 per cent of the families; children of parents in their forties and early fifties were usually still living in the parental home, while children of older parents rarely lived at home. For the most part, the families resided in single households, either in individual residences or in apartments. Only 13 per cent shared their homes with persons other than members of the nuclear family group, these extra persons being, in most instances, aged relatives or young children of relatives, but rarely boarders or nonrelatives. Socioeconomically, the families ranged from the wealthy with an annual income of $100,000 and more to the very poor eking out an existence on public welfare.

Impact of Illness on the Patient

Patients were classified into one of five categories according to our evaluation of the impact of their illnesses upon them. These categories, which were based upon the probable prognosis, the success of treatment, and the patient's subjective feelings, included:

1. Improved
2. Did not change
3. Became worse
4. Became much worse
5. Deteriorated catastrophically

Six of the patients (4 per cent) were classified as improved. Each of them suffered from a disease that was curable. Four were successfully treated by surgery and two improved with specific medical therapy. At the time of the home interview each had resumed his usual role in the home and on the job. The treatment they had received had relieved them of their symptoms and their worries over the illness.

Mr. Tischler is illustrative of the patients in the "improved" category. At the age of fifty-nine years he suffered progressive discomfort from a growing lump in his groin, and he began to fear it was cancer. He did not discuss it with his wife or anyone else until six weeks prior to his admission to the hospital. When Mrs. Tischler eventually learned of the lump, she too was fearful of cancer but did not mention this to her husband. However, she did discuss his condition with a close friend who was the secretary of a local surgeon. Through this friend, Mr. Tischler was introduced to the surgeon, who examined him, made a diagnosis of hernia, and recommended hospitalization. The surgeon scheduled Mr. Tischler's admission to the hospital for elective repair of the hernia. Both spouses thought the surgeon was trying to be kind to them, since in their fearful fantasies Mr. Tischler was afflicted with cancer.

After the surgical repair the hernia disappeared, the incision healed normally, and there were no complications. Mr. Tischler was free from pain and all disability; he resumed his usual functions at home, and he returned to his job in a few weeks. He was free from anxiety that the lump in his groin might be cancer. His state of mind improved just as the condition of his body did. He was pleased with the outcome and grateful for the services of his surgeon. Worry free, he approached his work with added vigor.

Forty-two patients (26 per cent) were classified in the "did not change" category. Prior to hospitalization these patients had usually suffered from acute illnesses that were sometimes very troubling. Hospitalization was indicated and a therapy was available to alleviate or cure their illnesses. Recovery from the episode of illness was accompanied by the restoration of their health. Over-all, individuals in this category exhibited few alterations in their feelings toward themselves, their work, and their families as a result of their illness. In general, they looked back upon the illness and the accompanying hospitalization as an historical event. It was over, and thankfully so.

To illustrate, Mr. Bickford, a fifty-one year-old businessman, developed abdominal pain suddenly. He telephoned his regular physician who told him to go immediately to the emergency service of the hospital. Mr. Bickford was met in the emergency room by his physician, and after examination he was admitted to the hospital. A need for emergency surgery was indicated, and he was taken to the operating room. A Meckel's diverticulum was found and removed, and he convalesced rapidly. After his return to work his view of the illness was that it had caused him temporary inconvenience, a moderate amount of suffering for a limited time, and a minimal economic loss, as his colleagues carried on his business during his illness. At the time of the home visit he thought his recovery was complete and he would probably have no complications from the illness or the treatment. Mr. Bickford's life changed very little from the onset of the illness to the time of his recovery and return to work. He felt the illness was now past and would not return. He was not burdened by unusual fears regarding his body, his ability to carry on his work, his home life, or his usual recreational activities.

Thirty-seven patients (23 per cent) "became worse" after hospitalization and convalescence than before. Some persons in this category were impaired by either disease or treatment. Whether their bodies were less whole or not, they felt disabled in various ways. Often the chief handicap was traceable to a belief that they had become peculiarly vulnerable to illness. They thought that they had been weakened by disease, the treatment, or both and that in the future they might undergo more suffering from the same disease or a different one. These individuals invariably exhibited symptoms of depression concerning themselves, their work, and their families.

Mrs. Dahlia illustrates this type of patient. For complications of her various maladies Mrs. Dahlia, age forty-one years, had been to numerous general practitioners, one of whom eventually referred her to a specialist who admitted her to the hospital for congestive heart failure. Over the years Mrs. Dahlia had suffered from hypertension, diabetes, obesity, and toxemia of pregnancy. She had known for ten years that she had diabetes, but she had denied its significance until this episode. While she was in the hospital Mrs. Dahlia belittled the severity of the condition by emphasizing to the interviewers that she was being treated as "queen for a day." She responded to medical treatment for diabetes and was soon discharged. However, during the hospitalization she became troubled by the thought that diabetes had killed her mother, and she was haunted by the idea that she would die of the same disease.

Although encouraged by her response to treatment and pleased with the new physician, whom she viewed as more competent than her previous one, she was uneasy about the relentless progress of her symptoms. She approached her household tasks and the supervision of her children with much less vigor. During the first home visit after discharge from the hospital she referred repeatedly to her body "falling apart." She told and retold the story of her mother's fatal illness and compared that story with her own unfolding experience with illness. She also recalled that several family members who had suffered from diabetes had died in their forties or fifties, and she said, "Time is running out. Diabetes gets you sooner or later, but in my family it gets you early." Although Mrs. Dahlia was not bereft either physically or emotionally, her feelings toward herself, her family, and her work became worse after her hospitalization.

Forty-four patients (27 per cent) were classified as "became much worse." These persons had strong feelings about their handicaps and their inability to carry on their work, their family life, and their future. Increasing disability was an overriding consideration in their efforts to cope with family and work situations. Sometimes it was physical disability that resulted in discouragement and depression; sometimes it was fear of illness (such as heart disease or malignancy) which made them feel much worse after hospitalization. As the illness progressed the handicaps became greater. The burdens of chronic disease were closing in on them, and the weakening persons often anticipated death.

An example of this type of patient is Mr. Stauffer who felt much worse after hospitalization. As a child he had believed that his parents compared him unfavorably with his brothers and sisters. He entered college hoping to go to medical school, but he did poorly and left. He then went to a technical school, successfully passed the courses and worked for a number of different companies.

Mr. Stauffer married and in due course had three children. The burden of family expenses over the years was so great that he had not been able to meet them even though Mrs. Stauffer went to work in a nearby store. Gradually, Mr. Stauffer came to view himself as a failure; his wife and children concurred in this view. The daughter married successfully, but the sons were having difficulty. The older son failed in college, as his father had done, and the younger son developed chronic osteomyelitis and had to leave school in the tenth grade.

At age forty-five, Mr. Stauffer had $2,000 saved, with which he hoped to buy into a small business, when he suddenly developed severe chest pains. He recognized the symptoms of a heart attack and called a doctor who sent him to the hospital. His diagnosis was coronary thrombosis. This illness experience confirmed Mr. Stauffer's conception of himself as a weakling and a failure. His life's savings had to be spent on his illness; this ended any possibility that his career ambitions would be achieved. He viewed the heart attack as heralding the beginning of old age and, perhaps, an early death. He had, for years, seen himself as inferior mentally; now he felt inferior physically. He told us that his sons were "failures too" and that he had "accomplished nothing he had set out to do." He became preoccupied with the fear that another heart seizure might occur and kill him. Mrs. Stauffer who had always dominated her husband and family began to belittle him even more and overpowered him with her open criticism. In brief, Mr. Stauffer's attitude toward himself predisposed him to interpret the illness in this way. Regardless of his physical recovery from the heart attack he was convinced that he would never feel healthy again.

The thirty-two patients (20 per cent) classified as "deteriorated catastrophically" were severely disabled by disease and each one had a poor prognosis. All were so weak that they were unable to engage in their usual work routines; some were wrenched away from their families and placed in institutions for custodial care, with the expectation that they would be there for the rest of their lives. They were physically devastated and emotionally severely depressed. Enmeshed in the impairment of their lives and powerless to alter the situation, these individuals were convinced that they were a burden to their families and to those who cared for them. A lingering death often contributed to the catastrophe for both the patient and the family. This is illustrated by the story of Mr. Deo, a victim of pulmonary tuberculosis.

Mr. Deo's first episode of tuberculosis began when he was thirty-eight years old. At that time the illness was controlled by medication after a brief sanitorium stay, and he continued working at his factory job until shortly before he entered our study at the age of fifty-one years. Now the illness had recurred, but the drugs which earlier had successfully controlled the infection were no longer effective. He was admitted to the hospital for evaluation and possible surgical treatment. The surgeons decided that removal of infected lung tissue would be the treatment of choice; however, removal of diseased tissue would mean the loss also of some functioning tissue which might result in such severe pulmonary insufficiency as to cause death. The surgeons, therefore, viewing him as a poor operative risk declined to operate; the patient was sent to the state tuberculosis sanitorium where different drug combinations were tried with little success. Mr. Deo viewed the sanitorium as a prison and found it difficult to endure the institutional controls. After a few months he signed out, against medical advice. He had resolved, for better or for worse, to take his chances at home.

Since the onset of his tuberculosis 13 years ago, Mr. Deo has suffered from many social and economic problems. His first wife committed suicide shortly after he became ill, leaving him with two children under ten years of age. His second wife reared the children. Mr. Deo was able to support his family and provide for the children's education through high school. During the course of his second stay in the sanitorium he gradually came to realize that he was a very sick man. He was discouraged and depressed, yet talked a great deal about wanting to get back to his job.

After he signed out of the sanitorium, Mr. Deo found life at home similar to what it had been in the public hospital. He was told not to sleep with Mrs. Deo, and he was separated from his children for fear of spreading the infection. At this point Mr. Deo viewed himself as an outcast from his family and an untouchable in society. He had only his wife to shield him from the public sanitorium. He was angry, depressed, and anxious. He felt there was nothing left for him. He could not return to work and he was isolated from society, particularly his wife and children. In brief, he had moved from the approved role of family head and wage earner to a sick role in which he was socially and physically bereft, stripped of his savings, and fully dependent on public welfare. As the disease process went on, his ability to function decreased and his anxieties rose until he was fully incapacitated physically and emotionally. During our last home visit a few days before he died, Mr. Deo expressed this final phase of hopelessness when he told us in a half-whisper: "I am just a little bit alive."

There were no significant differences in the patients' reactions to their illness experiences by sex, type of treatment received, or hospital service (medical or surgical). Instead, the person's subjective reactions were linked to the disease itself, its duration, and the degree of concomitant disability. A corrected contingency coefficient of 0.71 was calculated for the association between physical disability and subjective reaction to illness. This suggests that the physical effects of the disease process were the primary source of the sick person's feelings about his inability to perform his usual roles in the family and on the job.

Reactions of the Spouse to the Illness

Patient and spouse are linked to one another by generational and affective feelings, shared responsibilities, and years of living in their common home. The necessary removal of one responsible member of the spouse pair from the home for a shorter or longer time created situations which required adjustment to the changed situation by the patient, the spouse, the children, and others within the familial group. Prior to illness, the spouses had fulfilled their role responsibilities more or less successfully; now one of them had to carry on alone for an indefinite period of time, perhaps permanently.

In order to evaluate the emotional reactions of the spouse to the illness, his or her behavior toward the hospitalized person was studied, as well as statements made about adjustments in the family resulting from the illness. Assessments of the spouse's reactions to the illness statements made by other family members were utilized, as well as the behavior observed from the time the patient was selected for study, throughout the hospitalization, and during the home visits. The impact of the illness on the spouse was classified into four categories:

1. Minimal impact
2. Moderate impact
3. Extensive impact
4. Catastrophic impact

In the first category (minimal impact), the illness was either minor or of short duration, and the patient was left with no physical or emotional handicap at the end of convalescence. The family could and did cope successfully with the temporary adversity. For example, the illness of Mr. Cuffstat, who was hospitalized with an acute infectious disease, had little apparent impact upon his spouse. Although he was absent from the home for ten days he was hardly missed, as this couple and their children had lived with her parents from their marriage to the present time. He returned to his job in two weeks and there were no known aftereffects of the illness.

Mrs. Colten, who was afflicted with psoriasis, is another illustration of minimal impact of the illness on the spouse. Mrs. Colten's illness provided justification for an adjustment which both the husband and wife sought but which each was reluctant to act upon until her physician urged her to enter the hospital for treatment. Mrs. Colten was told the approximate length of her hospital stay and the expected outcome. Her absence from home did not seriously interrupt family routine because she had prepared meals in advance. Mr. Colten was relieved of the unpleasant task of caring for his wife's body, and Mrs. Colten escaped from her husband's sexual advances which she found distasteful. "It's a kind of vacation," Mrs. Colten told us in the hospital. Three weeks after her return home her condition was markedly improved and she was more cheerful than she had been in many months. Mr. Colten was pleased by his wife's improvement and her renewed efforts to meet her family responsibilities. Fifty-one (32 per cent) of the spouses were classified as having undergone reactions of minimal impact.

Forty-four (27 per cent) of the reactions were considered to be of moderate impact. This category includes cases in which the illness gave rise to reactions on the part of the spouse that were clearly discernible but did not seriously disrupt the adjustment the spouse pair had made to one another prior to the illness. Mrs. Roberts, who underwent a radical mastectomy for carcinoma of the breast, is illustrative of patients in this group. From childhood Mrs. Roberts had suffered from exposure to illness and death. She had assumed adult responsibilities for bringing up two brothers and a sister after her parents died at an early age. Since several persons in her family and among her friends had died of cancer, Mrs. Roberts thought she was doomed when she discovered a lump in her breast. Although her physician tried to reassure her by saying, "You've saved your life by coming in early for treatment," Mrs. Roberts's fears spread to Mr. Roberts and their son. Both became frightened by this development. Mr. Roberts and the son spent considerable time and energy discussing their fears and the prospects of Mrs. Roberts's early death with one another and with us.

After the surgery the family was pleased to hear the surgeon's assurances, but they were convinced that doctors do not always "tell the truth about cancer, and you just can't be sure." When she was discharged from the hospital Mrs. Roberts could not bear to look at her own body, and she would not allow Mr. Roberts to view her scars. In addition, since she had associated earlier uterine bleeding with her now established breast cancer, she refused to have sexual intercourse with her husband. Although Mr. Roberts accepted the enforced celibacy after Mrs. Roberts's hospitalization and convalescence from surgery, interspouse relationships became more tense than before.

Forty-two (26 per cent) of the families in the "extensive impact" category were faced with the necessity of coping with the disturbing influences of severe forms of physical diseases and emotional difficulties of the sick person. The occurrence of a heart attack, the existence of chronic alcoholism, advancing malignancy, and so on were very disquieting to the spouse. In all instances, the patients in this category could no longer carry out their usual family roles. Often they reversed their family position from dependability to dependency.

Mr. Ronco's illness provides an illustration of extensive impact on the spouse. Mr. Ronco had been a chronic alcoholic for many years and had been treated for bleeding esophageal varices, hepatic coma, meningitis, and renal complications arising from alcoholic cirrhosis of the liver. In the two years prior to the present hospitalization, Mr. Ronco had been admitted to the hospital 7 times for a total of 75 days. After liver failure developed he stopped drinking and accepted therapy in the outpatient department of the hospital, where he became almost a mascot. His adjustment to treatment was a kind of symbiosis in which he exchanged his body and its disease in return for limited therapy and the status the clinic physicians and nurses gave him for performing a superior role as a patient; he achieved a unique status in this situation and chose to make the most of it as long as he could.

Although Mr. Ronco had been a social problem to his family for several years, he had been able to produce an income to support them. However, at the age of sixty-two years, a few months before we began to study the family, he and his spouse became dependent upon the meager resources available through social security for total disability and the contributions of their three adult children. They were not eligible for public welfare as they had some savings and a house. Mrs. Ronco, at age sixty years, had no skills with which to earn money in the labor market. Besides, she was needed at home to prepare the menus in order to maintain the delicate balance of her husband's health. Financial problems, the daily worry of preparing special meals for Mr. Ronco, the necessity for his many trips to the hospital, home care, and medication created a new way of life that had an extensive impact on Mrs. Ronco and the related families in this kin group.

A catastrophic impact was judged to have occurred in 24 (15 per cent) of the families. This invariably followed upon the hospitalization of a severely disabled spouse or one who had a poor prognosis and faced an early death. When families in this category confronted untreatable disease, family functioning was altered initially because the patient was unable to perform his accustomed roles, but when death occurred the family structure was changed.

Mrs. Lottso illustrates the catastrophic impact of an illness upon the spouse. When the Lottso's general practitioner was asked for his permission to include Mrs. Lottso in the study, he characterized the Lottsos as "a roughhewn working class family." This physician was correct. Mr. Lottso is a subforeman in a local factory, earning $115 a week. He has been with this plant for 15 years and he has high seniority in his union. The Lottsos have three children, a married daughter living out of the country at an army post with her husband and two teen-aged sons.

Mrs. Lottso was suffering from metastasized cancer when she entered the study. During her first admission to this hospital some years ago a radical mastectomy had been performed. The surgeon told her, "You're one of the lucky ones. We got it all." Mrs. Lottso, who had attended school only through the ninth grade, was satisfied and returned home.

Four years later Mrs. Lottso complained to the family doctor of pain in her hip. The physician made an initial diagnosis of arthritis; three weeks later he changed this to bursitis. Some six weeks later Mrs. Lottso was brought to the hospital with a broken leg, and a third diagnosis was made—cancer of the bone. Mr. Lottso, when informed of his wife's condition, begged the physicians to keep the truth from her, and the interviewers were warned within one minute of their first contact with the family physician never to indicate to her that she had cancer. Mr. Lottso wanted to do everything possible for her. During the six subsequent hospitalizations Mrs. Lottso was treated for her "arthritis and bursitis" by chemotherapy and surgery to which she consented when her physician told her it would help alleviate the pain if it didn't actually make her better. In the course of treatment an orthopedic surgeon put a pin in her leg and repeated the operation a second time when the tissue failed to hold. He then had to remove the pin in a third operation.

During this long, complicated, and expensive series of hospitalizations, Mr. Lottso attempted to adjust to his domestic and economic problems. He sold the family's six-room home in a suburban town to help meet expenses entailed in his wife's illness. He moved with his family into a flat in a four-family house, owned by Mrs. Lottso's sister, in an area near the factory where he worked. In this way, the sister would be available to assist Mrs. Lottso when she was home from the hospital and Mr. Lottso would be nearer his place of work and would have more time for the family chores which now became his obligation. He told the interviewers that his sons were prepared for their mother's death: "My sons are men all the way." Yet, the sons seldom visited their mother in the hospital. Mrs. Lottso explained their absence by saying, "They're busy—one with his girl friend, and the other with his old car."

During the last months of Mrs. Lottso's life, her husband was frantic with fear that she would learn of her malignancy. His anxiety was the controlling factor in his relationships with her and with the physician. By entering into a conspiracy of silence with the physicians, he thought he was prolonging her life, since he was sure she would commit suicide if she learned she had cancer.

As time passed Mr. Lottso became increasingly worried about money. In the first year of the terminal illness he exhausted his Blue Cross-Blue Shield and major medical insurance coverage, spent an additional $2,500 of his earnings, and still owed over $1,000 in medical bills. Mrs. Lottso, ignorant of her impending death, worried most about the cost of her illness and its effects upon her husband and sons. She told us, "Doctors today charge lots of money. Everything is so expensive these days." However, she did not communicate her fears about expenses to her husband and he did not communicate his fears about her illness to her. By early fall of the second year of her illness Mrs. Lottso's hospitalizations had exhausted all of the family's medical benefits.

Upon his wife's final admission to the hospital, Mr. Lottso had an argument with the admissions officer. Mrs. Lottso had been brought into the hospital in an ambulance and was wheeled into the hall while Mr. Lottso, who had requested a private room for her, was parking his car outside. The admissions officer intercepted Mr. Lottso at the hospital entrance and challenged his ability to pay for a private room. Mr. Lottso was furious. He had always been able to pay the hospital bills for his wife's earlier admissions, and he could not understand the hospital's concern now that his wife was so ill. What Mr. Lottso had failed to realize was that his major medical policy was limited to $10,000 in a single year and the hospital had already collected $9,500 from it. As a consequence, the Lottsos accepted a multiple-bed room.

The day before the major medical insurance benefits expired completely, a hospital social worker came to her room and told Mrs. Lottso she had better have her husband arrange a transfer to a convalescent home. Mrs. Lottso was humiliated by what she thought was strange advice given in front of the other patients in her room, but she did not ask the reason for it, and the social worker did not explain. When Mr. Lottso came to the hospital Mrs. Lottso told him about the social worker's advice. He then questioned the social worker and was told that the hospital had done all it could for Mrs. Lottso. He said later, "I didn't believe them. I put two and two together and I realized that as long as the money lasted, the doctors and the hospital were interested in helping my wife, but my insurance was all gone." He knew, however, that the hospital would not "toss her out." Instead of looking for a convalescent home he went to the personnel officer in his factory and explained his predicament. The personnel officer made arrangements with the hospital for Mrs. Lottso to have credit for a month, with the assurance that the factory would underwrite the bill. The personnel officer then contacted the Cancer Society which agreed to pay $300 toward the medical expenses. Three weeks later Mrs. Lottso died.

Mr. Lottso had accumulated a total of $6,500 in medical bills after his insurance benefits were exhausted. Although Mrs. Lottso, while in the hospital, had been cared for by house staff, the family practitioner sent a bill for $1,700 for his calls. Mr. Lottso felt there was nothing he could do about this. He told us, "They just drain it out of a working man."

A year after Mrs. Lottso's death, the family was shattered. Mr. Lottso was living alone in a single room, "My bachelor quarters," he wryly commented. He was struggling with unpaid doctor and hospital bills. He was separated from his sons. One had dropped out of high school and enlisted in the army; the other had married, moved to another city, and was working part-time while he attended barber's school. Depressed and isolated, Mr. Lottso was alone with his memories.

The emotional impact of illness on the spouses of patients hospitalized in the wards was judged to be significantly greater than that on the spouses of semiprivate or private patients. There were relatively few differences from one type of accomodation to another in the proportion of spouses affected moderately or extensively, but there were sharp differences at the two extremes. There was a strong relationship between the kind of physical disability and the emotional response. In general, the emotional reaction of the well spouse was closely related to the level of the sick person's ability to perform his usual roles in the family. A strong relationship was also observed between family maladjustment and the expressed sense of relief at the death of the patient.

POTENTIALS

In the past 100 years, the most spectacular successes in treating disease have been based upon applications from the physical and biological sciences. At the same time, social influences upon health have been largely neglected. Our investigation represents one approach to the study of the interrelationships between sickness and society.

The sample was restricted to white persons living within a well-defined segment of the life arc and to functioning families residing in a single metropolitan area. This permitted us to concentrate our research around a variety of factors related to the illness in the hospital and in the post-hospital period as well.

By limiting the number of cases, we were able to study in depth the constellation of social factors revolving around the illness, rather than the illness per se. At the same time, the number of patients and families was large enough so that the assembled data could be quantified and then analyzed statistically. While we have not thrown any new light on the epidemiology of disease, we believe we have added to man's knowledge of the effects of social factors in the perception and treatment of disease. Our methodological approach offers a direct means for subjecting these factors to critical analysis.

A more comprehensive treatment of the material discussed here has been published elsewhere (Duff and Hollingshead 1968).

Reference

Duff, R. S. and Hollingshead, A. B. 1968. *Sickness and Society.* New York: Harper & Row.

EDITORIAL COMMENTS

1. This is not a community-based but, rather, a hospital-based study. It was included in the casebook to illustrate that not all epidemiological questions require a community approach for their resolution. Hospi-

talized persons, occupational groups, college students, and others, de-
pending upon the circumstances, may constitute appropriate populations
for sampling and study.

2. The author of the University-Community Hospital chapter was
a principal investigator in an earlier and classical community study of
social factors in psychiatric disease (Hollingshead and Redlich 1958).
It was found that there were significant associations between social
class status and the prevalence of psychiatric disorders, the types of
disorders, and the treatment modalities utilized by psychiatrists in the
New Haven area. In the present study, attention was to be intensively
focused upon illness (of all types) in its social setting. For this purpose,
a sample of patients and their spouses seen in one hospital is an appropriate study population.

3. The nonresponse was concentrated among higher social class
patients. This is the usual pattern in many studies. However, one
should note the recent emergence of minority group resistance to
interviews, as, for example, in Washington Heights.

4. The detailed observations made upon patients, spouses, doctors,
and other hospital figures are very illuminating. However, there are a
number of uncontrolled variables in this study. These include the
effects of the diseases, the prior mental health and spouse relationships of the patients, and, possibly, the social environment of the particular hospital studied. A subsequent study can be visualized in which
groups of demographically comparable patients with similar diseases
are followed through their hospitalization and post-hospitalization
period. The difficult problem of retrospectively ascertaining the pre-
illness mental status of patient and spouse would remain, of course,
even with this approach.

Reference

Hollingshead, A. B. and Redlich, F. C. 1958. *Social Class and Mental Illness: A Community Study*. New York: John Wiley & Sons, Inc.

PART V

NATIONAL HEALTH SURVEYS

National studies are a logical extension of community studies. The problems inherent in the epidemiological study of so large and heterogeneous a country as the United States are formidable. On the other hand, there are many methodologic and administrative advantages, some of which are discussed here.

THE UNITED STATES AS AN EPIDEMIOLOGIC
LABORATORY: AN OVERVIEW

Oswald K. Sagen

The concept that a nation as large as the United States of America can be regarded as a laboratory for epidemiological studies may be startling when first considered. It startled the writer when this was suggested as a theme. On reflection, this way of looking at epidemiology testifies to how we concern ourselves about the macrocosm as well as the microcosm and to how our tools of investigation have grown so as to enable us to deal with the large situation. This is certainly a far cry from the classical epidemiological investigation which could be carried out single-handedly.

What are the reasons for studying large populations as opposed to smaller, more tractable, population enclaves? One is that findings in a selected population group are not always generalizable to the entire population about which we are concerned. The selected population may be highly specialized without our being able to recognize this fact. In studies where effective control over important variables is either impossible or infeasible, using a large, heterogeneous population such as the nation as a whole will, in effect, neutralize the difficulty. This comes about because the uncontrolled variations in the national population tend to occur randomly. Therefore, they are, in a sense, self-compensating, and in a national sample they are absorbed within the sampling error instead of producing a bias of unknown magnitude or direction.

A second reason for using a national population is that a disease may not occur with sufficient frequency in a smaller subpopulation. Another cogent and practical reason is that epidemiological use can be made of existing national data, collected for other purposes, whereas sufficient detail on smaller localities is lacking. This applies particularly to basic demographic data, such as age and sex, for a study population. Since the United States population is counted only once every ten years, intercensal estimates of persons having selected characteristics of interest can be made better on a national basis than for individual geographic regions.

Not every epidemiological problem is suited for study in a national population. Physiological characteristics of persons are an appropriate subject. So, too, are the chronic diseases in which the pathological changes usually progress slowly enough so that observations may be extended over relatively long periods of time. Increasingly, concern over the utilization and distribution of health services has also led to the epidemiological study of these problems in the nation as a whole.

The communicable diseases continue to pose a problem to the entire nation. A national surveillance system has been developed in the United States, not only for administrative control purposes but also for epidemiological study of the diseases themselves, many of which are of such low incidence and prevalence that data from the entire population are required for their analysis.

For the most part, epidemiological studies based on the entire nation are necessarily in the form of descriptive statistics. Such studies are best suited to the development of epidemiological hypotheses rather than to hypothesis testing. In this sense, the nation as a whole is not quite a laboratory in that it is rather unsuitable for the kinds of controlled experiments that can be done on more limited populations. A notable exception to this was the nationwide trial of the Salk polio vaccine conducted some years ago. In any event, a nationwide experiment presents great difficulties in the maintenance of necessary controls and is very expensive.

An important consequence of employing the nation in epidemiological studies is that especially sophisticated statistical methods are required for the study design as well as for the collection, tabulation, and analysis of the data. All of this impels epidemiology toward a coordinated interdisciplinary approach on a large scale, a process which becomes more apparent when one considers the data collection devices used in studies of national populations.

There are two types of data collection methods for national studies:
1. Reporting mechanisms.
2. Population survey mechanisms.

The reporting mechanism is a system of gathering information on each event as it occurs at, or near to, the time of occurrence. Prime examples are the vital statistics system and the notifiable disease surveillance system. A feature of both systems is that data are sought on 100 per cent of the events. The 100 per cent reporting mechanism has the disadvantage that the reporting is often variable as to completeness, even when required by law.* Also, in trying to ascertain all events it is difficult to obtain uniformity in the reporting of many important characteristics of the event and in the application of a standard definition of the event itself. For example, the distinction between what constitutes a live birth and what constitutes a stillbirth is not easily made for borderline cases. Similarly, wide variations in both standards and procedures for establishing diagnoses are to be found over the nation as a whole. In both types of reporting mechanisms there is no practicable way to insure complete uniformity. Therefore, national data collected on a 100 per cent basis cannot furnish the refined information which is needed for many purposes. The great advantage of such data is that they relate to an entire population and can provide comparable statistics between the various regions of a country. It must be remembered, of course, that no large data collection mechanism escapes underreporting, the extent of which is difficult and costly to measure.

Population survey mechanisms are a purposeful elicitation of data, usually on a sampling basis. The oldest operating survey mechanism in the United States is the decennial census of population, which enumerates on a 100 per cent basis. On the other hand, the national surveys on health and disease are done on samplings of the national population. Modern sampling has the advantage of producing data at less cost and with a specified precision. Sample surveys generally permit more attention to and control over standardization of the information. A principal disadvantage is that the smaller the sample the less can be learned about low frequency events or classes, while the larger the sample the greater the cost and attendant difficulties. The problem of survey design, therefore, is somewhat delicate and requires a highly sophisticated approach. A manifest advantage is that surveys permit the investigation of a variety of subjects and can be specifically designed for the purpose at hand.

The data collection methods just discussed apply equally to epidemiological studies of smaller areas and to the nation as a whole. However,

---

* For both vital statistics and communicable disease surveillance the reporting is done under state laws and state administration. Data are furnished to the federal government on a co-operative basis, and, inevitably, there is a lack of full uniformity in the data collection process.

it is especially important to have their advantages and shortcomings in mind when thinking about the nation as an epidemiological laboratory and when using information derived from our national health surveys. While there have been various surveys of the nation as a whole on many health subjects, the only continuing program is the one established by the National Health Survey Act of 1956. This program has developed three approaches to the collection of data for epidemiological purposes:

1. *The Household Interview Survey*, collects data in personal interviews with a sample of the national population and obtains the kinds of information which people can, and are willing to give, about themselves.
2. *The Health Examination Survey*, collects data by a single visit, direct physical examination of sampled individuals in order to obtain physiological and physical measurements.
3. *Surveys based on health resources and facilities*, obtain data on these resources and also on such characteristics of the utilizers of health services as their personal attributes, health problems, and types of health services received.

These surveys are producing an abundance of data which are periodically summarized and published by the National Center for Health Statistics in its report series *Vital and Health Statistics* (see References).

The data from the national health surveys yield baseline information which have particular value in epidemiology. Reports from the Health Examination Survey, for example, provide population norms based on carefully standardized observations of body measurements, blood pressure, hearing levels, glucose tolerance, serum cholesterol levels, blood hematocrit, and visual acuity, among others. They also provide prevalence estimates for a variety of chronic conditions. One useful product was the analysis of data on age at menopause by MacMahon and Worcester (1966). This pointed up the value of the national sample, emphasized the epidemiological importance of these data, and called attention to the methodological problems of studying this important phenomenon. The fact that other studies on menopausal age have been conducted on specialized populations, primarily hospitalized women, was also noted.

Because the Household Interview Survey has been carried on continuously since its initiation in July 1957, it can provide useful trend data of epidemiological significance. These include annual reports on the incidence of various acute conditions and associated disabilities. The trend observed for measles, as an illustration, reflects the dramatic reduction in this disease subsequent to the extensive program of vaccination. This confirmed previous observations based on notifiable disease reports, which, because of their variable degrees of completeness, tend to distort the true situation.

Trends in the prevalence of diseases and in the bed disability and other limitations of activity associated with them are published annually in the Health Statistics series. In addition, a considerable amount of information on the characteristics of persons with chronic disease is made available. All these data pertain to noninstitutionalized persons, of which nearly one out of every two has a chronic condition of some kind. Data on institutionalized persons are now being collected in new surveys based on hospital and other institutional records.

The national statistics described here also serve epidemiology indirectly by making it possible to identify the health problems of greatest impact on the population. Even though epidemiological research necessarily focuses on one problem at a time, it is useful to know something about the totality of problems before selecting a particular one and before seeking support for its investigation.

Although our national health data system produces a wide variety of useful information and has many important implications for epidemiology, it must be recognized that there remain many deficiencies both in its operation and application. The natality and mortality data from vital statistics surveillance have been collected and used for many years but their potentials for epidemiological purposes have not been fully exploited. Improvement is needed in the quality of the information gathered and in the techniques of assembling, tabulating, analyzing, and reporting data. In the area of surveys, two particularly important developments are essential. First, larger samples must be drawn so as to provide statistics in greater detail. More geographic detail is needed, even for the higher frequency events. More detailed information on the demographic characteristics of the population (less broad age groupings, for example) is also needed. Second, and equally important, is the need for samples large enough to assess conditions which are of low frequency and which have too great a sampling error in samples of the sizes presently employed.

Another much needed development is to obtain data on patients who usually elude ascertainment at present, viz., from the solo practitioner, the group practice clinic, the industrial health facility, and the hospital outpatient department and emergency room. Investigation of methods for gathering such data is now under way but has not progressed to the point where a national data collection system can become a reality. We are still a long way from fully realizing the usefulness of the nation as an epidemiological laboratory.

References

MacMahon, B. and Worcester, J. 1966. *Age at Menopause.* National Center for Health Statistics, Vital and Health Statistics, P.H.S. Pub. No. 1000, series 11, no. 19. Washington: U.S. Government Printing Office.

The following is an outline of the Report Series for Vital and Health Statistics (P.H.S. Publication No. 1000):

Series 1. Programs and collection procedures. Reports which describe the general programs of the National Center for Health Statistics and its offices and divisions, data collection methods used, definitions and other material necessary for understanding the data.

Series 2. Data evaluation and methods research. Studies of new statistical methodology including: experimental tests of new survey methods, studies of vital statistics collection methods, new analytical techniques, objective evaluations of reliability of collected data, contributions to statistical theory.

Series 3. Analytical studies. Reports presenting analytical or interpretive studies based on vital and health statistics, carrying the analysis further than the expository types of reports in the other series.

Series 4. Documents and committee reports. Final reports of major committees concerned with vital and health statistics, and documents such as recommended model vital registration laws and revised birth and death certificates.

Series 10. Data from the Health Interview Survey. Statistics on illness, accidental injuries, disability, use of hospital, medical, dental, and other services, and other health-related topics, based on data collected in a continuing national household interview survey.

Series 11. Data from the Health Examination Survey. Data from direct examination, testing, and measurement of national samples of the population provide the basis for two types of reports: (1) estimates of the medically defined prevalence of specific diseases in the United States and the distributions of the population with respect to physical, physiological, and psychological characteristics; and (2) analysis of relationships among the various measurements without reference to an explicit finite universe of persons.

Series 12. Data from the Institutional Population Surveys. Statistics relating to the health characteristics of persons in institutions, and on medical, nursing, and personal care received, based on national samples of establishments providing these services and samples of the residents or patients.

Series 13. Data from the Hospital Discharge Survey. Statistics relating to discharged patients in short-stay hospitals, based on a sample of patient records in a national sample of hospitals.

Series 20. Data on mortality. Various statistics on mortality other than as included in annual or monthly reports—special analyses by cause of death, age, and other demographic variables, also geographic and time series analyses.

Series 21. Data on natality, marriage, and divorce. Various statistics on natality, marriage, and divorce other than as included in annual or monthly reports—special analyses by demographic variables, also geographic and time series analyses, studies of fertility.

Series 22. Data from the National Natality and Mortality Surveys. Statistics on characteristics of births and deaths not available from the vital records, based on sample surveys stemming from these records, including such topics as mortality by socioeconomic class, medical experience in the last year of life, characteristics of pregnancy, etc.

EDITORIAL COMMENTS

1. Countries as large as the United States are obviously not suitable for community studies such as for example, those conducted in Tecumseh or Rochester. On the other hand, there must be many clues to etiological factors in geographic and ethnic differences in disease prevalence or mortality. For the identification and description of such differences, national data can be very useful.

2. The author has pointed out a major problem with the National Health Survey at present. Although it rests upon a probability design which, in respect to sampling, is essentially unbiased, complete tabulations are possible only for the country as a whole. More limited statistics can be derived for each of four broad geographical regions and for selected large metropolitan areas, but estimates for individual states or smaller areas cannot be made. The utility of national data for epidemiological inquiries is, at least in part, a function of the availability of detailed statistics on geographical subregions. Unfortunately, the large expenditures necessary for making this possible by modifying the National Health Survey have not yet been considered justified. However, the National Center for Health Statistics has been exploring possible ways of producing crude state estimates from the national interview survey (Woolsey 1968). For diseases in which regional differences are relatively small, there does not seem to be much point in doing national studies at all.

3. The development of the Regional Medical Program, with its interest in standardized reporting systems, etc., may make it possible to conduct epidemiological studies in widely separated geographical regions without necessarily including the entire national population or a sample thereof.

4. The reader who is interested in detailed descriptions of the methods used in the National Health Survey will find these in the Report Series for Vital and Health Statistics, described in the author's References.

Reference

Woolsey, T. D. 1968. *Synthetic State Estimates of Disability Derived from the U.S. National Health Survey.* U.S. Department of Health, Education, and Welfare. P.H.S. Pub. No. 1759, 1–16. Washington: U.S. Government Printing Office.

CHAPTER 13

The Caribbean island of Puerto Rico, having succeeded in controlling infectious disease, is turning its attention to such problems as chronic disease, medical care, and health education. The development of an ongoing master sample survey makes it possible to include evaluation procedures in the planning of new public health programs. Another feature of the survey is that it encourages collaboration between administrators of public health policies and investigators of public health problems.

THE PUERTO RICO MASTER SAMPLE SURVEY OF HEALTH AND WELFARE

Raúl A. Muñoz and Guillermo Arbona

INTRODUCTION

Three decades ago the acute health problems of Puerto Rico were so overwhelming that almost any health service provided anywhere was bound to have an effect. Half of all deaths were attributed to diarrhea, enteritis, tuberculosis, pneumonia, and malaria. The latter has now been completely eradicated and such great progress has been made in the control of the other infectious diseases that they now account for less than one-fifth of the total mortality.

At present, the chronic diseases are predominant in Puerto Rico and efforts toward their prevention and control are gaining a higher priority. Thus, a substantial proportion of the Puerto Rico Department of Health budget is now devoted to chronic disease and especially to the care and maintenance of the chronically ill. In relation to the magnitude of the problem, however, funds are limited and difficult decisions are needed as to their optimal allocation.

In order to fully discharge its responsibilities for the health and

279

welfare of Puerto Ricans, the Commonwealth Department of Health required the systematic collection of data which would:

1. characterize the island-wide population, rather than a small portion thereof;
2. determine the magnitude of chronic illness and other health problems of the island as a whole;
3. evaluate the effect of existing programs in prevention, control, and clinical service;
4. document the effects of illness on family units as well as on individuals.

These objectives could not be attained utilizing the existing sources of health data, viz., mortality statistics, registries of reportable diseases, and routinely published bureau reports. Instead, a specially designed Master Sample Survey was undertaken; this dealt with all aspects of health in Puerto Rico but was primarily concerned with problems of the chronically ill and the elderly. It was intended to serve four main purposes:

1. As an aid in over-all planning, evaluation, and assessment of priorities, by providing quantitative island-wide information. The data collected and analyzed will highlight and place in perspective, the unmet needs in health and welfare services.
2. As a means for directors of health and welfare department programs concerned with various aspects of chronic illness and aging to secure essential information.
3. As a means for the Secretary of Health and Welfare and his staff to identify areas of health and welfare needs not adequately met by current programs, both public and private.
4. As an instrument for the planning and conduct of epidemiologic and social research investigations on chronic conditions, poverty, disease etiology, and related health and welfare programs.

THE COMMUNITY

Puerto Rico is the fourth largest island in the Caribbean. Discovered by Christopher Columbus on his second voyage to the New World, its colonization began in the early sixteenth century under the governorship of Juan Ponce de León. During its first three centuries under Spanish rule, Puerto Rico grew slowly as it was subject to frequent attacks by the great maritime powers interested in its strategic location on major trade routes. It was largely bypassed by the streams of immigrants moving to the more promising settlements in America.

Puerto Rico came under United States sovereignty by the Treaty of

Paris in 1898, and a civilian government was established two years later. By the Organic Act of 1917 U.S. citizenship as well as local suffrage were granted to the Puerto Ricans. The first and very limited public health services were also developed at this time.

The island underwent steady economic growth for a while, but its rapidly increasing population, underindustrialization, and scarcity of natural resources contributed to a severe economic depression in the 1930's. Operation Bootstrap, an economic self-help program was initiated in the 1940's; this, together with the development of local self-government and the creation of the Commonwealth in 1952, reversed the decline and brought about a remarkable economic, social, and political rejuvenation. The gross product has increased nine-fold since 1940, reaching $3,038 million by June 1966, according to statistics of the Government Development Bank. Net income has increased from $225 million in 1940 to $2,525 million in 1966, and per capita net income has risen from $121 to $1,047 per annum.

The Division of Vital Statistics in the Puerto Rican Health Department estimated the Island's population in 1960 as 2,360,300, or 687 persons per square mile. In that year, 55.7 per cent of the people were still rural dwellers. By 1965 the percentage fell to about 51.1 per cent and estimates for 1970, 1975 and 1980 were fixed at 46.3, 41.6, and 36.8 per cent, respectively. The present population has nearly identical proportions of males and females; approximately 42.6 per cent are under fifteen years of age, while only 5.2 per cent are over sixty-five years.

The health and social welfare of Puerto Ricans has improved in recent years, along with the economic standards. Life expectancy has increased from forty-six to seventy years and the crude death rate has declined from 18.2 to 6.5 per thousand, somewhat below that in the United States. All this has been accompanied by a fall in the birth rate from 39.0 per thousand in 1940 to 28.3 per thousand in 1966. During this period, public and private day school enrollment has increased from 286,000 to 716,986, covering 87 per cent of school age children, and the literacy rate has increased from 68.5 per cent to 86.2 per cent. Institutions of higher learning have also expanded, the University of Puerto Rico, for example, experiencing a six-fold rise in enrollment to 30,100 in 1967.

Accompanying the decline in mortality and morbidity and the improvements in socioeconomic conditions has been an increase in health insurance coverage and in specific demands for health services. This makes even more imperative the development of an efficient and effective system for the optimal utilization of health manpower facilities and funds.

Organization of Health Care Services in Puerto Rico

There are two systems of health care delivery in Puerto Rico: the private and the public or governmental. It is estimated that 40 per cent of the population utilize the private medical and hospital services and 60 per cent utilize the public services. Between 18 and 25 per cent of the population are now covered by some type of prepaid health insurance.

Private health services are provided in the home, office, and hospital, usually by a solo practitioner. Organized group practice has not yet developed on the island to any significant extent. However, there are physicians who, though not organized in formal groups, practice as such in their own privately owned hospitals. These proprietary institutions contain about 24.2 per cent of the island's general hospital beds, while another 17.2 per cent are found in private nonprofit hospitals. Together, the two types of private hospitals render a great volume of health services in the larger cities, where they are generally located, as well as in nearby municipalities. Puerto Rico is so small and the means of transportation so convenient that financially secure patients select the hospital they prefer irrespective of its location (Figure 13–1). There is even a traffic of patients to the mainland, especially New York, Miami, and Chicago, where there are large Puerto Rican communities. The extent of this traffic has not been determined.

The public health services of Puerto Rico are administered by the Commonwealth Department of Health, the municipal governments, and various state agencies such as the Workmen's Compensation Board. Individual municipalities, ranging in population from 7,000 to 500,000 people, have the principal responsibility for the medical care of their needy. The Commonwealth government complements the municipal public health programs, both preventive and curative, by assuming responsibility for technical and professional services in nearly all municipalities except San Juan. In each of the 75 municipalities there is a health center which includes a hospital (usually one bed per 1,000 inhabitants), outpatient clinics, and a public welfare unit. In 45 municipalities these health and social welfare facilities are presently housed in temporary structures.

Puerto Rico is administratively divided into five health and welfare regions, each directed by a regional health and a regional welfare officer. The offices of the regional health programs are located in the corresponding regional hospitals. Under an agreement between the school of medicine and the department of health, the northeast region is operated by the school, with the dean serving as regional director

Figure 13–1. Hospital and medical facilities in Puerto Rico.

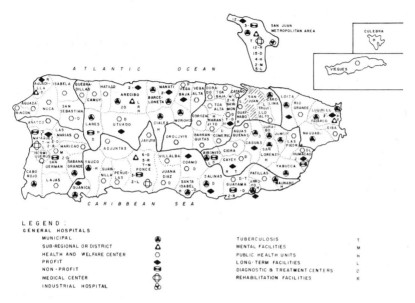

LEGEND :
GENERAL HOSPITALS

MUNICIPAL	◐◓	TUBERCULOSIS	T
SUB-REGIONAL OR DISTRICT	△	MENTAL FACILITIES	M
HEALTH AND WELFARE CENTER	○	PUBLIC HEALTH UNITS	H
PROFIT	◆	LONG- TERM FACILITIES	L
NON - PROFIT	⊟	DIAGNOSTIC & TREATMENT CENTERS	D
MEDICAL CENTER	⊕	REHABILITATION FACILITIES	R
INDUSTRIAL HOSPITAL	⊗		

and the chairman of the Department of Preventive Medicine and Public Health in the School of Public Health, serving as executive regional health officer. The clinical faculty of the medical school serves in the regional hospital and, through a continuing educational program, oversees the activities of the local and intermediate health centers.

Medical care services in Puerto Rico are closely co-ordinated with social welfare services. An individual in need of these services goes to the local health center in the smaller municipality or to the dispensary in the larger city. In instances where the patient's needs cannot be satisfied locally, the case is referred by the physician or social worker to an intermediate or regional center. The Northeast Regional Hospital (University Hospital) and the central offices of the Department of Health, function as referral centers of last resort when the patient's needs cannot be met at the regional level. All services in the governmental system are provided free of charge and all personnel, including physicians, are salaried.

The over-all health and social welfare systems are administered by a director of health and a director of welfare services, who are responsible directly to the Commonwealth Secretary of Health. Categorical program directors (in heart disease or cancer control, for example) work out of the central departmental offices, but in close co-ordination with the regional administrators.

METHODS AND PROBLEMS

A major requirement of a continuing population survey is a sampling scheme which will permit both the follow-up of a cohort of families or individuals over time and the periodic collection of cross-sectional data. The first approach is essential for the development of incidence statistics, while prevalence data may be derived from the latter. This double purpose created difficult sampling problems which were met with a rather sophisticated sampling design.

A multi-stage stratified area probability sample was constructed in such a way as to permit a series of representative samples of the population to be drawn, taking into account population changes due to slum demolition and new residential construction. Puerto Rico was divided into five regions, based on data from the Bureau of Regional Planning, and each region was divided into two zones, urban and rural. The resulting ten strata were supplemented by two special strata: one consisting of housing developments occupied after the date of the 1960 census and the other consisting of rural communities occupied after the same date. Within each stratum a systematic random sample of enumeration districts was selected with a probability proportional to the segment size.

Two previous samples of noninstitutionalized persons, drawn for other purposes, were incorporated, in part, into the Master Sample— the current labor force sample of the Puerto Rican Bureau of Labor Statistics and the 3,000 family sample interviewed in the 1958 "Study of Medical and Hospital Care in Puerto Rico" conducted in collaboration with Columbia University. This was done in order to make possible an early measurement of longitudinal changes in pertinent variables. The number of households sampled, by region, is shown in Table 13–1.

The final design allowed for annual interviewing of households in quarter samples of about 800 households each, which could be treated as independent samples or combined. During the survey's first year, approximately one-half of the households were drawn from the 1958

TABLE 13–1. POPULATION AND HOUSEHOLDS SAMPLED IN THE 1967 SURVEY, BY REGION

| Region | Population | Number of households | |
		Total	Sampled
Northeast	976,100	207,240	1,714
North	354,600	75,287	592
West	346,300	73,524	588
South	585,000	124,204	943
East	424,200	90,064	673

family sample and one-half from households not previously interviewed. In the second year the latter group was reinterviewed and a new subsample was selected to replace the 1958 family sample households. Thereafter, the design called for households to be interviewed twice and then be replaced by others in the same fashion every other year. This feature of reinterviewing and replacement after the second year was discarded in favor of drawing independent quarterly samples, because the cost of locating and reinterviewing households was found to be high in relation to the rather small changes observed over the year in the variables of interest. It appears that prospective designs are more productively applied to long-term than to relatively short-term studies.

Segment size in the Master Sample Survey averaged four or five households in rural areas and one to three households in urban areas. These numbers are half the size of those employed by the Bureau of Labor Statistics and were arrived at out of the following considerations:

1. In rural areas, after allowing for travel time, an interviewer can complete two or three interviews in one sample segment per day. An assignment of four or five households would, in general, permit the interviewer to locate all the respondents and to interview some. The remaining cases could be seen on the second day.

2. In urban areas, travel represents a relatively small proportion of the interviewer's work day; most of the time is spent in locating and interviewing households. Thus, no more than two or three interviews per day can usually be completed.

Interviews were conducted by a carefully selected field staff of eight college graduates and one field supervisor who were thoroughly trained in health survey techniques and familiar with local cultural traits. Three types of questionnaire schedules were employed:

1. A basic health questionnaire, dealing with the occurrence of illness, its care, and its disabling effects along with data on demographic variables such as age, sex, economic status, education, and residence.

2. Special questionnaires dealing with specific health problems, such as dengue, mental illness, cancer, and immunizations.

3. Special questionnaires dealing with health-related social issues and problems such as migration, family planning, happiness, and health insurance.

Completed interviews were coded by a staff of three coders and one supervisor and were prepared for computer processing by a statistician.

A major problem of the Master Sample Survey has been the delay in processing, analyzing, and reporting of findings. In large part this has been due to the scarcity of adequately trained personnel, but deficiencies in computer technology have also played a role.

Nonresponse has not been a serious problem, although a rather high percentage of households were found to be ineligible. Of 1,161 households selected in the first half of 1967, 961 were considered to be eligible for inclusion. However, on-site visits revealed that 158 of these (16.4 per cent) were either vacant or demolished. Of the remaining 803 units, interviews were completed on 761; a response rate of 94.8 per cent.

FINDINGS

Acute Conditions

Acute medical conditions were observed most often in young children, and the proportion of such conditions which received medical attention was higher in the young than in any other age group. More females than males reported acute conditions at all ages and a higher proportion of their conditions were medically attended. Acute conditions were slightly more frequent in lower income families, but a higher proportion of these were medically attended in the higher income families. Among low income families, those receiving public assistance were more likely to see a physician for acute conditions.

Chronic Conditions

The proportion of persons reporting one or more chronic conditions (Table 13–2) and the number of conditions reported (Table 13–3) were both found to increase with age in each sex. Prevalences were higher among females than in males aged 15 years and over. Slightly increased prevalences were also observed in urban dwellers as compared with rural dwellers, in families with annual incomes under $1,000, and in families of moderate income with health insur-

TABLE 13–2. PER CENT DISTRIBUTION OF PERSONS REPORTING ONE OR MORE CHRONIC CONDITIONS BY AGE AND SEX (1963–64)

Sex	All ages	Age (years)					
		0–4	5–14	15–24	25–44	45–64	65+
Males	36.1	16.9	21.5	23.7	46.2	65.9	82.7
Females	44.0	12.9	20.7	34.9	63.9	77.2	85.1
Total	40.1	15.0	21.1	29.3	51.6	71.3	84.0

ance as compared to those without coverage. The percentage of respondents who saw a doctor during the previous year increased slightly with income, regardless of whether chronic conditions were present or not (Table 13–4).

When the survey findings were compared with those of the U.S. National Health Survey of 1963–64, a somewhat greater prevalence of chronic conditions was observed in Puerto Ricans of all age groups (Table 13–5).

Mental Illness

In collaboration with the staff of the Mental Health Program of the Commonwealth's Health Department a special survey was conducted on the knowledge, attitudes, beliefs, and practices of Puerto Ricans relative to mental illness. A parallel study is being carried out* among Puerto Ricans living in New York City, and it is anticipated that useful comparisons between the natives and the migrant groups, in their attitudes and perceptions regarding mental illness and mental health services, may emerge.

TABLE 13–3. NUMBER OF CHRONIC CONDITIONS PER 100 POPULATION, BY AGE AND SEX (1963–64)

Age (years)	Sex		
	Both sexes	Male	Female
All ages	78	64	91
0– 4	17	20	15
5–14	26	26	25
15–24	44	30	56
25–44	109	78	134
45–64	168	139	200
65+	252	220	228

TABLE 13–4. PER CENT OF POPULATION SEEING A PHYSICIAN DURING THE YEAR PRECEDING INTERVIEW, BY FAMILY INCOME AND PRESENCE OR ABSENCE OF CHRONIC CONDITIONS (1963–64)

1+ Chronic conditions	Annual family income				
	All incomes	Less than $1,000	$1,000–$1,999	$2,000–$2,999	$3,000 or more
Absent	58	52	57	61	64
Present	73	71	73	75	74

* In co-operation with the Community Mental Health Board of New York City.

TABLE 13–5.　PER CENT OF THE POPULATION WITH ONE OR MORE CHRONIC CONDITIONS, BY AGE AND SEX, PUERTO RICO AND UNITED STATES (1963–64)

Age (years) and sex	Survey area	
	Puerto Rico	United States
Both sexes		
Under 25	27.0	24.8
25–44	59.8	53.1
45–64	74.8	65.4
65+	88.3	82.3
All ages	44.5	45.2
Age-adjusted[a]	50.3	
Males		
Under 25	26.7	25.2
25–44	51.1	50.0
45–64	72.5	63.2
65+	88.2	80.2
All ages	41.7	43.5
Age-adjusted[a]	47.6	
Females		
Under 25	26.8	24.4
25–44	66.6	56.0
45–64	80.2	67.5
65+	88.4	83.9
All ages	47.2	46.9
Age-adjusted[a]	53.0	

[a] Adjusted to the age distribution of the civilian population of the United States, as reported by the National Health Survey.

The attitudes of the Puerto Rican sample toward the mentally retarded were rated on a subjective scale by the respondents' age, sex, urban-rural residence, and schooling. Negative attitudes were somewhat more frequent than expected among older persons, females, rural dwellers, and the uneducated (Table 13–6).

Happiness

In responding to questions relating to their degree of happiness in life, Puerto Ricans were scored as being considerably less happy than a number of United States communities interviewed in comparable fashion. The differences were observed in comparisons with economically depressed as well as prosperous U.S. communities (Table 13–7). The reporting of happiness was clearly related to the state of perceived health, irrespective of age: persons reporting fair or poor health were much less likely to feel very happy (Table 13–8).

TABLE 13-6. DISTRIBUTION OF PERSONS BY SCALE OF ATTITUDES TOWARD THE RETARDED BY SCHOOLING, AGE, SEX, AND RESIDENCE (APRIL 1966)

Charac- teristic	Total		Scale of attitudes							
			Very positive		Somewhat positive		Somewhat negative		Very negative	
	Number	Per cent	Number	Per cent	Number	Per cent	Number	Per cent	Number	Per cent
AGE (years)										
20–34	328	43.9	56	42.4	152	48.4	80	41.4	40	37.0
35–49	268	35.9	58	44.0	103	32.8	70	36.3	37	34.3
50 or more	151	20.2	18	13.6	59	18.8	43	22.3	31	28.7
Total	747	100.0	132	100.0	314	100.0	193	100.0	108	100.0
SEX										
Male	315	42.2	59	44.7	135	43.0	78	40.4	43	39.8
Female	432	57.8	73	55.3	179	57.0	115	59.6	65	60.2
Total	747	100.0	132	100.0	314	100.0	193	100.0	108	100.0
RESIDENCE										
Urban	417	55.8	102	77.3	192	61.1	95	49.2	28	25.9
Rural	330	44.2	30	22.7	122	38.9	98	50.8	80	74.1
Total	747	100.0	132	100.0	314	100.0	193	100.0	108	100.0
Schooling (years)										
0–3	206	27.6	15	11.4	54	17.2	67	34.7	70	64.8
4–7	203	27.2	12	9.1	84	26.8	78	40.4	29	26.9
8–12	263	35.2	66	50.0	143	45.5	45	23.3	9	8.3
More than 12	75	10.0	39	29.5	33	10.5	3	1.6	—	—
Total	747	100.0	132	100.0	314	100.0	193	100.0	108	100.0

TABLE 13–7.   PER CENT OF RESPONDENTS BY DEGREE OF HAPPINESS AND COMMUNITY

		Population			
	Puerto	4 U.S. communities[a]			10 U.S. metropolitan
Happiness	Rico	Depressed	Improving	Prosperous	areas[a]
Very happy	17%	22%	30%	24%	32%
Fairly happy	50	58	57	63	56
Not too happy	33	20	13	13	12

[a] Source: National Opinion Research Center, Chicago.

TABLE 13–8.   PER CENT OF RESPONDENTS WHO SAID THEY WERE "VERY HAPPY," BY REPORTED HEALTH AND AGE

Reported	Age (years)			
health	20–29	30–39	40–49	50 and over
Excellent	29	40	38	22
Good	26	21	14	19
Fair, poor	6	5	13	13

Knowledge of Dengue

In August, 1963 an epidemic of dengue was reported in Puerto Rico. It lasted for about 6 months and 27,000 cases were reported, although the attack rate was believed to be much higher than the 1.1 per cent indicated by this figure. Shortly after the onset of the epidemic, an island-wide health education program was undertaken. A subsample of the Master Sample Survey population was interviewed in order to evaluate the effectiveness of this program.

Most respondents were worried about contracting the disease and most knew that it was spread by a mosquito. There was, however, considerable variation in this knowledge according to sex, age, education, and urban-rural residence. A greater understanding of the pathogenesis of dengue was observed among the young, the more educated, and the urban residents (Table 13–9). Interestingly, the occurrence of dengue in the family was not associated with much of an increase in knowledgeability. The survey also demonstrated that among these less knowledgeable groups health personnel played a relatively more important role in health education than was true among the more medically sophisticated respondents (Table 13–10).

The use of the Master Sample Survey in this manner illustrates its quick adaptability in meeting needs for health intelligence on topical questions. The findings in the dengue survey have led to an intensive educational and public health program to eliminate the dengue mosquito.

TABLE 13–9. KNOWLEDGE OF THE CAUSE OF DENGUE, BY SELECTED CHARACTERISTICS, FEBRUARY–APRIL, 1964 (PER CENT)

Selected characteristics	Total	Knowledge of cause		
		Mosquito	All other causes	Don't know
All persons	100.0	65.3	8.9	25.8
SEX				
Male	100.0	57.1	10.0	32.9
Female	100.0	68.9	8.4	22.7
AGE (years)				
Under 45	100.0	77.0	4.6	18.4
45–64	100.0	60.0	10.9	29.1
65 and over	100.0	29.0	22.0	49.0
EDUCATION				
Less than 4 years	100.0	47.2	12.8	40.0
4–7 years	100.0	66.5	9.2	24.3
8–11 years	100.0	78.3	4.6	17.1
12+ years	100.0	89.9	4.3	5.8
RESIDENCE				
Urban	100.0	74.5	8.3	17.2
Rural	100.0	52.9	9.7	37.4
DENGUE IN FAMILY				
Yes	100.0	68.9	8.9	22.2
No	100.0	61.4	9.0	29.6

Immunization Levels

In November, 1965 the Puerto Rico Department of Health undertook a vaccination campaign in an attempt to immunize the entire population against selected diseases. As part of an effort to evaluate the effectiveness of this program, an investigation of the immunization status of Master Sample Survey children was begun a few months before the vaccination campaign. A surprisingly small proportion of children under age nineteen years of age were reported to have been immunized: 40 per cent against smallpox and 46 per cent against diphtheria and tetanus. The proportion of children with recent (and presumably active) immunizations was highest at the youngest ages, in families with well-educated heads (Table 13–10), among urban residents and higher income groups. The immunization status of nearly one-quarter of the surveyed children was unknown, however, and this may have exaggerated the observed differences by social class.

Studies in Progress

At the behest of the Puerto Rico Planning Board, studies on migration patterns are in progress. These involve the collection of data on movements into and out of the island and are expected to be of value in economic and social planning. A special survey was recently undertaken on the incidence of cancer in women who had been surgically sterilized. Another study in progress is an investigation of the nutritional status of a population sample, with ascertainment based upon both medical examination and laboratory tests.

POTENTIALS

With the extension to Puerto Rico of the Comprehensive Health Planning Act, the Master Sample Survey is being called upon to perform a major role in an expanded Office of Research, Planning, and Evaluation of the Department of Health. When integrated with the data obtained from routinely collected vital statistics and from the records of health service programs it will provide the epidemiological

TABLE 13–10. PER CENT DISTRIBUTION OF CHILDREN, BY LEVEL OF DIPHTHERIA AND TETANUS IMMUNIZATION[a] ACTIVITY, AND BY AGE OF CHILD AND EDUCATION OF FAMILY HEAD (JANUARY–MARCH, 1965)

Age of child and education of family head	All levels	Level of immunization		Never immunized	Status unknown
		Immunized			
		≤3 years ago	3+ years		
0–5 years[a]					
All education levels	100.0	49.1	—	40.1	10.8
0–3 years	100.0	37.0	—	49.6	13.4
4–7 years	100.0	43.0	—	45.0	12.0
8–12 years	100.0	65.4	—	27.6	7.0
13+ years	100.0	85.4	—	10.4	4.2
6–10 years					
All education levels	100.0	30.7	23.1	23.6	22.6
0–3 years	100.0	23.0	14.0	33.6	29.4
4–7 years	100.0	36.1	21.7	22.8	19.4
8–12 years	100.0	36.6	33.8	13.4	16.2
13+ years	100.0	31.1	42.2	6.7	20.0
11–18 years					
All education levels	100.0	11.6	25.8	31.5	31.1
0–3 years	100.0	9.4	20.7	38.0	31.9
4–7 years	100.0	15.8	26.7	25.1	32.4
8–12 years	100.0	10.2	32.7	28.8	28.3
13+ years	100.0	20.0	40.0	12.0	28.0
Under 19 years					
All education levels	100.0	28.4	17.2	31.9	22.5
0–3 years	100.0	20.7	13.1	40.1	26.1
4–7 years	100.0	30.3	16.7	30.8	22.2
8–12 years	100.0	34.8	22.9	24.0	18.3
13+ years	100.0	50.8	24.6	9.3	15.3

[a] For children under six, includes immunization for pertussis.

base for modern health planning in Puerto Rico. This potential will be realized particularly after the staff shortages and budgetary problems of the project have been remedied.

An effort is now being made to alter the survey methodology so as to make it more consistent with that of the U.S. Health Interview Survey. This will, of course, add to the value of the studies.

Another approach to realizing the full potential of the Master Sample Survey is to encourage closer and more systematic contact between the major governmental or agency users of the survey with the survey staff. This will better acquaint the users with the problems amenable to study by the survey method. At the same time, it will help to inform the survey staff of public health problems in need of investigation. Examples of such problems which have been suggested for study are listed in Table 13–11.

Bibliography of the
Puerto Rico Master Sample Survey of Health and Welfare
(Processed)

Series 1, No. 1. Acute and Chronic Illness, Medical Care and Insurance, Puerto Rico, 1963 (October–December 1963).

Series 1, No. 2. Acute and Chronic Conditions and Medical Care, Puerto Rico, October 1963–November 1964.

Series 2, No. 1. Knowledge of Dengue in Puerto Rico, February–April 1964.

Series 2, No. 2. Immunization Level of Children in Puerto Rico, Preliminary Findings, January–March, 1965.

Series 2, No. 3. The Demography of Happiness.

Unnumbered Series

Mental Retardation in Puerto Rico, Knowledge, Beliefs and Attitudes, April–June 1966 (Spanish).

Knowledge and Attitudes About Cancer, Puerto Rico, May–July 1964 (Spanish).

Patterns of Utilization of Dental Services in Puerto Rico, 1966. Special presentation before the Society of Government Dentists of Puerto Rico (Spanish).

TABLE 13–11. PUBLIC HEALTH PROBLEMS SUGGESTED FOR THE MASTER SAMPLE SURVEY

Problem area	Study variables
1. Aid to the permanently and totally disabled and 2. Medical assistance to the aged	a. Proportion receiving services, e.g., home nursing or homemaking b. Changes in family composition over time c. Effect of program on family relationships, living arrangements, and socioeconomic conditions
3. Crippled children and 4. Maternal and child health	a. Types of defects among children b. Preventive and rehabilitative services rendered and/or received c. Types of pregnant women receiving and not receiving prenatal care d. Children receiving and not receiving pediatric services
5. Preventive medical services	a. Utilization patterns b. Characteristics of vaccinated and nonvaccinated subpopulations
6. Nutrition	a. Description and variation of Puerto Rican diets b. Attitudes about nutrition among parents, teachers, doctors, and others c. Utilization and effectiveness of specific nutritional programs, such as school lunch, surplus food distribution, and preschool child breakfasts
7. Environmental sanitation	a. Public knowledge, attitudes, and practices regarding latrine use, river bathing, clothes laundering, potable water sources, etc.
8. Oral hygiene	a. Characteristics of recipients and nonrecipients of dental care b. Distinctions between public and private dental care
9. Control of cancer, tuberculosis and other chronic diseases	a. Public knowledge of prevention and control of chronic diseases b. Public practices in prevention and control
10. Mental health	a. Public awareness of available services for mental illness b. Public utilization of services, normative or deviant c. Family attitudes toward ambulatory care for mental illness
11. Health education	a. Interrelations between knowledge, attitudes, and practices in various program areas

EDITORIAL COMMENTS

1. The island-wide surveys of Puerto Rico were patterned after the Master Sample Survey of Washington Heights. With the increasing importance of comprehensive health planning in the commonwealth, the methodology has been modified to conform more closely with that of the U.S. Health Interview Survey. This calls attention to the possible effect of illiteracy upon questionnaire responses in such countries as Puerto Rico and Colombia.

2. The close working relationship between the survey staff and personnel of the vital statistics and public health departments of Puerto Rico resembles the situation evolving in Rhode Island. Such collaboration is desirable in all population laboratories but it may be essential in small countries with limited resources, high illiteracy rates, and serious unmet health needs. Little can be left to private medicine in these countries: the monitoring and preservation of health is and will probably remain a major governmental responsibility there.

3. The Puerto Rico surveys lost the inherent advantage of the prospective approach when it was decided to discontinue reinterviewing the same samples "because the cost of locating and reinterviewing households was found to be high in relation to the rather small changes observed over the year in the variables of interest." This is a valid reason but, of course, it might not apply to a future investigation in which the longitudinal approach was advantageous. Presumably, prospective follow-up could then be reinstituted.

4. A rather unusual feature of the Puerto Rico master sample is that it is a hybrid composed of one newly drawn sample and the survivors from two earlier samples selected for studies of medical care and the labor force. The old samples permit certain longitudinal trends to be measured after the first round of survey interviews have been completed. However, this advantage must be weighed against the difficulties inherent in making inferences from such a composite sample.

CHAPTER 14

Colombia, South America, a developing country with abundant poverty and illiteracy, is the site of a statistically sophisticated national health survey modeled after that in the United States. Among the problems posed by this study is whether a detailed health interview questionnaire is the most appropriate research instrument for a population three-quarters of whom have no more than a primary school education.

THE COLOMBIA, SOUTH AMERICA, NATIONAL HEALTH SURVEY

Alfonso Mejía Vanegas,* Robin F. Badgley, and Richard V. Kasius

INTRODUCTION

The Charter of Punta del Este, in which the objectives of the Alliance for Progress were established in 1961, recommended that member nations should give high priority to the education and training of health workers and that efforts should be directed "to determine the number of experts required in the various categories for each activity or profession" (Arreaza-Guzman et al. 1964). Two years later the Pan American Health Organization and the Milbank Memorial Fund sponsored a Round Table on Health Manpower and Medical Education in Latin America. The charge to the experts convened at this Round Table was "to design an appropriate research approach to the problems of physician needs and of medical education, to discuss the methodologies to be used and to define the appropriate emphases and parameters of the studies" (Arreaza-Guzman et al. 1964). The participants at the Round Table drafted a report describing the concepts and methods for a National Health Manpower Study and recommended

* Dr. Mejía is presently Medical Officer for Health Manpower and Medical Education, at the World Health Organization in Geneva.

that pilot studies based on this report be undertaken in a Latin American country.

In Colombia, which was selected in 1964 as the site of the health manpower study, the Ministry of Public Health and the medical schools had been concerned for many years with the quality of medical education and the supply and distribution of health personnel. A program of rural medical service had been established in 1950 which required medical and dental graduates to work for a year in areas designated by the ministry. In 1956, in co-operation with several international agencies, a program for the progressive improvement of public health services in Colombia was undertaken and, subsequently, several national health plans were drafted. For their part the medical schools had reviewed all phases of medical education in a series of seminars and conferences during the 1950's. In 1963, shortly after the Round Table Conference in New York had been convened, the newly organized Colombian Association of Medical Schools at its first general assembly discussed the types of physicians needed in Colombia, the role of medical auxiliaries, and the health needs of the nation.

The Study of Health Manpower and Medical Education in Colombia was directed by one of us (A.M.V.), then of the Ministry of Public Health, and Doctor Raul Paredes Manrique of the Colombian Association of Medical Schools. For operational purposes the project was divided into nine study areas (Table 14–1), of which the National Health Survey was one. This represented the first attempt to study the extent of illness in a Latin American population on a national scale.

TABLE 14–1. STUDY AREAS OF THE STUDY ON HEALTH MANPOWER AND MEDICAL EDUCATION IN COLOMBIA

Study area	Study objectives
1. Demography	Attributes and dynamics of the population of Colombia
2. Mortality	Analysis of death rates by cause, age, and sex
3. National morbidity survey	Estimates of health needs (see text)
4. Medical resources	Number, geographic distribution, and other characteristics of physicians
5. Nursing resources	Census of nurses and trained nursing auxiliaries
6. Medical education	Resources and characteristics of medical education
7. Nursing education	Resources and characteristics of nursing education
8. Medical care institutions	Number, utilization, needs, and costs of medical care facilities
9. Socioeconomic aspects of health	Relationship of socioeconomic factors to health and assessment of national expenditures for health

The general objectives of the National Health Survey were described at the Round Table on Health Manpower as follows:

A picture should be obtained of present unmet health needs and demands. It should be noted that perception of a need may be made by the population or by the health experts themselves and that these two estimates will seldom precisely coincide. The data required would come from hospitals, clinics, and other health services as well as from special surveys and studies. From another angle, the geographic distribution of resources and facilities alongside demographic data and knowledge of the nature of the areas in question will serve to indicate unmet needs even in the absence of accurate field data although, of course, the establishment of priorities for services in these areas will require more precise information. Comparisons of the health levels in groups covered by social security or insurance programs with the health of populations without such coverage would also reveal unmet needs. This step, in effect, defines the maximum level for future planning (Arreaza-Guzman et al. 1964).

The specific objectives of the health survey were:

1. To determine the causes, magnitude and severity of morbidity, and to identify the most influential ecological factors.
2. To study the economic and social impact of disease on the individual, the family, and the community.
3. To ascertain the availability and use of medical care and other health services and arrangements for the financing of such services.
4. To verify the completeness and reliability of certain vital statistics records (Mejía and Paredes 1967).

THE COMMUNITY

Colombia is a country of social, economic, and geographic contrasts. It was settled in the sixteenth century by Spanish immigrants who soon dominated the Indians and introduced large numbers of Negro slaves. The result was a multi-racial nation which has grown from 4.3 million in 1900 to a current population of over 18 million inhabitants. During the past decade the average annual rate of growth has been 3.2 per cent, a rate which, because of rural-urban migration and changing population policies, may be expected to decline in the future. The profile of Colombia's population has all of the characteristics of a developing nation—a high birth rate, a high death rate, and almost half (47.8 per cent) of its population under age fifteen years. In 1965–66 the birth rate was 40.0 per 1,000 and the death rate, allowing for underregistration, was 10.5 per 1,000.

The majority of the population lives in the Andean highlands of the western half of the country and in the tropical lowlands of the northern coastal region. These two areas encompass 53 per cent of

Colombia's land and 99 per cent of its population, leaving the arid Llanos Orientales in the east and the jungle of the southeast virtually unpopulated. Transportation and communication are serious problems in many parts of the country, and in some of the heavily settled mountainous regions travel is only possible by air. The rugged terrain of a country which equals France, Spain, and Portugal in size (439, 519 square miles) was a factor which had to be considered in designing the National Health Survey.

Prior to the National Health Survey of 1965–66 there was little up-to-date valid information about the Colombian people. The most recent census data were for 1951. The results of the 1964 census were not available when the design of the National Health Survey was being developed and the existing information on morbidity and mortality was largely inaccurate or incomplete. It was known, for example, that the total number of deaths from tetanus in 1965 was much greater than the number of cases reported by doctors in institutions (1,997 vs. 754), and the number of deaths from rabies was fewer than the number of reported cases (47 vs. 109) (Agualimpia 1968).

When the preliminary findings of the 1964 census and the 1965–66 National Health Survey became available in 1967, it was possible for the first time to present a comprehensive national social and health profile of the Colombian people. The results presented here are drawn primarily from the National Health Survey.

Two divergent worlds coexist in Colombia, the world of the city and the countryside, of the rich and the poor, of the educated and uneducated. The customs and social values of the traditional peasant economy mold the lives of most Colombians. Half of the population live on farms or in small villages. Three out of four have either no education or only a primary education, and two out of five families have a monthly income of less than 300 pesos or the equivalent of $21.50. Half of the rural inhabitants live in huts or shacks, usually without running water or sanitary facilities.

The affairs of the nation are managed by a cosmopolitan, urban minority conversant with modern developments in technology and production. The leaders of government, business, the professions, and the military are drawn from a small educational pool consisting of some who have completed elementary or secondary schooling and others with university or professional training. It is this professional and entrepreneurial group which has developed modern industries in Medellin, Cali, and other cities, successfully promoted international trade, and introduced modern agricultural techniques in the rich farmlands of the Andean valleys. Representing less than one-third of the country's labor force, these manufacturers, businessmen, and allied workers account for some 80 per cent of the country's total economic output (Zschock 1967).

During the past two decades the exodus from the countryside to the cities has gained momentum and has resulted in widespread unemployment and in the rapid growth of barrios or slums in many of the large cities. The gap between the rich and the poor may be widening because these migrants lack the skills required for employment in factories and offices. An estimated 20 per cent of the labor force is currently unemployed or grossly underemployed. Because of rapid population growth and projected future levels of employment needs in the productive sectors of the economy, it is estimated that perhaps 25 per cent of the labor force may be unemployed by 1980. With these economic prospects the government is faced with the agonizing dilemma of balancing two major needs in Colombia: on the one hand, of raising the standard of living by increasing production and developing more employment opportunities; on the other hand, of providing costly health and welfare services in an attempt to alleviate widespread poverty and disease.

For many years Colombia has suffered from the divisive effects of mass insurrection and banditry. La violencia, as this phenomenon is known, evolved from the fierce rivalry between the nation's two major political parties but soon spread throughout the country. According to conservative estimates, la violencia has claimed the lives of over 200,000 Colombians since 1946, a proportion of the population which is larger than the total of Americans killed in World War I, World War II, and the Korean War. An additional 400,000 persons may have been injured, and it is estimated that la violencia has directly affected the lives of one out of five individuals in the country. In 1957 the leaders of the nation's two major political parties, the Liberals and the Conservatives, called for a period of national unity. Since then the government has alternated between the two parties, with administrative posts being assigned equally. Although la violencia is now largely contained, through the years it has hindered the execution of national censuses and other surveys and has probably compromised the accuracy of those surveys which were completed.

METHODS

The Colombian National Health Survey was modeled in many respects on the U.S. National Health Survey, and experts drawn from the latter served as consultants during the several phases of the Colombian study. The population of interest was the civil, noninstitutionalized population of Colombia's 18 *departamentos* (states or provinces). These *departamentos* contain 98.7 per cent of the country's population and 52.7 per cent of its land area. The remaining 1.3 per cent of the population, who live in the sparsely settled eastern half of the country, were excluded from the study. Long-term hospital patients and other institutionalized groups were also excluded.

The sample was a multi-stage probability sample of land areas (Mejía and Paredes 1967). The universe to be sampled was the civilian noninstitutional population of the 18 *departamentos* existing in 1964. The country was initially divided into four regions, one of which includes the capital, Bogota. The actual sampling required two major steps. The first was the identification of 716 primary sampling units and the selection of 40 of them. The second involved the selection of 24 segments of approximately 10 dwelling units each in each of the 40 primary sampling units.

The primary sampling units were defined as those *municipios* of the 18 *departamentos* which had populations of over 5,000 and a hospital, health center, or other medical service. *Municipios* of under 5,000 population or lacking health services were annexed to the nearest accessible and contiguous *municipio*.

The 716 primary sampling units were classified into 40 strata, each with a population of about 450,000. Bogota comprised four of these strata, Cali and Medellin, two each, Barranquilla and Bucaramanga one each. This yielded a total of ten "certainty strata" in which the sample area and the strata were the same. In the other 30 strata, one health district (primary sampling unit) was selected to represent each stratum. The classifications of health districts into strata were made so as to maximize the homogeneity within strata and the heterogeneity between strata. The criteria for stratification were, in order of their application:

1. Total population of each primary sampling unit, based on preliminary data from the 1964 census.
2. Per cent of urban population.
3. Average altitude.

One primary sampling unit was selected from each of the 30 non-certainty strata. The selection was made with a probability of selection proportional to the 1964 population. Thus, a health district of 150,000 residents had twice the chance of being selected as one with 75,000 residents. The ten units corresponding to the certainty strata were selected in the same manner. The 40 sampling units comprised 2 independent subsamples of 20 units each, selected in such a manner that results generalizable to the entire country could be obtained from either subsample. This provided an insurance mechanism for the study, in case it were not possible to complete the total survey either because of the complexity of the study or because of *la violencia*. It also made it possible to estimate the reliability of the findings economically and rapidly.

The sample in each primary unit consisted of 24 segments distributed into urban and rural areas according to population distribution. Each segment contained an average of 10 dwellings with 55 persons. The household interview sample, therefore, was intended to comprise approximately 1,300 persons per unit, with 52,000 persons in the entire sample. Approximately 130, or 10 per cent, of the persons interviewed in each unit were randomly selected for clinical examination. The clinical subsample was planned to include 5,200 persons.

As a first step in the sampling procedure the census sectors containing the 24 random segments were identified at the central level. The sectors consisted of selected blocks in the municipalities and well-defined rural areas. Urban segments which had more than 15 dwellings were randomly subsampled by the interviewers. Rural segments had been checked, and, if necessary, subsampled by trained environmental sanitation staff, prior to the field work. The subsample of persons to be clinically examined was selected as the interviews were held, at constant intervals established prior to the field operations. The age distribution of this subsample was controlled on three groups, under fifteen years, fifteen to forty-four years, and forty-five years and over. One person interviewed represented 340 persons, and one person examined represented 3,400 persons in the total population.

A total of 8,920 households with 52,964 individuals were sampled and 8,669 households with 51,473 individuals (or 97.2 per cent) were actually interviewed. Of the 5,258 individuals selected for clinical examination, 5,027 (or 95.6 per cent) were examined. In comparison with other health surveys these constitute unusually high completion rates.

The questions on the interview schedule were adapted from those used in the U.S. National Health Survey. They sought to elicit six categories of information:

1. Household composition: number, age, sex, and relationships.
2. Housing conditions: type of home, water supply, and waste disposal facilities.
3. Family income.
4. Personal data: occupation and education.
5. Personal health: illnesses, accidents, dental problems, disability, selected chronic conditions, receipt of medical and dental care, hospitalizations, medical costs, and methods of payment.

6. Obstetric and pediatric history: pregnancies, deliveries, and deaths of children under five years of age.

Before the actual field work began, working manuals were prepared and extensive pretests undertaken. Five field teams were organized, each consisting of:

1. One field supervisor: a public health physician who directed all local operations.
2. One clinical co-ordinator: a public health dentist who co-ordinated the work of the clinical unit and made the dental examinations.
3. One field administrator: an environmental sanitation inspector who served as administrative assistant to the supervisor.
4. Six interviewers: medical students in their final years of study.
5. Two examining physicians: residents in internal medicine and pediatrics.
6. One laboratory technician.
7. One X-ray technician.
8. One nurse.
9. One receptionist.

Medical students were chosen as interviewers in order to take advantage of their relatively sophisticated training; in turn, their participation in the survey served as a valuable practical experience for them.

All members of the field teams underwent an intensive period of preliminary training. After working in the field their performances were periodically reviewed. Wherever possible the supervisor observed the conduct of interviews and selected respondents were reinterviewed for studies of questionnaire reliability.

Comparison of population figures from the 1964 census with those of the national health survey revealed differences between 0.1 and 2.7 per cent for particular age and sex classes. These differences may be explained by the exclusion from the survey of institutionalized persons and military personnel.

PROBLEMS

Definition of Household

The basic unit of analysis was the household, defined as "a group of persons sharing the same home and food and hence exposed to similar environmental influences"; and as "a house, apartment, flat, or room occupied, or destined to be occupied, by a family or group of persons living together or by a person living alone." In the analysis of survey results it was assumed that household and family are the same. This assumption is not always valid because more than one family may occupy a given household, and because households may contain variable numbers of unrelated persons, such as servants, etc. The extent to which such confounding has occurred is unknown.

Illiteracy of Respondents

One-quarter of the surveyed population over age fifteen years had no formal schooling and more than three-quarters had a primary education or less. Such a population might be expected to respond differently to a health questionnaire than a more literate group and one with more extensive knowledge about illness. For this reason, although the survey was modeled along the lines of the U.S. National Health Survey, a comparison of findings in the two studies would be misleading. In Colombia, much more so than in the United States, the findings do not measure the actual frequency of disease or the utilization of health services as much as perceptions of illness and attitudes toward medical care. The high prevalence of reported illness and the shortage of health personnel observed in Colombia must, therefore, be interpreted with caution.

Reliability of Social and Economic Data

The reliability of the data collected on occupation, education, and income is not known. The International Classification of Occupations, which was used to code occupation, is based upon both occupational and industrial categories. This system precludes a complete and accurate occupational classification of individuals or families. The reliability of the information on education and income was also compromised by nonresponse, which amounted to 16.5 per cent on income questions and 5.ō per cent on education questions asked of persons over the age of fifteen years.

Unequal Periods of Recall

In the questions on personal health and on obstetric and pediatric history (see Methods) the respondents were asked to recall their experiences since Holy Week. For example, they were asked: "During the period between Holy Week last year and today, have you given birth to any living child, had a miscarriage, an abortion, or still birth?" Since the survey was conducted over a period of ten months (September 1965 to June 1966), the respondents were being queried about a reference period of varying length. This unequal period of recall ranged from a time span of a few weeks to several months and probably affected the comparability of the responses.

Another problem relating to interview timing stemmed from the questions asked on illnesses during the two weeks preceding the interview. This two-week prevalence period refers to illnesses reported by various respondents at different times of the year. The calculated rates might, therefore, be affected by seasonal differences in climate, employment cycles, or other factors. However, since the whole survey was carried out during a calendar year, the results may be counter-balanced, allowing for variations in the country as a whole.

Operational Problems

In addition to methodological problems a number of operational difficulties were also encountered. One was the demand from several administrative sources for a premature disclosure of the survey findings while the data were still being tabulated and analyzed. The analysis itself was complicated by the fact that some members of the research team resigned early.

The research team concluded, in retrospect, that more attention should have been paid to the design of interview schedules, pretesting, and programming of the analysis. It was noted that bottlenecks occurred in the programming and subsequent analysis of the data which might have been avoided with the full-time assistance of statistical consultants and skilled programmers.

A significant problem was posed by the fact that the National Health Survey was conducted in conjunction with the other component studies of the Health Manpower Study. The co-ordination of these studies was essential if duplication of effort were to be minimized.

A major operational problem was topographical. Many areas selected for survey were relatively inaccessible and could only be reached by airplane. In other instances, survey teams had to travel by jeep over hazardous mountain roads or on horseback and in canoes.

FINDINGS

The findings in Colombia confirm the tragic association between disease and poverty which has been universally documented. Where and how men live are related to the amount of sickness which they experience and to the availability and type of medical care which they subsequently receive. More specifically, the findings confirm that:

1. Sharp regional differences occur in the utilization of health services.
2. The amount of reported illness varies by occupation, education, and income.
3. Physicians and related health workers treat only a fraction of the illnesses reported by the population (16 per cent approximately).
4. The demand and use of health personnel and services varies according to social circumstances (Badgley et al. 1968).

Each respondent was asked whether he was sick during the previous two weeks. Approximately 4 out of 10 individuals (387 per 1,000) gave affirmative answers. Among males the reported illness rate was 363 per thousand, and among females 410 (Table 14–2). This sex differential held for all age groups. Rates were lowest for children five to fourteen years old, but increased with age thereafter. Reported illness prevalence was about the same in urban and rural dwellers, but was universally associated with income (Table 14–3) and education (Table 14–4).

TABLE 14–2. PREVALENCE OF ILLNESS REPORTED DURING TWO WEEKS BEFORE SURVEY, PER 1,000 POPULATION, BY AGE AND SEX (1965–66)

Age	Illness rate		
	Both sexes	Male	Female
All ages	387	363	410
Under 1	432	429	435
1–4	403	403	404
5–14	294	289	300
15–24	319	284	349
25–44	439	389	482
45–64	531	489	572
65+	654	630	674

Source: Badgley, R. F. 1968. Social science and health planning: culture, disease and health services in Colombia. Milbank Mem. Fund Quart. 46:1–348. New York: Appendix B.

TABLE 14–3. PREVALENCE OF ILLNESS REPORTED FOR A TWO-WEEK PERIOD, BY RESIDENCE AND INCOME PER 1,000 POPULATION (1965–66)

Residence	Total	Income (pesos)			
		3,600 or less	3,601– 6,000	6,001– 12,000	12,001 or more
Total	387	415	389	370	305
Urban	378	436	386	374	304
Rural	398	407	393	360	312

Source: Badgley, R. F. 1968. Social science and health planning: culture, disease and health services in Colombia. Milbank Mem. Fund Quart. 46:1–348. New York: Appendix B.

For all persons over the age of six years it was determined whether they had been prevented from carrying out their ordinary activities during the previous two weeks because of sickness or accident. The activities of approximately one person out of ten (108 per thousand) were so restricted, especially among the poor (Table 14–5).

Variations in the rate of activity restrictions by age, sex, and income were similar to those found for illness prevalence (Table 14–6).

TABLE 14–4. RATE OF ILLNESS PER 1,000 POPULATION, BY EDUCATION AND RESIDENCE

Education	National	Urban	Rural
None	411.3	418.9	407.2
Primary	385.8	373.3	400.7
Secondary	323.4	322.4	332.3
Superior	198.7	200.7	161.0
Don't know	436.6	404.1	475.7
No information	391.4	400.2	383.3
Total	381.1	377.0	397.8

Source: Badgley, R. F., Agualimpia, C., Kasius, R. V., Mejía, A., and Schulte, M. 1968. Illness and health services in Colombia: implications for health planning. *Milbank Mem. Fund Quart.* 46:146–64.

TABLE 14–5. RATE OF RESTRICTED ACTIVITY DURING A TWO-WEEK PERIOD, BY RESIDENCE AND FAMILY INCOME PER 1,000 POPULATION, AGE SIX OR ABOVE (1965–66)

Residence	Total	Income (pesos)			
		3,600 or less	3,601–6,000	6,001–12,000	12,001 or more
Total	108	127	112	105	73
Urban	104	142	113	100	73
Rural	115	120	111	119	75

Source: Badgley, R. F. 1968. Social science and health planning: culture, disease and health services in Colombia. *Milbank Mem. Fund Quart.* 46:1–348. New York: Appendix B.

TABLE 14–6. RATE OF RESTRICTED ACTIVITY DURING TWO WEEKS BEFORE SURVEY, PER 1,000 POPULATION, BY AGE AND SEX (1965–66)

Age	Restricted activity rates		
	Both sexes	Males	Females
All ages (6 and over)	108	103	113
6–14	76	74	78
15–24	83	74	90
25–44	125	111	138
45–64	157	160	154
65+	222	250	198

Source: Badgley, R. F. 1968. Social science and health planning: culture, disease and health services in Colombia. *Milbank Mem. Fund Quart.* 46:1–348. New York: Appendix B.

Six per cent (63.2 per thousand) of the individuals surveyed had consulted a physician during the two weeks prior to the survey (Table 14–7). Consultation rates varied with residence from 93.3 per 1,000 among urban dwellers to 31.3 per 1,000 among rural residents.

Contacts with physicians constituted 72 per cent of all visits to health personnel. Among those in need of medical care, almost all persons with a higher education (96.2 per cent) visited a doctor in contrast to only about half (54.3 per cent) of those with no formal education. The latter, together with the poor and those in isolated rural areas, frequently sought help from pharmacists, nurses, midwives, bone setters, and medical quacks or *teguas*.

TABLE 14–7. RATES OF CONSULTATION WITH HEALTH PERSONNEL, PER 1,000 POPULA-
TION, BY INCOME IN PESOS AND BY ZONE

Income[a]	M.D.	Phar- macist	Nurse	Tegua	Other	Total
NATIONAL						
Under 3,600	38.6	8.8	2.7	9.8	7.2	71.1
3,601–6,000	57.4	10.9	1.6	7.3	5.6	85.8
6,001–12,000	86.9	10.7	2.1	4.1	6.0	112.1
12,001–30,000	107.6	10.3	1.9	1.4	3.1	127.7
30,001+	105.7	5.5	.8	3.1	3.4	125.0
No information	55.9	6.4	2.2	6.9	5.8	83.4
Total	63.2	9.2	2.2	6.7	5.9	91.0
URBAN						
Under 3,600	65.8	14.0	4.5	9.3	9.3	104.3
3,601–6,000	85.8	12.9	1.5	4.5	5.6	110.8
6,001–12,000	102.5	12.1	1.8	2.2	6.4	125.4
12,001–30,000	120.0	10.1	2.1	1.4	3.0	136.7
30,001+	116.1	6.2	.9	1.0	3.3	127.6
No information	82.6	7.2	3.2	3.7	6.3	105.3
Total	93.3	11.1	2.5	4.0	6.1	117.7
RURAL						
Under 3,600	27.2	6.6	1.9	10.0	6.2	54.0
3,601–6,000	32.8	9.2	1.6	9.7	5.5	59.4
6,001–12,000	43.0	6.6	2.9	9.2	4.8	67.0
12,001–30,000	46.8	11.4	.9	1.7	3.8	66.3
30,001+	48.9	1.4	—	14.6	3.8	68.6
No information	29.5	5.7	1.3	10.1	5.3	53.1
Total	31.3	7.1	1.8	9.6	5.7	56.8

[a] These findings refer to the median income or the income in the midpoint of each group and not to the mean or average income. Medians were calculated with households with unknown income excluded. During the period of the survey the value of the peso fluctuated between 11 and 19 U.S. dollars. For purposes of calculation the rate used here is 15 pesos to the dollar.

Source: Badgley, R. F., Agualimpia, C., Kasius, R. V., Mejía, A., and Schulte, M. 1968. Illness and health services in Colombia: implications for health planning. *Milbank Mem. Fund Quart.* 46:146–64.

Residents of towns and cities visited all types of health workers with a frequency twice that of the rural population (118 versus 57 per thousand). In part, this was a reflection of the differential availability of health services. The majority of hospitals, public health facilities, doctors and nurses are located in the major cities. Less than 10 per cent of the physicians practice in cities of less than 20,000 persons and 68 per cent of the trained nurses who are currently active, practice in the 3 largest cities of the country.

An effort was made to obtain information about 12 specific chronic conditions which were thought to be easily recognizable. These included: deaf mutism, deafness, blindness, harelip, defective feet, other deformities, loss of extremity, paralysis, asthma, epilepsy, mental retardation, and ulcers. The reported prevalence for all these conditions was 67.2 per thousand, a rate which increased sharply with age. Almost one out of four in the population over sixty-five years of age (240.7 per thousand) reported one or more of these conditions. Asthma ranked first out of the 12 chronic conditions, with a prevalence of 30.1 per 1000, with no variation by residence. This must be interpreted as a prevalence of respiratory conditions which increases with age.

Another objective of the household survey was to verify the completeness and reliability of birth and infant death registration. Questions were asked concerning the pregnancy history of all adult females and the deaths of children under five years of age during the previous year. The responses have not yet been completely analyzed, but it is estimated that there is probably a 10 per cent or higher underregistration of births and a similar underreporting of infant deaths in Colombia.

The more general contributions which the survey has already made to the promotion of public health research in Columbia have been summarized as follows:

1. The large (and successful) ad hoc technical assistance program.
2. Development of the nucleus of a health statistics center in Colombia.
3. Benefits to the scientific community of Colombia—a new awareness of surveys as a scientific tool in medical and social fields.
4. The innovations of the sample design—having the clinical sample as a subsample of the household sample was one: another was the use of two half-samples and application of two-stage controlled selection.
5. The carrying out of this complex operation, starting with no staff and no organization, in two years (West 1968).

POTENTIALS

Well-established statistical procedures and pretested questionnaires were utilized in the Colombian National Health Survey. Accordingly, it represents an important first step in the development of quantitative health research studies in Latin America. Until recently, a full appreciation of the scientifically rigorous approach in the social sciences has been lacking in Latin America. The situation has been described as follows:

A researcher, in many cases, must still devise his own samples, draw his own maps, make his own census tabulations, and calculate his own production indices before carrying out original field work. Very often his training, either at home or abroad, has not adequately prepared him for these activities, and both time and scarce resources are devoted to matters which are sometimes not part of the research problem itself. Matters have been made more difficult because no tradition of interdisciplinary research exists in Latin America. Very often the sociologist or anthropologist does not know what the economist or the geographer can offer him and is equally ignored by them (Stavenhagen 1966).

The Health Survey may foster the development and refinement of valid indices of education, income, occupation, and other social variables. In this connection it has been observed that:

As far as is known, not a single country in this part of the world [Latin America] has a profile of social stratification and/or class on a national level. A careful analysis of the three dimensions, occupation, income, and education, and their interrelations can be a great help for further studies, since social scientists doing research in that country will not have to validate the variable each time it is used (Iutaka 1968).

At a recent conference convened to examine the methods and selected findings of the Colombian National Health Survey, the potential utility of this type of survey was sharply challenged. Several observers contended that few unanticipated findings were discovered, that definitions of several key variables were imprecise, and that the findings in general would make only a limited contribution to the development of a national health plan in Colombia. This assessment appears to be widely held because, of the several countries which have undertaken national surveys, only the United States has not discontinued them. Even the once continuous British health survey has been dropped.

The Colombian survey followed the general procedures which had been developed for the U.S. National Health Survey during the past decade. Two technical innovations included the division of the total sample into two balanced subsamples and the incorporation of a simultaneous subsample for clinical evaluation to permit cross-tabulations of variables from both types of study. It will thus be possible to analyze national data on questions which have hitherto been studied on limited cross-sections of population. The value of studying inconsistencies between patient responses on health and medical reports is not inconsiderable:

Until now the emphases in methodological studies have been on determining how well the household interview reports mirror the reports of physicians. But if this relationship should, on study, prove to be a poor one, the need to know what it is that survey information does in fact reflect, will still remain. Through followback studies of physicians and patients, some understanding could be obtained regarding the influence on respondent reporting of doctor-patient communication, the assessment and interpretation the patient made of his illness, and the circumstances that made the respondent aware of and ready to report a given condition in an interview situation (U.S. National Health Survey 1961).

The Colombia survey data are very suitable for such analyses.

The salience of a given disease and the accuracy with which it is reported for others in an individual's family are important considerations in health surveys. In studies of the Eastern Health District in Baltimore, distinctions were drawn between sickly and healthy families (Downes 1949). A correlation between the mother's report of her own health status and that of her child was found in a study of 350 mother-child pairs (Mechanic 1964). The findings of the Colombian Health Survey could be used to study the extent to which the health status of a respondent affects the reporting for other members of the family. All persons over age fifteen were interviewed, but information about the health of children under fifteen years of age was obtained from the mother or another responsible adult. It should be possible, then, to determine the patterns of reporting on their families by healthy mothers and unhealthy mothers.

In a review of morbidity studies, Mechanic and Newton (1965) concluded:

All of the methodological studies appear to support the general principle that accurate reporting occurs when the illness in question is salient, and social and psychological barriers to reporting are absent. Degree of saliency is inferred from the following distinctions which are related to quality of reporting: self reports versus proxy reports; conditions requiring single physician consultation versus conditions requiring more attention; short versus long hospital stays; episodes involving surgery versus those not involving surgery; and the length of time for which recall is required.

A scale incorporating these various items could be developed and tested against the findings of the Colombian Household and Clinical Examination Surveys.

To establish priorities in health and welfare one must rely upon accurate assessments of the available resources and the relative effectiveness of alternative systems of health services. For this and other reasons there has been an increasing momentum in the growth of comparative studies in the provision and utilization of health services and social welfare. The International Collaborative Study of Medical Care Utilization is the current spearhead of efforts to develop a standardized survey instrument which can be used in various countries. Because the general design and interview protocols of the Colombian Health Survey were modeled after those of the United States National Health Survey, it may be possible to compare the health experience of these two nations in terms of traditional health indices, such as reported morbidity, restricted activity, days confined to bed, and utilization of health services.

The National Health Survey may also provide the means for developing a conceptual framework for the formulation of health policies in Colombia and, perhaps, elsewhere in Latin America. Health priorities must be evaluated in the context of the total picture of health needs and demands. The direct costs of illness can be calculated from estimates of the demand for health services, the costs of medical care, and capital investment in medical facilities. However, much needs yet to be done in developing cost estimates based on the illnesses reported by the population, or better still, on the actual prevalence of disease. The development of a methodology of cost-benefit analysis is a necessary step before the morbidity findings of national health surveys can be effectively translated into a set of health priorities for a nation.

Acknowledgments

Responsibility for the design and execution of the survey was shared by a team headed by Doctor Alfonso Mejía Vanegas and Doctor Raúl Paredes-Manrique which included Doctor Carlos Agualimpia, Doctor Aldemar Gómez, Doctor Ricardo Galán, Mr. Luis Carlos Gomez, Doctor Aurelio Pabón, Doctor Pablo Solano, and Doctor Guillermo Torres of the Ministry of Public Health of Colombia. Consultants from the U.S. Public Health Service included two of us (R.F.B. and R.V.K.) as well as Mrs. Margaret West, Mr. Garrie J. Losee, and Doctor Philip Lawrence.

References

Agualimpia, C. H. 1968. The clinical examination. Round table on social science and health planning. *Milbank Mem. Fund Quart.* 46:86–92.
Arreaza-Guzman, A. A., Alarcon, D., Cibotti, R., MacLead, J. W., Payne, A.M.-M., Pedreira de Freitas, J. L., Sepulveda, O., and Sheps, C. G.

1964. Health manpower and medical education in Latin America. *Milbank Mem. Fund Quart.* 42:19–136.
Badgley, R. F., ed. 1968. Social science and health planning: culture, disease and health services in Colombia. *Milbank Mem. Fund Quart.* 46:1–348.
Badgley, R. F., Agualimpia, C., Kasius, R. V., Mejía, A., and Schulte, M. 1968. Illness and health services in Colombia: Implications for health planning. *Milbank Mem. Fund Quart.* 46:146–64.
Downes, J. 1948. Social and environmental factors in illness. *Milbank Mem. Fund Quart.* 26:366–85.
Iutaka, S. 1968. Commentary. *Milbank Mem. Fund Quart.* 46:97–100.
Mechanic, D. 1964. The influence of mothers on their children's health attitudes and behavior. *Pediatrics* 33:444–53.
Mechanic, D. and Newton, M. 1965. Some problems in the analysis of morbidity data. *J. Chronic Dis.* 18:569–80.
Mejía Vanegas, A., Paredes Manrique, R. et al. 1967. *Study on Health Manpower and Medical Education in Colombia I. Methodology.* Washington: Pan American Health Organization.
Ministry of Public Health of Colombia and the Colombian Association of Medical Schools. 1967. *Study on Health Manpower and Medical Education in Colombia. II. Preliminary Findings.* Washington: Pan American Health Organization.
———. 1967. *Study on Health Manpower and Medical Education in Colombia. III. Proceedings of the International Conference on Health Manpower and Medical Education.* Washington: U.S. Government Printing Office.
Stavenhagen, R. 1966. Behavioral science in Latin America. *Milbank Mem. Fund Quart.* 44:17–26.
U.S. National Health Survey, 1961. *Health Interview Responses Compared with Medical Records,* series D, no. 5. Washington: U.S. Government Printing Office.
West, M. 1968. The Colombian National Health Survey. *Milbank Mem. Fund Quart.* 46:45–53.
Zschock, D. K. 1967. *Manpower Perspective of Colombia.* Industrial Relations Section, Research Report Series No. 110, Princeton University.

EDITORIAL COMMENTS

1. The Colombia National Health Survey was modeled closely after the U.S. National Health Survey, although conditions in the two countries are markedly different. The illiteracy of a major portion of the Colombian population and the possible effect of this upon interview responses is a serious problem, not only for this survey but for any that may subsequently be undertaken in Colombia. It seems doubtful that much valid information on the prevalence of specific diseases or conditions can be obtained by questioning illiterate people who are

ignorant of medicine. A direct ascertainment of disease by mass screening may be an alternative.

2. As in Alameda County, the Colombia interview responses reflect perceptions of illness and not the prevalence of disease per se. Of course, the health perceptions of an urbanized population in a developed country may bear an entirely different relationship to objective health indices than those of a rural people in a less advanced country.

3. The rather unusual administrative problems encountered during the study were, at least in part, due to the novelty of the survey technique in South America. The unequal recall periods stemmed from the necessity to date the respondents' health experiences from the previous Holy Week, presumably in consideration of their illiteracy.

4. The whole question of whether questionnaires and other survey instruments designed for use in relatively advanced countries can be adapted for use among illiterate populations is worthy of study. The problem is somewhat analogous to that of modifying psychometric tests to make them independent of language or culture.

INDEX